Infertility

A Clinician's Guide to
Diagnosis and Treatment

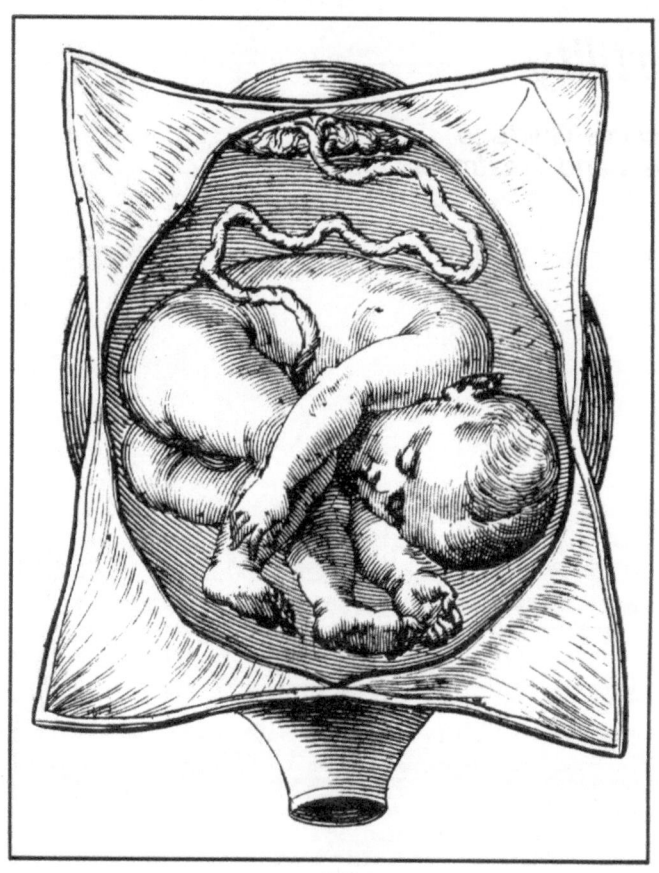

An artist's conception of a normal fetus at term.

Woodcut from "Traites des Maladies des Femmes Grosses"
by Francois Mauriceau, Paris, 1681.

Infertility

A Clinician's Guide to Diagnosis and Treatment

Melvin L. Taymor, M.D.

Professor of Life Sciences and Technology
Massachusetts Institute of Technology
Cambridge, Massachusetts
and Clinical Professor Emeritus of Obstetrics and Gynecology
Harvard Medical School
Boston, Massachusetts

Plenum Medical Book Company
New York and London

Library of Congress Cataloging-in-Publication Data

Taymor, Melvin L.
    Infertility : a clinician's guide to diagnosis and treatment /
  Melvin L. Taymor. -- Rev. and expanded ed.
      p.   cm.
    Includes bibliographical references.
    Includes index.

    1. Infertility.   I. Title.
    [DNLM: 1. Infertility--diagnosis. 2. Infertility--therapy.   WP
  570 T247ia]
  RC889.T34   1989
  616.6'92--dc20
  DNLM/DLC
  for Library of Congress   90-7659
                                                                      CIP

ISBN-13: 978-1-4612-7899-3   e-ISBN-13: 978-1-4613-0627-6
DOI: 10.1007/978-1-4613-0627-6

This volume is a revised and expanded edition of *Infertility*
by Melvin L. Taymor, M.D., published in 1978 by Grune & Stratton, Inc.

© 1990 Plenum Publishing Corporation
233 Spring Street, New York, N.Y. 10013

Softcover reprint of the hardcover 1st edition 1990

Plenum Medical Book Company is an imprint of Plenum Publishing Corporation

To Betty

Preface

A little over 12 years ago I wrote a small volume entitled *Infertility.* It seemed to me at that time that significant advances in the field called for the publication of such a volume. The following is from the preface to that volume:

> During the past 15 years considerable progress has been made in the field of infertility diagnosis and management. It is perhaps a paradox that much of this increased knowledge has come about because of Western medicine's preoccupation with the search for a means to control reproduction. As a result, we have achieved new insights into the physiologic mechanisms involved in reproduction, and we have found better methods for measuring physiologic changes in reproductive health and disease. To these advances can be added improvements in the utilization of endoscopic and surgical techniques, in the diagnosis and treatment of infections and endometriosis, and in the treatment of hormonal disorders.
>
> During this period, too, through workshops and conferences and in journals and texts, these latest advances have been made available to physicians, an outstanding example being the two volumes of *Progress in Infertility,* edited by Drs. Jan Behrman and Robert Kistner. As necessary as these publications are, they do not offer an overall view of infertility diagnosis and management. Although the articles are usually written by the outstanding specialists in the field, who set forth their particular interest with scientific precision, for those primarily interested in the practice of infertility, there is often more fine detail than can be absorbed or utilized. The causes of infertility are often treated as single, isolated units and the physician–reader's view tends to become fragmented.
>
> The main purpose of this book is to provide the practicing physician,

the resident, and the interested medical student with an overview that will help guide him or her in caring for patients. This text combines the new with the old. I have attempted to evaluate the significance and potential of some new achievements in the light of the perspective of older literature. I hope not only to provide a sequential unity to the recent advances in the field, but to synthesize this progress with the many significant accomplishments of the past.

This holistic approach, reflected through my 25 years of experience in infertility diagnosis and management, is consistent with what I believe to be the very essence of the management of the infertile couple: the need to look at the couple as a whole throughout the course of treatment, and to avoid concentrating on one partner, or one organ system within one partner. To emphasize further this sense of unity, the chapters are presented, insofar as possible, in the order in which the physician might approach the problem of the infertile couple.

Since 1978 there has been an accelerated accumulation of knowledge of reproductive science and a remarkable increase in our ability to help our infertile patients. Much of this new knowledge and practice has come from the science and technology developed in relation to in vitro fertilization. Once again, there is a need for a volume that will present to the practicing physician the new science and technology, but weaving into it the still important basic holistic approach to the infertile couple.

Much of the first part of this book is taken from the earlier volume, *Infertility.* New developments in the subject areas covered by the earlier volume are touched upon. However, chapters on immunology, endoscopy, ovulation induction, endometriosis, and infertility surgery have been virtually rewritten. Chapters on in vitro fertilization, gamete intrafallopian tube transfer, and unexplained infertility have been added. Extensive references are available for the reader who wants to explore an area in depth. It is hoped that this volume will provide the practicing obstetrician–gynecologist with a complete view of the field as well as a sound approach to diagnosis and therapy.

I am indebted to Dawn de Freitas and Nancy Soverino for their invaluable help in the preparation of the manuscript.

Melvin L. Taymor, M.D.

Brookline, Massachusetts

Contents

Part IV   Management of the Infertile Couple

Part V   Special Areas and Special Diagnostic Tests

Part VI   Therapy

Contents

PART I

Introduction

CHAPTER 1

Historical Review

The problem of infertility has been with us as long as the recorded history of mankind. The ancient civilizations of Babylonia, Persia, and Greece had their goddesses of fertility, fertility rites and a whole body of superstition surrounding the process of birth. The Bible is replete with references to the fertility or infertility of many of its patriarchs and their wives: Abraham and Sarah; Jacob, Leah, and Rachel; and the mother of Samson.[1] It is reported that the use of the mandrake restored Leah's fertility after a period of sterility. In most instances there is little scientific rationale for the remedies utilized. Rather, they do attest to the importance of emotional factors in infertility. However, that the Israelites knew about the optimum time for fertilization is confirmed in the orthodox law that forbids coitus until 7 days after the end of the menses.

Early Western physicians were also cognizant of the mechanical barriers to conception. Roman and Byzantine gynecologists related sterility to obesity; they used pessaries to treat sterility associated with a retroverted uterus.[2] Soranus of Ephesus, who practiced medicine in first-century Rome during the reign of the Emperors Trajan and Hadrian, contributed greatly to our knowledge of obstetrics and gynecology; he described the pelvic organs, the process of labor, the uses of vaginal speculae, and methods for contraception. He noted that the most favorable time for conception was shortly after the menstrual period, and he felt that staying in bed after coitus would improve fertility.[2]

The Middle Ages contributed little new knowledge either to medicine in general or to infertility in particular, since the ancient manuscripts preserved in the monasteries were still being consulted. While the rise of scientific knowledge in the 17th century brought isolated contributions to medicine, little was added to the understanding of the problems of infertility. It is remarkable, however, that in the 18th century, artificial insemination with husband's semen was carried out by John Hunter for hypospadias.[3] The development of the microscope by Leeuwenhoek in the 17th century allowed Lazzaro Spallanzani to demonstrate that spermatozoa are essential to fertilization, and also allowed Karl Ernst von Baer to describe the mammalian ovum in 1827.

The investigation of late 19th- and early 20th-century scientists widened the horizons of embryology, physiology, and cellular pathology and established the foundations of modern medicine, but the basis for the modern era of infertility may be said to have been laid down only in this century with the studies of Huhner on sperm survival in the cervical mucus,[4] the test for tubal patency described by Rubin in 1920,[5] the development of the modern concepts of menstruation by Allen and Doisy in 1924,[6] and a description by Moench in 1931 of semen characteristics associated with infertility and fertility.[7] These studies, encompassing the areas of the cervix, the endometrium, the ovulatory factor, and the male factor, remain today the backbone of diagnosis and therapy.

Of still great significance today, although proposed by Meaker in 1934, is the recognition of the complex nature of infertility diagnosis and treatment.[8] Meaker wrote about the "multiple nature of causation" and "division of responsibility between male and female partners." These two principles and their utilization in practice still continue to provide the greatest impetus to success in diagnosis and therapy.

In the past 30 years, we have seen virtually an explosion of both knowledge and technology for the diagnosis and treatment of the infertile couple. The first area to yield to developing scientific investigation was that of gynecologic endocrinology.[9] First came the availability of the ovulatory-inducing medications, pituitary gonadotropin in 1958, clomiphene citrate in 1960, and menopausal gonadotropin in 1961. The development of radioimmunoassay for polypeptide and steroid hormones in the 1960s allowed reproductive physiologists to unravel many of the secrets of the normal and abnormal menstrual cycle. Improvements in endoscopic techniques were taking place at the same time. Although Decker's culdoscope had been utilized since the mid-1940s, the availability of fiber optics and sophisticated carbon dioxide insufflators in the 1960s brought about a resurgence of interest in laparoscopy, which soon proved to be a fundamental part of the infertility workup and of therapy. Increased knowledge of the function of the hypothalamic–pituitary axis, microsurgery, and new therapies for endometriosis were the significant advances of the 1970s.

Finally, in the 1980s, we saw a synthesis of many of these scientific and technology advances into the procedures of in vivo fertilization, gamete intra-fallopian tube transfer, and intrauterine insemination procedures that are at present adding to our treatment potential, and that also hold even greater promises for the future.

Although these past 30 years have brought significant improvements in diagnostic and therapeutic techniques in many parts of the world, the problem of infertility still has not been lifted completely out of the realm of magic and superstition. Ancient rituals persist; even today, fertility rites are practiced in many of the developed and underdeveloped countries of the world. Statuettes of pregnant females or of males with outsized phalluses are used as fertility fetishes and symbols in Africa, Central American, Indonesia, and Polynesia (Fig. 1-1). Successful outcomes following these approaches undoubtedly have their modern counterpart in our constantly increasing awareness of the importance of emotional factors of infertility. Modern endocrinology confirms the folkloric practice of Hungarian peasant women who bite their own afterbirth to continue their fertility, and of Chinese women who are given dried placenta to eat to improve their fertility.[3] In these cases, it is perhaps we who have learned from the old midwives' practices, for placenta contains chorionic gonadotropin, one of the hormones used in the present-day treatment of ovulatory failure.

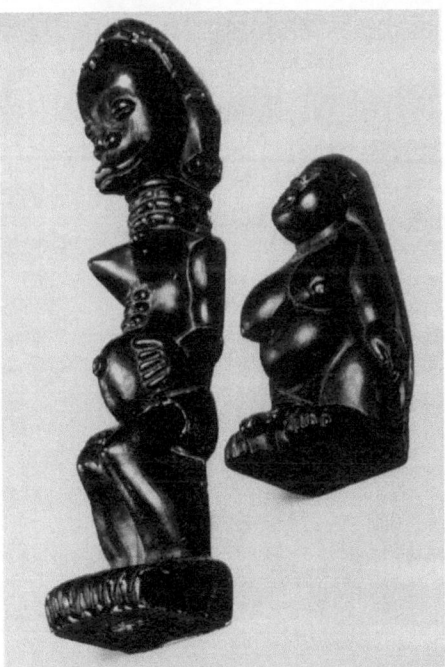

Figure 1-1. Fertility dolls from the South Seas and Africa.

REFERENCES

1. Ober W: Reuben's mandrakes: Infertility in the Bible. *Int J Gynecol Pathol* 3:299, 1984
2. Graham H: *Eternal Eve*. Garden City, NY, Doubleday, 1951
3. Johnston RJ: The history of human infertility. *Fertil Steril* 14:261, 1963
4. Huhner M: *Sterility in the Female and its Treatment*. New York, Rebman, 1913
5. Rubin IC: The non-operative determination of patency of fallopian tubes. *JAMA* 75:661, 1920
6. Allen E, Doisy EA: The induction of sexually mature condition in immature females by the injection of ovarian follicular hormone. *Am J Physiol* 69:577, 1924
7. Moench GL: The sperm morphology in relation to fertility. *Am J Obstet Gynecol* 22:199, 1931
8. Meaker SR: *Human Sterility*. Baltimore, Williams and Wilkins, 1934
9. Taymor ML: Advances in endocrinology: A ten-year review. *Clin Obstet Gynecol* 10:667, 1967

CHAPTER 2

The Specialty of Infertility

Medical articles for the laity, as well as journals of medical education, deplore the modern tendency toward specialization. Much can be said for the criticism that the superspecialists, focusing their attention on one aspect or one organ system of their patients, often lose sight of the whole person. But the onus of overspecialization cannot be leveled at the physicians who devote themselves to the care of the infertile couple, for these physicians are concerned not only with the female organs of reproduction, but with the interplay of other endocrine systems as well as systemic disease on these organs, with the influences of the wife's emotional state, with the fertility of her husband, and with the all important relationship between the two partners.

Indeed, the specialty of infertility may be unique in medicine, because in no other medical situation does a combination of factors in two individual human beings — each essentially healthy and each perhaps capable of producing children with another partner — produce a pathologic condition. A physician interested and trained in all aspects of this complex human and medical situation is best qualified to unravel the causes, to institute indicated therapy, and to bring the problem to a successful solution.

Because the defect in one organ system is usually not a straightforward, black-and-white situation, and because of the frequent occurrence of multiple factors, a fertility specialist must constantly weigh the significance of findings in one system against the findings in another. This is especially true in the evaluation of the male factor, where a sharp line of normality does not exist.

It is ideal if one physician can so develop a relationship with both husband and wife that the concept of a "partnership" is established. In investigating and

7

treating the important aspects of sexual adjustment, such cooperation is especially vital. In the management of therapy, as well, one physician is also more effective. Multiple deficiencies or defects in both partners can be treated simultaneously; this not only increases the chances of bringing the problem to a successful solution, but ensures that a thorough workup and course of therapy have been undertaken within a shorter period of time, and with a minimum of emotional and economic strain.

Few physicians have had the opportunity to receive comprehensive training in endocrinology, surgery, psychiatry, marriage counseling, and male infertility. Even with such training, physicians often do not have the time to devote to all of these aspects of the infertile couple. A fertility clinic, where specialists pool their particular knowledge for diagnosis and therapy, is an improvement over the independent obstetrician–gynecologist working with a urologist. Even in a clinic, however, the concept of the couple as a whole can be lost unless one of the specialists is considered the *personal* physician of the couple.

The fertility specialist or the clinic may be the ideal, but most patients with an infertility problem will seek help from an obstetrician–gynecologist. If these individuals elect to treat this patient, they should have a thorough understanding of the tests necessary for a complete workup, be competent in the field of gynecologic endocrinology, be aware of the emotional implications of what the patient reveals, and of what they tell the patient. Above all, they must be aware of any limitations of their expertise or of their time available, and be ready to refer the patient to an appropriate specialist when it appears indicated.

If the obstetrician–gynecologist cannot care for the male, a close liason should be maintained with a urologist who is trained and who is interested in male infertility. When two physicians are taking care of the separate partners, each physician must understand the relative nature of their individual fertility findings. They should have a good working relationship and consult each other frequently. This will avoid a situation in which the urologist, who considers a sperm count of twenty million the lower limit of normal, may report independently to the husband that all is well. The gynecologist, noting a poor postcoital test, may report to the wife that her husband is "at fault." The husband, who has no way of judging the relative significance of the findings, is all too ready to accept the favorable opinion of his own physician rather than that of his wife's physician, who, in addition to disputing his manhood, is also possibly sending him the bills! Such a "rivalry" between husband and wife, each with his or her own physician, can be avoided by the physicians sharing their findings and their implications. By pooling the results of their therapy, the two can ensure that when the relative fertility of the two individual partners can be increased simultaneously, the overall fertility of the couple will be augmented.

CHAPTER 3

The Science and Art of Infertility

> To start off with the observation of facts, to draw from them
> predictions which are verifiable by other facts; that is the
> modest endeavor of scientists today.

So wrote Bernfeld about scientific objectivity.[1] The physician caring for the infertile couple should, whenever possible, utilize the latest that science has brought to the care of the infertile couple. In such areas as therapy for anovulation and endometriosis, and in the use of microsurgery, intrauterine insemination, and in vitro fertilization, there has been an accumulation of scientific data to provide appropriate guidelines.

However, in infertility management, in addition to the many verifiable scientific advances, of which Bernfeld would have approved, many empirical approaches have been utilized by physicians for decades. They have been employed so extensively that they are now an integral part of the physicians' armamentarium, so culturally ingrained that it is extremely difficult to eradicate them. When Buxton and Southam evaluated fertility practices in 1958, they were rightfully skeptical of many procedures they felt lacked scientific objectivity.[2] Yet, I feel there are still areas of fertility investigation and treatment that are of value although they appear to be beyond the scope of precise scientific evaluation. I agree that some practices do need to be discarded, but others I would place in the category of the *art of infertility* management.

One form of art, I feel, is to utilize approaches in diagnosis or therapy that appear to be effective, but that as yet do not conform to the rigidities of statistical evaluation. Into this category fall such procedures as the evaluation

9

of immune factors, the relative importance of a mycoplasma infection, the use of homologous insemination, and the diagnosis and treatment of the inadequate luteal phase. While these methods appear to be effective in individual cases, the complex nature of infertility often makes it difficult to set up objective studies that will give statistically valid answers. *In rejecting methods just because they do not conform to statistical evaluation, we may be rejecting approaches that may be of some benefit.*

Art in the management of infertility also brings us far beyond where pure science can take us—to a consideration of emotional factors, particularly the relationship between the patient and the fact of his or her infertility, how this affects him or her as an individual and, ultimately, how this affects the outcome of the problem, itself.

Our management of the couple, as we help them work their way through these problems, make up the very essence of the art of infertility.

REFERENCES

1. Bernfeld S: The facts of observation in psychoanalysis. *Soc Psychiatry* 12:289, 1941
2. Buxton CL, Southam AL: *Human Infertility.* New York, Hoeber-Harper, 1958

CHAPTER 4

General Principles

DEFINITION

As medical science probes deeper into the causes of human reproductive failure, it becomes increasingly difficult to develop an all-encompassing definition for the term "infertility." Infertility as a diagnosis applied to an individual or couple must be considered to be a relative term. In some situations, infertility merely means "reduced infertility."

"Fertility" denotes the ability of a man and woman to reproduce. Recently, the term "fecundity" has been used to denote the ability to reproduce. Infertility, conversely, implies a lack of fertility or the inability to produce children. However, because fertility requires a variable time factor for establishment and development of the zygote, the term infertility, unlike other medical conditions, has a time element in its definition. The definition proposed by the American Fertility Society, and one that is widely accepted, states, "a marriage is to be considered barren or infertile when pregnancy has not occurred after a year of coitus without contraception."

This definition has been based on studies such as those of Tietze and coworkers who found that in 1727 planned pregnancies, 90% of couples became pregnant after the 1st year following discontinuation of birth control methods.[1] Such a study suggests that if a couple has not achieved pregnancy after 1 year, there is a 90% chance that they are outside of the norm, and have a problem that is reducing their fertility. A fertility survey of these individuals would have an excellent chance of uncovering a significant factor, perhaps a correctable one.

11

On the other hand, the results of several studies caution the physician against too early an intervention. In their text on *Human Infertility* Buxton and Southam review 12 demographic studies concerning the length of time required for conception to occur.[2] In a collective series including 9595 subjects of various environments and economic groups, it was found that 65% of the women were pregnant at the end of 1 year; 90% required more than 2 years for conception to occur.

From these figures it follows that if patients were considered to have an infertility problem after only 6 months, a large "cure" rate could be obtained without any treatment. As one moves toward 1 year or 2 years, the chances of pathology being uncovered are increased. However, in the final analysis it is difficult to define fertility in terms of time alone; each couple must be taken as an individual problem.

THE COUPLE AS A UNIT

An additional reason for the difficulty in defining infertility is the relative nature of the problem in so many cases. Individuals themselves are often neither "fertile" nor "infertile." Because of many reasons, their individual fertility potential may be reduced to a varying degree. Here the significance of the couple as a unit plays an important role as to whether or not each individual will or will not be considered as having a "fertility problem." A male with a somewhat lowered fertility potential, if married to a very fertile woman, may not come to the physician's attention. On the other hand, a male with a similar sperm count, but married to a woman with somewhat lower fertility potential, will have an infertility problem. Similarly, a woman with olio-ovulation, a condition that might reduce fertility, married to a very fertile male, will not be aware that she has a problem, and instead, as a couple, this man and woman do not have an infertility problem.

This all-important principle has many ramifications. First, this indicates the need for evaluation of the husband in all cases of infertility, a practice that even at this time is not always carried out. It further indicates that when two physicians are taking care of the separate partners, a close liaison must be maintained; they must both understand the relative nature of their infertility conclusions and must have a knowledge of the findings in the opposite partner to evaluate the significance of their own findings. This close relationship between the two physicians must be maintained during therapy so that the relative fertility of the two partners will be increased simultaneously and thus serve to augment the overall fertility of the couple.

The physician's awareness of the importance of the couple as a unit, while helping his or her search for the cause of infertility, also brings psychological benefits to both partners involved. Neither the man nor the woman feels it is entirely his or her "fault"; guilt and recriminations are minimized. Some of the devastating effects of infertility on a partner's self-esteem and personal life remain unmitigated if each must deal separately with the problem.

Working together as a team may help sustain a couple through what may be a long battery of inconvenient and painful tests and treatment. Even if the most desirable result of treatment, conception, is not realized, the couple will more readily accept that they have tried their utmost, and, in active cooperation with their physician, were offered the best of medical science as well as compassionate understanding.

MULTIPLICITY OF FACTORS

Another important principle to be kept in mind in approaching the infertile couple, in regard to both diagnosis and treatment, is the knowledge that reduced fertility in many cases is brought about by a number of individual factors, each in themselves probably not significant enough to block fertility, but sufficient to cause reproductive failure when added together. A detailed analysis of the causes of fertility is outlined in Part II. Some of these causes are frequently found, some infrequently found; and in some cases the exact relationship to the problem of infertility remains to be proved or disproved; it took two years for 90% to achieve conception.

Taken into consideration the knowledge that some factors are fairly common and that there may be a number of these more common factors present, a rational approach to the infertile couple has been to put each partner through a basic minimum workup that may uncover from 80% to 90% of the possible deleterious factors. Simultaneous therapy for these factors, often in both the male and female partners, increases the chance of success in a larger portion of couples. It will diminish the number of individuals who will have to undergo more complicated and expensive testing, particularly tests that require hospitalization. On the other hand, considerable time and effort can be consumed by testing for and treating one factor at a time, ignoring others until a later time.

The basic workup as stated by the American Fertility Society and followed by most specialists consists of (1) history and examination of the female partner; (2) evaluation of the insemination factor (postcoital test); (3) evaluation of tubal patency (hysterosalpingogram); (4) evaluation of the hormonal factor (ovulation); (5) history and examination of the male partner; and (6) semen analysis.

THE VICIOUS CYCLE:
INFERTILITY–EMOTIONAL FACTORS–INFERTILITY

Emotional factors are well known to be among the many causes of infertility and will be dealt with in Chapter 7. What is less understood is that the *state of infertility, itself* is a factor; it precipitates emotional responses that, in turn, can play a destructive role on fertility. When minor organic problems are added to these emotional factors, the state of reproductive failure is firmly established, or continues.

The physician should be aware that many people look on failure to conceive as their personal failure, their failure as a sexual being, and they bring these feelings of inadequacy to their first medical interview. By the time the physician sees the man or woman, the patient may also be experiencing anxiety, anger, depression, guilt, or obsession with his or her plight. The fact of infertility, itself, and the resultant testing and treatment, with its precise concentration on coitus, on the quality of ovulation, and the sperm count, often leads to further anxiety and depression. The treatment, interfering as it does with normal sexual and interpersonal relationships, with spontaneous love-making deteriorating to "sex on a schedule," may prevent the maturation of what often is still a young and tenuous emotional bond between two people. Demands on the patient's time and the financial burden of extensive tests also increase already existing tensions. Thus, no physician should undertake caring for patients with infertility problems without being keenly aware of the potential seriousness of this vicious cycle.

AN APPROACH TO INFERTILITY INVESTIGATION AND TREATMENT

Any approach to the management of an infertility problem should take into consideration the four principles elucidated in this chapter: (1) a definition of infertility, (2) the couple as a unit, (3) the multiplicity factors, and (4) the vicious cycle of infertility-emotional factors-infertility.

In most cases the infertility investigation should not be initiated until at least 1 year of coitus without contraception has passed. There are, of course, exceptions to this rule. It is often considered advisable to initiate investigation after only 6 months when the female partner is over 35 years of age, since the amount of time available for diagnosis and treatment is limited. If there is a diagnosis or potential diagnosis of disease, such as endometriosis or ovarian cysts, a rapid investigation before surgery is justified and advisable so that corrective measures toward the infertililty problem, if present, can be carried out concomitantly. If for various reasons the male partner is known to have a significant semen deficit before marriage or early in the marriage, studies may be promptly initiated before the usual waiting period.

However, *institution of an infertility investigation, or even a partial investigation, prior to 1 year, generally does more harm than good*. Since approximately 35% of couples who conceive do so after 6 months of unprotected coitus, for many couples time is their greatest ally. In addition, we know that some couples have only a relative infertility problem. Secondary emotional factors, aroused by the infertility investigation, can often tip the delicate balance betwen fertility and infertility in a couple for whom only additional time was needed. A single semen analysis, putting the patient on a temperature chart, prescribing fertility drugs, and recommendations concerning coitus are often worse than doing nothing at all at this premature stage. Too often this couple will have been started off on years of testing–treatment–testing that sometimes ends in conception only after all investigation and therapy have ceased. Physicians must be firm and confident in their position concerning the importance of the necessary time element.

On the other hand, once a year or more has passed, the chances of organic disease being present have increased sufficiently so that the potential benefits of investigation and treatment are enough to outweigh their negative influences. A thorough course of investigation and therapy, utilizing all available techniques, should be carried out promptly. The male factor should be fully evaluated. The concept of multiplicity of factors should be kept firmly in mind. At this point much time and effort can be wasted by merely giving advice concerning time of coitus for a few months, then at a later date checking an xray, or at some future point carrying out a semen analysis. *Once a physican has accepted that there is a problem the workup should be complete.*

As with any rules there are exceptions. The woman with irregular cycles who is not ovulating can be given a 3-month trial of ovulation-inducing drugs after serious causes of anovulation have been ruled out, and prior to the extensive investigation of other factors of infertility. Once severe oligospermia or aspermia has been uncovered, further investigation of the female can be halted unless insemination therapy is to be considered.

At all times the therapist should be aware of the psychologically harmful effect of the tests and treatment, and one should be prepared to discontinue these when more harm than good is being produced. A confident, caring approach will do much to help the couple carry through to the termination of the tests and therapy.

REFERENCES

1. Tietze C, Guttmacher AR, Rubin S: Time required for conception in 1727 planned pregnancies. *Fertil Steril* 1:338, 1950
2. Buxton CL, Southam AL: *Human Infertility.* New York, Hoeber-Harper, 1958

PART II

Causes of Infertility

The physician investigating the causes of infertility should first have an understanding of the prerequisites for normal fertility. These are diagrammed in Fig. II-1. In summary these are production of an adequate number of motile and normal spermatozoa by the male partner; transport of these spermatozoa and deposition of an adequate number in the portio of the cervix and uterine fluid; transport of the sperm to the distal portion of the fallopian tubes, growth and development of a normal follicle, ovulation of a normal ovum, transport of the ovulated ovum to the distal portion of the fallopian tube; fertilization (indicating that coitus occurred during a required time interval); transport of the fertilized gamete down the fallopian tube by the ovary to ensure nidation and further development of the embryo.

This relatively complicated mechanism can be affected in a number of ways. The areas where infertility can be blocked or diminished are shown in Fig. II-2. These specific areas and problems will be briefly described in more detail in the workup of each anatomical area.

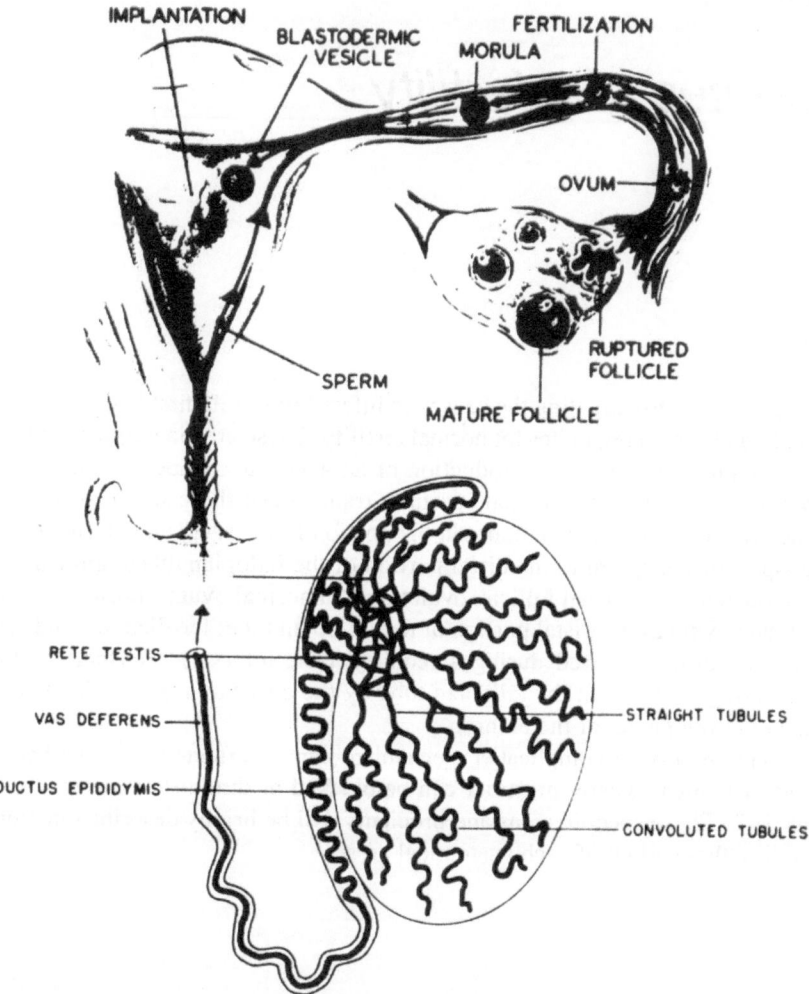

Figure II-1. Pathways to conception (adapted from Roland M: *Management of the Infertile Couple.* Springfield, IL, Charles C. Thomas, 1968; and Amelar R: *Infertility in Men.* Philadelphia, FA Davis, 1966).

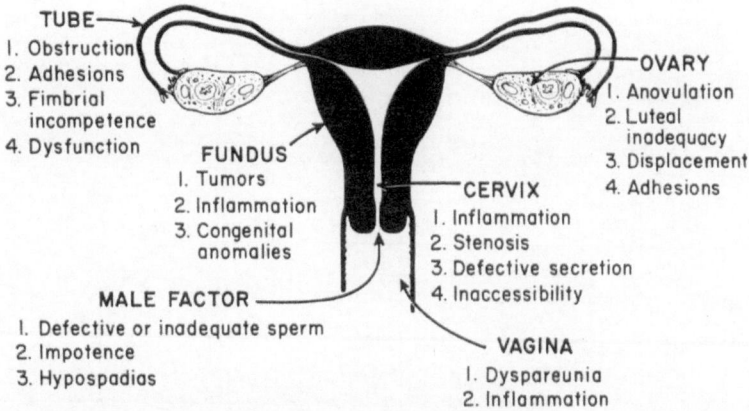

TUBE
1. Obstruction
2. Adhesions
3. Fimbrial
   incompetence
4. Dysfunction

FUNDUS
1. Tumors
2. Inflammation
3. Congenital
   anomalies

OVARY
1. Anovulation
2. Luteal
   inadequacy
3. Displacement
4. Adhesions

CERVIX
1. Inflammation
2. Stenosis
3. Defective secretion
4. Inaccessibility

MALE FACTOR
1. Defective or inadequate sperm
2. Impotence
3. Hypospadias

VAGINA
1. Dyspareunia
2. Inflammation

Figure II-2. Causes of infertility.

CHAPTER 5

Causes in the Male

Impaired fertility in the male is caused by either faulty sperm production (spermatogenesis) or faulty delivery of sperm.

IMPAIRED SPERMATOGENESIS

Sperm maturation or the process of spermatogenesis consists of a series of steps of division and then differentiation by which the spermatogonia progress to mature sperm. Sperm maturation is under endocrine control and depends on a delicate balance of hormones from the pititary gland, thyroid, adrenal, and testes.

The endocrine relationships are shown in Fig. 5-1. Luteinizing hormone (LH) stimulates testosterone production by the Leydig cells. Testosterone, in turn, exerts a negative feedback effect on the release of LH at the level of hypothalamus and pituitary. Follicle-stimulating hormone (FSH) stimulation results in the production of a substance called either "inhibin" or "Sertoli cell factor," which in turn, has a negative feedback effect on the production and release of FSH.

Testosterone is the primary spermatogenic hormone, at least at the level of the spermatid. At this point FSH also appears to be necessary, but even the FSH appears to exert its effect through the Sertoli cell by providing the spermatid with the correct concentration of testosterone.[1] These concepts, as well as the molecular mechanisms involved in the hormonal control of the spermatogenesis, have been extensively reviewed by Steinberger.[2]

21

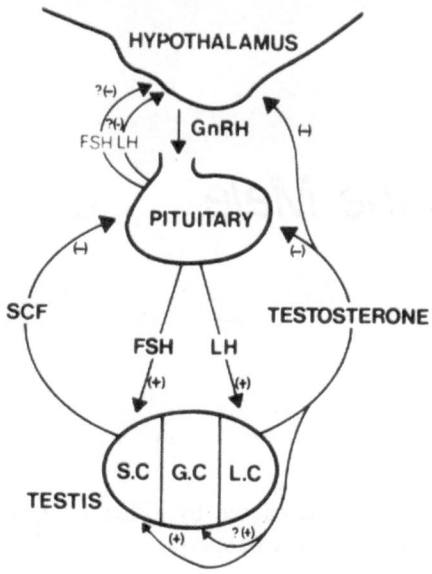

Figure 5-1. The hypothalamic–pituitary testicular axis.
S.C. = Sertoli cell; G.C. = germ cell; L.C. = Leydig cell (from Steinberger[2]).

An important feature of spermatogenesis is that the time required for development of mature sperm from spermatogonia is approximately 64 days.[3] Thus, 64 days must pass before any therapy can be evaluated.

Endocrine Causes

Endocrine deficiencies, as a cause of impaired spermatogenesis, are relatively rare. These may be primary gonadotropin lack, destruction of the pituitary tissue by a tumor or cyst, or destruction by surgical or radiation treatment for tumor or cyst. Thyroid deficiency, although rare, may affect spermatogenesis adversely. Congenital adrenal hyperplasia, relatively common in females, is very uncommon in males; when present, however, the elevated androgen from the adrenal suppresses the gonadotropin, which results in an arrest of spermatogenesis. If recognized and arrested by appropriate treatment, the impairment can be corrected. Some have suggested the presence of a mild form of adrenal hyperplasia acquired in adulthood. The diagnosis of this is based on the finding of elevated 17-ketosteroids.[4] However, such a condition is often difficult to document. Hyperprolactinemia is another, but extremely rare, cause of impaired spermatogenesis.

Genetic Effects

Genetic effects of spermatogenesis invariably result in complete azoospermia. Conditions such as true hermaphroditism, pure gonadal dysgenesis of the familial XX type, and congenital absence of testis have been reported. Fortunately, the conditions are rare, and they are not likely to find their way initially to a fertility specialist.

A relatively more common problem is Klinefelter's syndrome. Characterized genetically by 47 chromosomes, with an XXY karyotype, Klinefelter's syndrome affects 1 in 400 live born males. The internal and external genitalia are normal until puberty, and then the testes fail to develop. Although many are capable of erection and ejaculation, the ejaculate is without sperm. Gynecomastia is present in 80% of the individuals. Gonadotropins are elevated, but adrenal androgens are normal. There is no treatment to increase fertility.

Another important problem is cryptorchidism. Leydig cell function is normal, but spermatogenesis is disturbed. This results in varying degrees of oligospermia.

Nonendocrine Effects on Spermatogenesis

Spermatogenesis is more commonly affected by nonendocrine adverse influences. Many of these are related to the environment of the individual, and some are related to general disease processes. Some of these are well documented, and some of these are on a more tenuous basis. Because endocrine deficiencies as a cause of disturbed spermatogenesis are quite uncommon, I have always felt that an inquiry into the health habits of the male partner would yield more positive information than the routine investigation of endocrine disturbances. Yet, this is an area that is ignored by those physicians who rely solely on a single semen specimen and even by those who do carry out a historical and endocrine survey.

Nutrition. Nutrition is important in normal spermatogenesis. Only rarely, however, does an individual have a diet sufficiently deficient in protein so as to result in an impaired spermatogenesis. Vitamin deficiencies such as E and B have been shown to cause infertility in rats, but this has been difficult to document in humans.

Smoking. Until recently it had been difficult to document the harmful effects of tobacco on male infertility. For years, working on the concept that nicotine is a tissue poison, I have always recommended that my patients with low sperm quality give up smoking. In the last few years a number of scientific studies have confirmed this adverse relationship. Significantly abnormal morphology and decreased motility in sperm counts have been found in smokers as opposed to nonsmokers.[5,6] The mechanism of action seems to be a direct effect of nicotine on Leydig cell function. Actual decline in fertility has also been reported by others.[7,8] Marijuana intake has a smaller effect, a decline in testosterone levels and a possible decline in fertility.[9]

Alcohol. Similarly, for many years alcohol has been assumed to have a deleterious effect on sperm production, but only recently have there been studies documenting this relationship. Decreased sperm production has been demonstrated in chronic alcoholism,[10] and it would be safe to assume that lesser degrees of alcohol intake would cause lesser but still significant effects on sperm production. William Shakespeare's observation that "alcohol increases the desire but taketh away the performance" has also been scientifically confirmed.[11]

Heat. Excess heat is one of the common, well-accepted elements known to adversely affect spermatogenesis.[12,13] The testicles are situated in the scrotum and are, on the average, 2.2 degrees cooler than intra-abdominal temperature.[14] If the testicles are exposed to higher temperatures, sperm maturation is affected. This is reversible in most cases. Men whose occupations involve long hours of sitting, such as taxi or truck drivers, travelling salesmen, and business executives, may develop excess scrotal heat. Skin-tight underwear or frequent hot baths also play an adverse role. In cryptorchidism the testicle develops in an environment with excess heat, and there is serious impairment of spermatogenesis.[15] Unfortunately, this is not reversible.

Varicocele. The association of varicocele with fertility has been well documented.[16,17] However, the mechanism by which a varicocele affects sperm production remains unclear. Most studies suggest that a varicocele causes infertility by increasing the heat to the testes.[18,19] Other studies on heat transfer have thrown some doubt on this theory of causation.[20,21] Studies by MacLeod[22] and by Brown and his co-workers[23] indicate that there is considerable mixing of blood between the two sides of the testes. The theory further goes on to state that there is a lack of valves on the left spermatic vein and consequently there is pooling of venous blood in the varicocele and, as a result of mixing, in both testes. The blood is not cleared, and there is an accumulation of "toxins" in both testicles, which in turn has a deleterious effect on sperm production bilaterally. Catecholamines have been specifically incriminated.[24] A theory of increased cortisol concentration in the left internal spermatic vein as a causative agent has not been confirmed by studies of Agger.[25]

In addition to the above controversies, there are some who doubt the significance of varicocele in relation to infertility.[26,27]

Hypospadias. Hypospadias occurs in about 1% of infertile males and can result in faulty deposition of the sperm at or near the external cervical os.

Diethylstilbestrol. Another possible cause for infertility may be the effect on the male offspring of diethylstilbestrol taken by the mother during pregnancy. An increase in the incidence of congenital anomalies of the epididymis and a suggestion of deficiencies in serum quality has been reported.[28]

Generalized Illness. In taking the history from a man with a poor semen specimen, it is important to know about a past history of any febrile episode. Men who have had an acute febrile illness may well have a diminution of sperm production.[27] Usually the effect of the febrile illness persists for a 3-month period.

Physical and Chemical Agents Affecting Spermatogenesis. Spermatogenesis can also be affected by chemotherapy. Furadantin®, which is used frequently for urinary tract infections, caused degenerative changes in the spermatic tubules that apparently are reversible.[29] Other fairly common medicinal drugs that may suppress sperm quality are antidepressants, antimalarial drugs, and antihypertensives.

In severely disturbed spermatogenesis, the physician should also inquire about a history of radiation therapy.

Infections. Mumps orchitis, in which there is marked swelling of the testicle followed by atrophy, is a rare but well-documented cause of complete absence of spermatogenesis. The role of prostatitis is controversial[30] as well as is the role of mycoplasma infections.

The Immune Factor. The precise role of male autoimmunity in infertility is difficult to assess. Much of this difficulty has been due to the variability of types of testing for antibodies that have been available throughout the years. Also, there is very often a discrepancy between antibodies present on the sperm and levels of serum antibody. A fundamental principle to keep in mind is that the antibody effect, particularly in infertility, is not an all-or-none effect. Some men with a degree of positive antibody reaction can become fathers, while those with more severe degrees of immunity are indeed infertile.[31,32] The mechanism of action of infertility is the severe clumping of the sperm[33] and the possible decreased abilities to penetrate the ovum.[34] The incidence is about 5% and even that is relative.

The Effect of Continence or Coital Frequency on Semen Quality. The relationship between periods of continence and the various aspects of semen quality have been reported by MacLeod and Gold.[35] An increase in the period of continence is, in general, associated with a rise in the ejaculate volume and sperm count, and with a depression in the percentage of active forms. However, these qualities all level off after 10 days. Lampe and Masters, on the other hand, by studying daily ejaculation, found that frequency of intercourse is of little consequence in the normally fertile male, but that the relatively infertile male suffers a marked reduction of his fertility potential by too frequent ejaculation.[36]

SPERM TRANSPORT

After spermatogenesis, mature sperm are released into the lumen of the seminiferous tubules. From these tubules, they traverse the rete testes, a collecting network of fine tubules, to the convoluted ducts of the epididymis. Sperm moves through the epididymal ducts by a combination of muscular contraction and hydrostatic pressure. Ejaculation plays a role. Rowley and her co-workers studied the average time of sperm transport in the human. They concluded that it takes 12 days from the time of release in the seminiferous tubules to ejaculation.[37]

The fine tubules of the epididymis can be blocked by infection or injury. Gonorrheal infection is the most common, but epididymal infections may also be caused by other bacteria and rarely by tuberculosis.

Congenital absence of the lower end of the vas, or of the entire vas, may occur. Injury to these structures, due to trauma or surgery, can result in destruction and blockage. The vas may also be blocked subsequent to infection.

Retrograde ejaculation of semen into the bladder may follow surgery, injury, nerve interruption, spinal cord injury, or it may be idiopathic.

Impotence is an important cause of failure to transport spermatozoa to the vagina and cervix. Impotence may be a symptom of neurologic or general disorders such as diabetes, lumbar disc lesions, acute prostatitis, or drug ingestion. In most instances, the condition is psychogenic in origin. Masturbation is possible in such cases, and this is an important point in diagnosis, as well as allowing for therapy by means of homologous artificial insemination.

REFERENCES

1. Steinberger E, Root A, Fisher M, Smith KI: The role of androgens in the initiation of spermatogenesis in man. *J Clin Endocrinol Metab* 37:746, 1973
2. Steinberger E: Male reproductive physiology. In Crockett ATK, Urry RL (eds): *Male Infertility.* New York, Grune & Stratton, 1977, pp 1-25
3. Heller CG, Clermont Y: Spermatogenesis in man: Estimation of its duration. *Science* 140:184, 1963
4. Amelar R: *Infertility in Men.* Philadelphia, FA Davis, 1966, p 83
5. Evans JH, Fletcher J, Torrance M, Hargreave TB: Sperm abnormalities and cigarette smoking. *Lancet* 1:627, 1981

6. Vogt HJ, Heller WD, Borelli S: Sperm quality of healthy smokers, ex-smokers anad never smokers. *Fertil Steril* 45:106, 1986
7. Baird II, Wilcox AJ: Cigarette smoking associated with delayed ejaculation. *JAMA* 253:2979, 1985
8. Howe G, Westhoff C, Vessey M, Yeates D: Effects of age, cigarette smoking, and other factors on fertility: Findings in a large projective study. *Br Med J* 290:1697, 1985
9. Hembree WC, Zeidenberg P, Nahas GG. GG Nahas (ed): Marijuana's effect on human gonadal function in Marijuana: Chemistry, Biochemistry, and Cellular Effects. New York, Springer-Verlag, 1976, p 521
10. Farbas M, Rosen RC: Effect of alcohol on elicited male sexual response. *J Stud Alcohol* 37:265, 1976
11. Lester R, Van Thiel DH: Gonadal function in chronic alcoholism. *Adv Exp Med Biol* 85A:399, 1977
12. MacLeod J, Hotchkiss RS: The effects of hyperpyrexia upon spermatozoa counts in men. *Endocrinology* 28:780, 1941
13. Rock J, Robinson D: Effect of induced intrascrotal hyperthermia on testicular function in man. *Am J Obstet Gynecol* 93:793, 1965
14. Harrison RG, Weiner JS: Abdomino testicular temperature radiance. *J Physiol* 107:48, 1948
15. Steinberger E, Dixon WJ: Some observations of the effect of heat on the testicular germinal epithelium. *Fertil Steril* 10:578, 1959
16. Scott LS: Varicocele: Treatable cause of subfertility. *Br Med J* 1:788, 1961
17. Charney CW: Effect of varicocele on fertility. *Fertil Steril* 13:47, 1962
18. Agger P: Scrotal and testicular temperature: Its relation to sperm count before and after operation for varicocele. *Fertil Steril* 22:286, 1971
19. Zorgniotti AW, MacLeod J: Studies in temperature, human semen quality and varicocele. *Fertil Steril* 24:854, 1973
20. Tessler AN, Krahn HP: Varicocele and testicular temperature. *Fertil Steril* 17:201, 1966
21. Stephenson J, O'Shaughnessy E: Hypospermia and its relationship to varicocele and intrascrotal temperature. *Fertil Steril* 19:110, 1968
22. MacLeod J: Seminal cytology in varicocele as related to fertility. *Fertil Steril* 16:735, 1965
23. Brown J, Dubin L, Hotchkiss R: The varicocele as related to fertility. *Fertil Steril* 16:735, 1965
24. Comhaire F, Vermeulen A: Varicocele sterility: Cortisol and catecholamines. *Fertil Steril* 25:88, 1974
25. Agger P: Plasma cortisol in the left spermatic vein in patients with varicocele. *Fertil Steril* 22:270, 1971
26. Johnson DE, Puhl DR, Rivera-Correa H: Varicocele: An innocum condition? *South Med J* 63:34, 1970
27. Kursch ED: What is the incidence of varicocele in a fertile population. *Fertil Steril* 48:510, 1987
28. Bibbo M, Gill WB, Azizi F, et al: Follow-up study of male and female offspring of DES-exposed mothers. *Obstet Gynecol* 49:1, 1977
29. Albert PS, Salerno RG, Kapoor SN, et al: The nitrofurans as sperm-immobilizing agents, their tissue toxicity and their clinical application in vasectomy. *Fertil Steril* 26:485, 1975
30. Makler A, Urbach Y, Lefler E, Merxbach I: Factors affecting sperm motility: VI. Sperm viability under the influence of bacterial growth in human ejaculates. *Fertil Steril* 35:C66, 1981
31. Alexander NJ, Bearwood D: An immunoadsorption assay for antibodies to spermatozoa: Comparison with agglutination and immobilization tests. *Fertil Steril* 41:270, 1984
32. Wilkins SS, David SS: Effect of sperm antibodies vs. frequency outcome in a subfertile population. *Obstet Gynecol* 158:69, 1988
33. Fjallbrant B: Interaction between high levels of sperm antibodies, reduced penetration of cervical mucus by spermatozoa and sterility in man. *Acta Obstet Gynecol Scand* 47:102, 1968

34. Brown RA, Cooper GW, Rosenfeld DL: Sperm specific antibodies inhibit the bonding of human sperm to zona pellucida. *Fertil Steril* 38:724, 1982
35. MacLeod J, Gold R: The male factor in fertility and infertility: Effects of continence on semen quality. *Fertil Steril* 3:297, 1962
36. Lampe E, Masters W: Problems of male fertility: II. Effects of frequent ejaculation. *Fertil Steril* 7:123, 1966
37. Rowley MG, Teshima F, Heller CG: Duration of transit of spermatozoa through the human male ductular system. *Fertil Steril* 21:390, 1970

CHAPTER 6

Causes in the Female

THE VAGINA

Obstruction of the vaginal orifice can be a cause of infertility. The obstruction may be caused by a still unruptured hymen, or it may be functional, due to hypertrophy of the levator-ani muscles or to constriction of these muscles at the time of coitus. Most of the failure to penetrate the hymen, as well as the contractions of the levator-ani muscles, is psychological in origin. The female often offers primary resistance to coitus that brings about pain or dyspareunia, and further discomfort follows. Subsequent to this, male impotence often occurs. In a study reported in 1957, partners with the dyspareunia-and-impotence cycle made up 25% of our fertility clinic population.[1] Today, with improved sex education, and the resultant lessening of inhibitions, the incidence of this unfortunate cycle seems to be declining.

One might mention here the spermicidal effect of lubricants, since they are often used where there is difficult entry. Goldenberg and White confirmed the spermicidal effects of K-Y Jelly® and Surgilube®, but concluded that petroleum jelly and glycerine had little detrimental effect on sperm motility.[2]

Vaginitis, by itself, is not a serious cause of infertility, except as it serves as a temporary deterrent to coitus.

The most common congenital anomaly of the vagina is a complete septum. Usually the septum is pushed aside, and coitus occurs regularly on one side without difficulty. Narrowing of the upper vagina may be due to a congenital anomaly, but occasionally it may be due to scarring from trauma or infection. This may cause infertility by limiting coitus because of dyspareunia, or there maybe inadequate penetration and insemination.

29

THE CERVIX

The cervix is one of the important areas of obstruction to the passage of the sperm. During the few days prior to ovulation, in the normal menstrual cycle, under the influence of rising levels of estrogen, the endocervical glands secrete a thin watery mucus that is beneficial to sperm survival and migration. The sperms survive for many hours in the glands or crypts. At intervals they make their way to the uterus. Infection may destroy these glands or contaminate the mucus with leukocytes. Estrogen deficiency may decrease the volume and quality of the mucus. Overzealous cauterization of endocervical glands can be a factor by reducing the quality and quantity of mucus. The result is a dry, stenotic cervix, hostile to sperm survival and migration. There may be congenital anomalies of the cervix, the most common one being hypoplasia. Finally, a retroverted uterus keeps the cervix out of the seminal pool when the female is in the recumbent position, and thus may be a relative factor in faulty cervical insemination.

UTERINE FACTORS

The uterus is not a common cause of infertility. Congenital anomalies, such as a bicornuate uterus, are more likely to result in repeated abortion rather than in the initial inability to conceive, although, on occasion, lack of conception can be attributed to this cause. True double uterus is compatible with normal conception, pregnancy, and delivery, but it, too, on occasion, can be a factor in infertility. A unicornuate uterus is also compatible with normal pregnancy, but it is also associated with a relatively high risk for ectopic pregnancy.

Subserous and intramural fibroids usually do not interfere with fertility. Occasionally, growth during pregnancy may cause some problems. A submucosal fibroid is also more often associated with repeated abortion, but, on occasion, can possibly be a cause of infertility.

Intrauterine adhesions (Asherman's syndrome) are an increasing cause of infertility, and they are accompanied by oligomenorrhea or amenorrhea.[3,4] This syndrome is associated with a dilation and curettage following abortion or pregnancy, one in which infection is present. The increased incidence of therapeutic abortion has made this condition more common. Tuberculous endometritis, once quite common, is a rare cause of infertility in this country.

The female offspring of women who took diethylstilbestrol (DES) during their pregnancy have a high incidence of cervical and uterine abnormalities. Whether or not these abnormalities lead to infertility is controversial, but there is little doubt that the classic T-shaped uterus associated with DES intake results in almost a doubling of fetal loss.[5]

FALLOPIAN TUBES

The fallopian tubes act as a conduit for the sperm to reach the ovum and for the fertilized ovum to reach the uterus, but because the fertilized egg remains in the tubes for approximately 3 days, they must also provide nourishment for this developing zygote. Thus a tube that is not completely blocked by disease, but severely damaged with destruction of cilia or secretory cells, can contribute to infertility.

Complete blockage is usually a sequela of salpingitis of gonorrheal origin. This usually results in complete agglutination of the fimbria, as well as destruction of the endothelial lining of the tube and hydrosalpinx. Bacterial salpingitis, secondary to pelvic peritonitis, appendicitis, abortion, or instrumentation, usually results in a less severe blockage at the fimbriated end of the tube and less destruction of the endosalpinx. Blockage at the cornual end of the tube may be functional in nature because of spasm or congenital narrowing. It may also be caused by salpingitis isthmica nodosa, which is believed by some to be due to endometriosis, which may also result in complete blockage, and to salpingitis by others. Medical treatment of endometriosis has been shown to alleviate the blockage in some cases, and this suggests an etiologic role.[6]

Nongonorrheal infections are also more likely to result in what is called the *peritoneal factor*. The tubes are patent, but because of adhesions between the tube and ovary, or fixation of the ovary or tube to the pelvic peritoneum or broad ligament, there is an interference with the normal tubo-ovarian relationships required for tubal pickup. Acute pelvic inflammation, if treated properly, does not necessarily result in sterility; in a recent review, 63.4% of women with such inflammation ultimately became pregnant.[7] However, the frequency of ectopic pregnancy was 6 times that of a control group. However, there is increasing evidence that the prevalence of tubal disease has been on the rise in industrial nations, and it is further postulated that 2.5% of reproductive women in these countries will be infertile due to salpingitis by the time they reach 35 years of age. This increase appears to have started in association with an increased incidence of pelvic infections starting in the early 1970s. Furthermore, whereas in past years the gonococcus was a chief infectious agent, *Chlamydia trachomatis* is now responsible for 30% of cases.[8-10] T-mycoplasma has also been incriminated as a cause of salpingitis, but the relationship has not been fully established.[11] Intrauterine contraceptive device (IUD) users, particularly if nulliparous, are at increased risk of infection.[12,13] This may be due to the IUD itself, or due to reduced resistance to infectious agents when the IUD is in place. Later generations of IUDs, smaller and relying on copper as well, appear to be less harmful.

In addition to infection, a peritoneal factor can be caused by endometriosis. Although it is well recognized that moderate to severe degrees of endometriosis can cause infertility, the precise role of minimal and mild degrees of this disorder in causing infertility remains controversial. When the ovary is significantly enlarged with an endometriotic cyst, when it is adherent to the broad ligament, or when there are adhesions interfering with tubo-ovum pickup, there is an obvious relationship between the endometriosis and the infertility. It is much more difficult to establish a causal relationship with those degrees of endometriosis, mild and minimal, where there are only peritoneal or ovarian implants without interference with tubo-ovum pickup. Various explanations have been suggested, such as an increased number of prostaglandins[14] or CA-125,[15] an increased number of macrophages,[16] or an immunologic effect.[17] It is thought that the excess prostaglandins can affect ovulation and tubal motility, promote sperm phagocytosis, retard egg penetration, and induce uterine contractility. These theories are all speculative at best, and their significance is really put to the test by the number of studies that have shown that no treatment of minimal and mild endometriosis is as effective as medical therapy.[18-20]

THE OVARY

Ovarian factors in infertility are usually those associated with an endocrine imbalance. Occasionally, a large cyst of the ovary, usually of a benign nature, distorts tubo-ovarian relationships. However, the more common problem is interference with ovulation. Complete absence of ovulation, manifested by either amenorrhea or anovulatory cycles, can be caused by a disturbance of the normal pathways between the hypothalamus, pituitary, and ovary, and requires a thorough hormonal investigation of hypothalamic, pituitary, adrenal, and ovarian functions. These will be covered in chapter 19.

Overt hypothyroidism can result in complete anovulation,[21] and subclinical hypothyroidism in luteal phase deficiency.[22] Failure of the mature follicle to rupture despite relatively normal hormonal relationships, a condition called the luteinized unruptured follicle syndrome, is another possible cause of ovarian infertility.[23]

Premature ovarian failure can be caused by previous mumps infection,[24] radiation, chemotherapy, and autoimmune disorders.[25]

Another situation exists wherein ovulation occurs, but because of faulty corpus luteum function, there is an inadequate secretion of progesterone and inadequate stimulation of the endometrium. Hypothalamic, pituitary, and adrenal factors may be behind this relative effect as well.

GENERAL FACTORS

Tobacco has been noted to be a well-documented cause for lowering male fertility. In the last 6 to 7 years there have been a number of studies suggesting a causal relationship between female infertility and smoking, although only a few studies have shown a significant statistical relationship.[26,27] The mechanism of action appears to be the adverse effects of nicotine on tubal transport and implantation.

It is difficult to document that generalized systemic disease can play a significant role in infertility in the female other than those conditions that can cause obvious disruption of the ovulatory process at the level of hypothalamus, pituitary, or ovary; that virus infection or vitamin deficiencies ever play more than just a transient role remain speculative. The dangers of radiation have always been appreciated.[28] Recent animal studies document the incidence of congenital anomalies following radiation.[29] Genetic factors also play a role, but they are usually associated with conditions that result in amenorrhea.[30] A rare cause is toxoplasmosis.[31]

We are now becoming increasingly aware that age plays a significant role in fecundability, a term now often used to indicate chances of conceiving. Studies involving a large series of women undergoing donor insemination show a drop in fecundability from 74.1% before the age of 30 to 53.6% after age 35.[32]

Dietary deficiencies, particularly of calories and proteins, adversely affect the production and secretion of pituitary gonadotropins and lead to ovulatory defects of varying degrees.[33] Strenuous exercise such as jogging has been incriminated as producing ovulatory problems, either by direct effect of endorphins on the pituitary or because of an accompanying caloric deficiency. However, the amount of exercise has to be significant, about 10 miles of jogging per week according to one study.[34]

CONTROVERSIAL FACTORS

The role of mycoplasma infection and immune factors remain controversial and will be discussed in more detail in subsequent chapters. The weight of evidence suggests that these two can be causative agents in infertility, although this relationship has not yet been supported by valid statistical studies.

The relationship of emotional factors to infertility is also difficult to establish within a scientific framework, but such a relationship is well accepted and will also be dealt with in more detail.

REFERENCES

1. Sturgis SH, Taymor ML, Morris TA: Routine psychiatric interviews in fertility investigation. *Fertil Steril* 8:521, 1957
2. Goldenberg RL, White R: The effects of vaginal lubricants on sperm motility in vitro. *Fertil Steril* 26:873, 1975
3. Asherman JG: Traumatic intrauterine adhesions and their effects on fertility. *Int J Fertil* 2:49, 1957
4. Klein SM, Garcia C: Asherman's syndrome: A critique and current review. *Fertil Steril* 24:722, 1973
5. DeCherney AH, Naftolin F: Diethylstilbestrol-effect on fertility. In Behrman SJ, Kistner RW, Patton GW Jr (eds): *Progress in Infertility,* 3rd ed. Boston, Little, Brown, 1986, pp 227-236
6. Claman P, Taymor ML, Berger MJ, Seibel MM: Proximal obstruction of the oviduct: A possible role for medical therapy with danazol. *J Reprod Med* 3:687, 1986
7. Westrom L: Effect of acute pelvic inflammatory disease on fertility. *Am J Obstet Gynecol* 121:107, 1975
8. Westrom L: Incidence, prevalence and trends of acute pelvic inflammatory disease and its consequences in industrialized countries. *Am J Obstet Gynecol* 138:880, 1980
9. Sellers JW, Mahoney JB, Clernesby MA, Rath DJ: Tubal factor infertility: An association with prior chlamydial infection and asymptomatic salpingitis. *Fertil Steril* 49:451, 1988
10. Treharne JD, Ripa KT, Mardh PA, Svenson L, Westrom L, Darougan S: Antibodies to *Chlamydia trachomatis* in acute salpingitis. *Br J Vener Dis* 55:26, 1979
11. Mueller BR, Freundt EA, Mardh PA: Experimental pelvic inflammatory disease provided by *Chlamydia trachomatis* and *Mycoplasma hominis* in grivet monkeys. *Am J Obstet Gynecol* 138:990, 1980
12. Westrom L, Bengetsson LP, Mardh PA: The risk of pelvic inflammatory disease in women using intrauterine contraceptive devices as compared to non-users. *Lancet* 2:221, 1976
13. Serranyake P, Kramer D: Contraception and the etiology of pelvic inflammatory disease: New perspectives. *Am J Obstet Gynecol* 138:852, 1980
14. Badawy SZA, Machall L, Quenco V: Peritoneal fluid prostaglandins in various stages of menstrual cycle in infertile patients with endometriosis. *Int J Fertil* 30:48, 1984
15. Masahashi T, Matsuzawa K, Ohsawa M, Narita O, Ajai T, Ishuhara M: Serum CA 125 levels in patients with endometriosis: Changes in CA 125 levels during menstruations. *Obstet Gynecol* 73:328, 1988
16. Chacho KJ, Chacho MS, Anderson PJ: Peritoneal fluid in patients with and without endometriosis and their effect on the spermatozoa penetration assay. *Am J Obstet Gynecol* 154:1290, 1986
17. Wild RA, Shivers CA: Antiendometrial antibodies in patients with endometriosis. *Am J Reprod Immunol Microbiol* 63:51, 1985
18. Seibel MM, Berger MJ, Weinstein F, Taymor ML: The effectiveness of danazol in subsequent fertility on minimal endometriosis. *Fertil Steril* 88:534, 1982
19. Schenkeh RS, Malmak LR: Conservative surgery versus expectant management for the infertile patient with mild endometriosis. *Fertil Steril* 37:183, 1982
20. Thomas EJ, Cooke IE: Successful treatment of asymptomatic endometriosis: Does it benefit infertile women? *Br Med J* 294:1117, 1987
21. Thomas R, Reid RL: Thyroid disease and reproduction. *Obstet Gynecol* 70:789, 1987
22. Bohnet HG, Fiedler K, Leidenberger FA: Subclinical hypothyroidism and infertility. *Lancet* 2:1278, 1981
23. Donnez J, Thomas K: Incidence of luteinized unruptured follicle syndrome in infertile women and in women with endometriosis. *Eur J Obstet Gynecol Reprod Biol* 14:187, 1982

24. Morrison J, Givens J, Wiser WL, et al: Mumps oophoritis: A cause of premature menopause. *Fertil Steril* 26:658, 1975
25. Coulam EB: The prevalence of autoimmune disorder among patients with primary ovarian failure. *Am J Obstet Gynecol* 4:63, 1983
26. Phipps WR, Cramer DW, Schiff I, Belisle S, Stillman R, Albrecht B, Gibson M, Berger MJ, Wilson E: The association between smoking and female infertility as influenced by cause of the infertility. *Fertil Steril* 48:377, 1987
27. Stillman RJ, Rosenberg MJ, Sachs B: Smoking and reproduction. *Fertil Steril* 46:545, 1986
28. Kirsh IE: Radiation dangers in diagnostic radiology. *JAMA* 158:1420, 1955
29. Rugh R, Budd R: Does x-radiation of preconceptional mammalian ovum lead to sterility and/ or congenital anomalies? *Fertil Steril* 26:560, 1975
30. Miller J: Some genetic factors in human infertility. *Fertil Steril* 16:455, 1965
31. Eckering B, Neri A, Eylan E: Toxoplasmosis: A cause of infertility. *Fertil Steril* 18:883, 1968
32. Federation CECOS, Schwartz D, Mayaux MJ: Female fecundability as a function of age: Results of artifical insemination in 2,193 nulliparous women with azoospermic husbands. *N Engl J Med* 306:404, 1982
33. Pirke KM, Schweiger U, Laessle R, Dickhaut B, Schweiger M, Waechtler M: Dieting influences the menstrual cycle: Vegetarian vs. nonvegetarian diets. *Fertil Steril* 46:1083, 1986
34. Feicht CB, Johnson TS, Martin BJ: Exercise-related amenorrhea. *Lancet* 2:1145, 1978

CHAPTER 7

Emotional Factors

The role of emotional factors in infertility has been widely accepted for many years. A review of the subject was published by Kelly as far back as 1942.[1] Since that time, the literature has contained numerous reports and reviews.

Despite these reports, there are still many physicians who fail to appreciate the role of the psyche in infertility and who maintain that the failure of union of ovum and sperm is a mechanistic one in all cases. In a recent extensive review of infertility for a textbook, no mention of emotional factors was made other than as a possible cause of anovulation.[2] Perhaps the root of this skepticism, which is warranted to a degree, lies in the fact that psychiatric studies are usually inadequately controlled, and that the number of cases are few. Authors have often made extensive claims inconsistent with the available facts.

In a review of 75 references, Noyes and Chapnick concluded that (1) the authors assumed or stated the hypothesis that psychological factors altered fertility per se, (2) the evidence presented was scant, poorly organized, and poorly analyzed, (3) the literature was quoted unsystematically, (4) approximately 50 different psychological factors were said to relate psyche to fertility, (5) conclusive evidence was found that frigidity does not decrease fertility, and adoption does not increase fertility, and (6) no conclusive evidence was found that a specific, psychological factor can alter fertility in the normal infertile couple.[3] However, Noyes and Chapnick concluded that because such factors exist, extensive objective studies should be undertaken to isolate them.

The present methods of investigating these factors scientifically may be inadequate, but the importance of demonstrating how emotions affect fertility warrants the renewed efforts of gynecologists, behavioral scientists, and developmental biologists to develop new diagnostic and therapeutic tests.

Another difficulty in evaluating the significance of emotional factors may be because a situation is rarely one of psychogenic infertility, or organic infertility, alone. A combination of factors makes it hard to assess the relative importance of the emotions in any one patient.

Some physicians question the role of emotional factors as a *primary* cause of infertility, yet experienced therapists have little doubt that the state of infertility, itself, can provoke varying degrees of psychological symptoms. They know that psychic tension can, in turn, contribute to the state of infertility and may even be the decisive factor in a couple with marginal infertility. From the time of the initial interview with the couple, the physician should keep in mind the potential role of emotions. He or she should be sensitive to emotional clues from both partners, and throughout the course of diagnosis and therapy, the physician should maintain this heightened awareness.

INCIDENCE

Because we now lack controlled studies, and because of the complex and involved nature of the diagnosis and therapy (which means that only a limited number of patients can be studied), it is difficult to know the exact incidence of significant emotional factors among a group of infertility problems. Stone and Ward, reporting upon the etiologic factors in 500 cases of infertility, noted that apparent organic causes were absent in 24.4%.[4] Two-thirds of these patients conceived fairly promptly after reporting to the clinic. It is possible that a number of these conceptions could have occurred because of chance, but this figure suggests that so large a percentage of conceptions occurred because, once the patients placed themselves under a physician's care, their emotional factors lost their negative implications. Ford and co-workers reported that 9 patients of 38 had "functional" causes for infertility.[5] In a study at our clinic, 9 of 40 patients had significant neurotic problems, either alone or associated with organic factors.[6] These studies strongly suggest that emotional factors play a not insignificant role in the total problem of infertility.

PSYCHOPHYSIOLOGIC PATHWAYS

The mechanisms by which emotional tensions and neurotic problems might interfere with reproductive functions are fairly well documented in some cases; in others the mechanisms remain obscure. It is universally understood that the ovulatory process can be influenced adversely by emotional stimuli through the hypothalamic–pituitary–ovarian axis[7]; this may take the form of complete anovulation, or of milder defects such as progestational deficiency or irregular ovulation. Emotional tension has been shown to produce tubal spasm. Stallworthy reported that 50% of the tubal blockage diagnosed by insufflation was due to spasm.[8]

Vaginismus, dyspareunia, and frigidity are usually of psychic origin. Aside from limiting coitus, and thus the exposure of ovum to sperm, these conditions themselves appear to be associated with reduced fertility. Some physicians believe that the lack of sexual satisfaction results in sterility because of the failure of uterine contractions or because of chronic uterine congestion or cervical hypersecretion. I believe, however, that the role of orgasm in promoting fertility should be de-emphasized, because the symptoms of dyspareunia and frigidity are usually the symptoms of a psychic conflict, which by itself may impair fertility.

In the male, decreased libido and impotence are obvious sequelae of psychological problems. In addition, sham ejaculation, retrograde ejaculation, and premature ejaculation can be the result of psychic disturbances.[9] Fisher and Dorfman have suggested that impaired spermatogenesis may result from emotional conflict,[10,11] and still others have reported an improvement in sperm motility in a patient undergoing psychoanalysis.[12] Such isolated reports require further documentation.

PSYCHODYNAMICS

A number of studies have demonstrated psychological differences in infertile women or couples as compared with controls. Eisner found that infertile women showed more emotional disturbances in the Rorschach test.[13] Carr found more neurosis, neurotic dependency, and anxiety in infertile women.[14] Grimm reported on the increased presence of emotional instability, overt dependency, tension, hostile feelings, and guilt in chronic aborters as opposed to nonaborters.[15] Platt and his co-workers noted that couples with infertility perceived the locus of control over events in their lives as being exterior to themselves.[16] In addition, infertile females, but not infertile males, showed more neurosis, anxiety, and emotional disturbances than controls. Although these studies were well controlled, they cannot determine whether the emotional problems caused infertility or the infertility caused the emotional symptoms.

Other psychoanalytic studies of functional sterility have postulated that even though many women actively seek help for infertility, this overt action is really a strong, unconscious opposition to pregnancy. Psychoanalysts cite as examples the aggressive "masculine" type, who unconsciously may be rejecting her feminine role, and the immature "dependent" type who is attempting to make a child–parent relationship of the marriage.

Many physicians find it difficult to accept these theoretical psychoanalytic concepts because so many women conceive who do not want to become pregnant, as do vast numbers of women who are "overly aggressive" or "sexually immature." One can answer this paradox in three ways: first, the conscious expression of attitudes is less likely to result in psychosomatic disturbances than are repressed conflicts; second, psychological conflicts need not always manifest themselves through the generative tract; and third, the pluralistic nature of the etiology of infertility means that emotional factors must often be associated with significant organic defects before infertility occurs.

This should suggest to the therapist that even when emotional factors seem obvious, he or she should not attach such undue importance to them that the physician fails to treat potential organic problems.

The role of adoption in allaying emotional tensions has been considered classic evidence of how treating emotional factors can alleviate infertility, but even this supposition is not without its skeptics. Although Sandler concluded that adoption facilitates conception in those women whose organic factors have been adequately treated and where there is continuing emotional tension,[17] three other studies fail to show a statistically significant relationship between adoption and subsequent conception.[18–20] If psychiatrists and psychiatrically oriented gynecologists were to exercise restraint in emphasizing emotions to the exclusion of other pertinent factors, the overall importance of the emotional role would be more readily accepted.

A recurring emphasis in this book is that the state of infertility, the diagnostic tests, and the therapy involved are as likely to produce emotional factors as emotional factors are to produce infertility. Infertility brings with it feelings of frustration and depression.[21] The tests and treatments often engender anxiety and fear.[22] The involvement of a third party, even a sympathetic therapist, in a discussion of private sexual activity is not without serious emotional implications. These tensions, through the hypothalamic pituitary pathways, through autonomic smooth muscle systems, or through pathways not yet fully understood, add their inhibiting weight to whatever organic factors are already present; of this every therapist should be constantly aware. The physician should be understanding and sympathetic and so conduct diagnostic and therapeutic tests and treatment to minimize their adverse effects.

THERAPY

Is there a need for routine psychiatric evaluation in the management of the infertile couple? Is the ideal infertility specialist a gynecologist who has also been psychiatrically trained? Unfortunately, few gynecologists have the time, or inclination, for such intensive emotional exploration with each patient; but the infertility specialist or gynecologist should at least be sufficiently aware of the importance of emotional factors and recognize the patient who needs psychiatric help. Surely, these are the minimal qualifications for all those who attempt to treat the infertile couple.

The therapist should take the time for a careful initial history. The rapport established between therapist and couple should be maintained and strengthened in subsequent sessions. Sympathetically reviewing the patient's previous sexual history and investigating childhood family relationships will make the therapist more receptive to signals or clues that indicate underlying emotional disturbance. Thus, the gynecologist knows when a diagnostic step or therapy will do more harm than good.

With such an approach, the conscientious specialist can care for a large portion of the patient's emotional factors. In the past, I participated in a study in which routine psychiatric interviews were recommended. I could see the wisdom of such an interview, but many patients refused and viewed it as a threatening procedure. Therefore, I feel it is often more practical for the fertility specialist to serve as the screening physician, to practice preventive psychiatry by singling out the patient with significant emotional conflicts for whom psychiatric consultation can be arranged, and, finally, to urge psychiatric consultation for all patients with unexplained infertility.

REFERENCES

1. Kelly K: Sterility in the female with special reference to psychic factors: Review of the literature. *Psychosom Med* 4:211, 1942
2. Warren JC: Reproductive failure. In Romney S (ed): *Gynecology and Obstetrics*. New York, McGraw Hill, 1976, p 616
3. Noyes R, Chapnick E: Literature of psychology and infertility: A critical analysis. *Fertil Steril* 15:543, 1964
4. Stone A, Ward ME: Factors responsible for pregnancy in 500 cases. *Fertil Steril* 7:1, 1956
5. Ford ES, Forman I, Wilson WM, et al: A psychodynamic approach to the study of infertility. *Fertil Steril* 4:456, 1953
6. Sturgis SH, Taymor ML, Morris TA: Routine psychiatric interviews in infertility investigation. *Fertil Steril* 8:521, 1957
7. Igarishi M, Tahma K, Ozawa M, et al: Pathogenesis of psychogenic amenorrhea and anovulation. *Int J Fertil* 4:31, 1965
8. Stallworthy J: Facts and fantasy in the study of female infertility investigation. *J Obstet Gynecol Br Commonw* 55:171, 1948
9. Palti Z: Psychogenic male infertility. *Psychosom Med*, 31:326, 1969
10. Fisher IC: Psychogenic aspects of sterility. *Fertil Steril* 4:466, 1953
11. Dorfman W: Psychosomatics, psychopharmacology, psychotherapy and sterility. *J Reprod Med* 3:201, 1969
12. Heiman M, Klegman S: Insemination: A psychoanalytic and infertility study. *Fertil Steril* 17:117, 1966
13. Eisner BG: Some psychological differences between fertile and infertile women. *J Clin Psychol* 19:39, 1963

14. Carr GG: *A Psychological Study of Fertile and Infertile Marriages.* Unpublished doctoral dissertation. University of Southern California at LA, 1963
15. Grimm SR: Psychological investigation of habitual abortion. *Psychosom Med* 24:369, 1962
16. Platt JJ, Fisher I and Silver MJ: Infertile couples: Personality traits and self-ideal concept discrepancies. *Fertil Steril* 24:972, 1973
17. Sandler B: Conception after adoption: A comparison of conception rates. *Fertil Steril* 16:313, 1965
18. Tyler ET: Occurrence of pregnancy following adoption. *Fertil Steril* 11:581, 1960
19. Aronson HG, Glienke CF: A study of the incidence of pregnancy following adoption. *Fertil Steril* 14:547, 1963
20. Rock J, Tietze C, McLaughlin HB: Effect of adoption on infertility. *Fertil Steril* 16:305, 1965
21. DeWattsville H: Psychologic factors in sterility. *Fertil Steril* 8:12, 1957
22. Bullock JC: Iatrogenic impotence in an infertility clinic. *Am J Obstet Gynecol* 120:476, 1974

PART III

The Basic Workup

CHAPTER 8

History and Examination of the Couple

Because the initial interview sets the tone for the whole course of treatment, it is especially important that this first encounter should be with the couple. This immediately imparts both to the husband and wife not only the importance of the couple as a unit, but also the relative nature of infertility. Meeting with the couple creates the environment for a more complete and honest discussion of sexual and emotional factors; if necessary, it lays the groundwork for future counseling. It is also a time to banish fears and dispel general misconceptions about infertility and reproduction. So important is sensitive history taking that it should never be delegated to an aide, and, least of all, to a stereotyped questionnaire. With the physician's reassurance, the feeling of fault resting with one partner or the other is diminished. With the proper explanation, even if the sperm count later proves to be adequate, the maintenance of a supportive role by the husband is exceedingly helpful.

The perceptive physician can learn much from the nuances, the dynamic interplay between husband and wife. A basically strained relationship may become apparent. The relative indifference of the husband to the problems may surface. When taking the sexual history, the remarks of each partner may prove especially significant. Since one partner may be somewhat reticent about being completely honest in front of the spouse, it is often helpful to pursue questions later when the individuals are seen separately. Usually, the couple has already heard about infertility and reproduction, and about the temperature chart, and may have been attempting coitus by the chart with disastrous results. The initial interview is merely the first crucial step in what must be a process of continuing education between the therapist and couple.

HISTORY AND EXAMINATION OF THE FEMALE

Present Illness

Initial questioning determines (1) the age of the couple, (2) the years of marriage, (3) the history of previous marriages and pregnancies, (4) the previous use of contraceptives to determine the length of exposure to the possibility of pregnancy, and (5) the results of previous studies. An evaluation of these results and the decision to stand by these tests or have them repeated depend on the experience of the previous physician.

Menstrual History

The presence of marked menstrual irregularity and, of course, amenorrhea indicate the presence of an endocrine factor. Staining prior to menses and irregular cycles suggest a progesterone deficiency. The presence of secondary dysmenorrhea should raise the suspicion of endometriosis.

Obstetric History

The obstetric history is obviously pertinent only in cases of secondary infertility. Of special interest would be the presence or absence of a postpartum hemorrhage associated with secondary amenorrhea, which suggests the possibility of Sheehan's syndrome. Postpartum infection or a cesarean section might result in pelvic adhesions.

Past History and Review of Symptoms

A review of symptoms may reveal generally poor health in the present or the past. A history of previous pelvic infection or of surgery involving either the ovary or tube is pertinent. Adhesions involving either the ovary or tube should be viewed with suspicion, as should a history of a ruptured appendicitis. Varying degrees of interference with a hypothalamic–pituitary–ovarian axis may be caused by acute or chronic systemic infections. Of particular importance is a history of excessive weight gain or loss. Obesity may cause, or be associated with, anovulatory problems. This should be followed up with questions that might suggest hypofunction of the thyroid gland. True hypothyroidism can cause anovulation and amenorrhea, but is a rare cause when the relative frequency of such disturbances is taken into consideration. More commonly, amenorrhea is associated with severely underweight women, and a careful dietary history may reveal significant protein or caloric deficiency.

Diet, Habits, Exercise, Sleep

Disturbance of diet, use of excess tobacco or alcohol, and excess exercise or the lack of sleep either alone or together may have some effect upon fertility. In the female, unless there are extreme variations, especially in diet and exercise, it is difficult to document significant effects. One of the main results of questioning in this area is that it leads logically and naturally to a detailed investigation of coital habits.

Coital History

One can begin the investigation of the coital history with questions concerning the frequency of intercourse, the degree of satisfaction, and the absence or presence of orgasm. It is best that the physician explain at this point that questions concerning orgasm do not necessarily imply that the female orgasm is required for conception, but rather that the therapist is searching for any disturbances that might engender emotional tension. If orgasm does not occur regularly, but reasonable satisfaction is otherwise achieved, reassurance can be given. If one or both partners are concerned that the lack of orgasm means a degree of inadequacy, the time should be taken to place this in its proper perspective. Further questioning may also reveal a degree of ignorance and ineptness that may be corrected. Discussions concerning the frequency of coitus will often disclose that the pattern of intercourse is being dictated by a temperature chart or by other previous erroneous advice. Temperature charts are not only inaccurate in pinpointing the optimum time for coitus, but for most patients who volunteer such information, sexual activity has already become less and less pleasurable. Such information may form the basis for future counseling sessions.

At this point in the interview, sufficient rapport should be established so that the physician can question the patient concerning her emotional state. Is she excessively tense or worried? What are her relationships with her husband, family, and employer? What special fears does she have concerning pregnancy? Most patients will volunteer the information that if they do have present emotional problems, they are related to the fact of infertility itself. If such a statement is not volunteered or strongly implied, it is an area that should be explored further by the therapist. Such investigation of emotional factors should not stop with the initial interview but should be continued through the total period of management.

Physical Examination

The examination should be both general and gynecologic. In the general examination, stigmata of endocrine disturbances may be noted, such as changes in body habitus, degree of breast development, or hirsutism. General examination should include evaluation of thyroid enlargements and a thorough breast examination.

The pelvic examination starts with the examination of the vulva for normal proportions. The ability of the patient to relax during the pelvic examination and the amount of pain she experiences offer some clues about the individual's emotional makeup. Relaxation at the introitus is carefully evaluated as it might be related to problems during coitus. The vaginal length and depth are estimated. The cervix is inspected for polyps and infection and the stigmata of diethylstilbestrol exposure. The location of the cervix in relation to the seminal pool and its mobility are evaluated. Tenderness on motion is evaluated, and the cervix is inspected for erosion and possible endometriosis.

The uterus is examined for size, symmetry, and position. The presence of retroversion is noted for future evaluation of the postcoital test and also for future fertility tests where an instrument need be placed within the endometrial canal. In amenorrhea and oligomenorrhea, one looks for a hypoplastic uterus, where the uterus is small and the proportion of the cervix to the fundus is relatively increased. However, this condition is often overdiagnosed. The presence or absence of fibroids and other abnormalities in the fundus is noted.

The adnexa are examined for evidence of tenderness and enlargement. The diagnosis of endometriosis is best made by palpation of the uterosacral ligaments and posterior cervix rectal examination.

HISTORY AND EXAMINATION OF THE MALE

Although semen analysis provides the overwhelming signpost of the male partner's degree of fertility or infertility, much can be learned from a thorough history and physical examination that will lead to correction of deficiencies in semen quality.

Past History

The male's history should be reviewed to learn both routine childhood diseases and severe atypical ones. A sustained chronic illness or dietary deficiency during the critical time of childhood or puberty may have adversely affected testicular development. Routine childhood diseases may have been associated with severe febrile episodes. The presence of mumps orchitis should be investigated. Was growth and development normal? Is there anything to suggest a childhood endocrine disorder that would affect development?

Were the testicles descended at the time of birth? If not, was there any corrective surgery? Operations, particularly in the genital area, should be reviewed. Any x-ray treatment for tumors of the lower part of the body? In addition to chronic illness, an acute viral infection within the past 3 months could affect spermatogenesis. Injuries and instrumentation in the scrotal area are also important.

System Review

Questions concerning the cardiorespiratory and gastrointestinal systems will determine general health. Difficulties with urination, a history of a ureteral stone, bladder infections, and prostate infections are taken up in a review of the genitourinary system. Any past history of venereal disease is also ascertained at this time. Answers to questions about weight gain, the amount of energy, and intolerance to hot or cold weather can lead the physician to suspect the presence of an under- or overactive thyroid. When the dietary history is taken, the physician should note whether the diet is well balanced, particularly in reference to protein intake.

Habits

Perhaps among the most important questions the physician can raise pertaining to the male are to his occupation and other habits that might relate to sperm production. Excessive cigarette smoking and alcohol consumption is determined. Factors that might produce excess heat to the scrotum are investigated, such as frequent hot baths and skin-tight underwear. Whether the patient be a business executive or a taxi driver, a truck driver, or a traveling salesman, all these occupational situations involve prolonged sitting. Does the man take any exercise to compensate for these primarily sedentary occupations? Occupational exposure to chemicals is also sought.

Finally the *sexual history* is reviewed once again with the husband alone to be certain that he has nothing to correct or add to the previous joint history taken while the couple was seen together.

Physical Examination

With the patient's body stripped, the physician obtains a general impression of possible endocrine stigmata by viewing the body habitus, muscular development, and hair and fat distribution. The heart, lungs, and abdomen are routinely examined to rule out problems in these areas. The inguinal areas are examined. The testes are palpated for size, consistency, and the presence or absence of tumors, hydrocele, and spermatocele. The vas deferens is palpated on either side. The presence of a varicocele is determined; a Valsalva maneuver may often make a small varicocele more apparent. Finally, the prostate gland is palpated. If boggy or tender, a gentle massage is carried out to produce fluid for microscopic examination.

CHAPTER 9

Evaluation of the Cervical Factor

The importance of the survival of the sperm in the cervix after coitus was first described by Sims, the pioneer gynecologist, in 1866. In 1888 he further amplified the various causes for failure to find surviving sperm.[1] In 1913, further details of testing were expounded by Huhner,[2] and since that time the Sims–Huhner postcoital test has been widely accepted as an important tool in infertility diagnosis.

During recent years, as a result of more critical evaluation of the test in relation to pregnancy outcome, the prognostic value of the postcoital test has come under question.[3] It is true that pregnancies can occur in some women with poor postcoital tests and that all women with an excellent postcoital test do not conceive, but the extremes of the test correlate well with pregnancy outcome. Much of this discrepancy undoubtedly comes from inadequate studies and from the multifactorial nature of infertility, but possibly the failure to standardize the test in terms of time of performance after coitus adds to the lack of clarity of results. Recent investigations into the function of the cervix has placed the postcoital test on a firmer physiologic basis.[4-6]

FUNCTIONS OF THE CERVIX

The three main functions of the cervix in relation to fertility are (1) to serve as a passageway for spermatozoa, (2) to filter spermatozoa, and (3) to store spermatozoa.

Sperm storage and concomitant sperm migration are essential because the ovum is only fertilizable over a 6-hour period,[7] but sperm retain motility and fertilizing ability in all parts of the female genital system for at least 50 hours.[8] This increases the chances of there being normal sperm available for each ovulated oocyte.

The first two functions, *sperm migration* and the *filtering effect* are under the influence of the ovarian cycle. Under the influence of the rising level of estrogen, the endocervical epithelium increases the secretion of a thin, watery substance rich in mucin, glycoproteins, and salts, and relatively free of endocervical cells.

Spermatozoa survive well in the preovulatory mucus, and are probably stored in the crypts of the endocervical glands, and continuously make their way up the endocervical canal during the preovulatory period.

There are specific physical characteristics of preovulatory mucus that can be observed and measured.[9] The mucus develops elasticity (spinnbarkeit) (Fig. 9-1). The drying of the mucus at this time results in the development of cervical mucus arborization or ferning.[10] (Fig. 9-2) In addition, the cervical os and probably the endocervical canal are dilated at this time. During the luteal phase, as a result of progesterone secretion, the cervical canal narrows, and the secretions become scant, thick, gelatinous, and cellular; ferning and spinnbarkeit are absent or diminished (Fig. 9-3).

Studies have demonstrated that estrogen increases sperm transport through the cervix.[11] Observations on the structure of the cervical mucus reveal that under the influence of estrogen, the microfibrils of cervical mucus are arranged in longitudinal fashion with considerable space between the fibrils, thus aiding sperm migration.[12] Without estrogen, the fibrils form a dense network, impenetrable to the sperm (Fig. 9-4). Other factors in sperm migration may be enzymes[13] and pH.[14,15]

That cervical mucus also has a filtering function is suggested by studies in animals showing that (1) there is a leukocytic response to sperm in the cervix, (2) these do not reach the uterine cavity,[1] and (3) the leukocytes aid in the degradation of the sperm.[16] Presence of nonmotile and abnormal sperm in the cervical mucus 24 hours or longer after intercourse or insemination is additional evidence that cervical mucus acts as a filter that prevents ascent of abnormal sperm.[17]

The concept that the cervix has *storage* function, rather than just being a conduit, has important connotations from both the point of view of the fertile period and the timing of the postcoital test. Since coitus is rarely timed to coincide with ovulation in most instances, successful fertilization depends on a constant supply of sperm at the site of fertilization for many hours before and after ovulation. Motile sperm are commonly found in the cervix 58 hours after coitus.[18] Numerous studies have shown that viable sperm can be found in cervical mucus as long as 8 days after coitus.[18] One study showed that if there

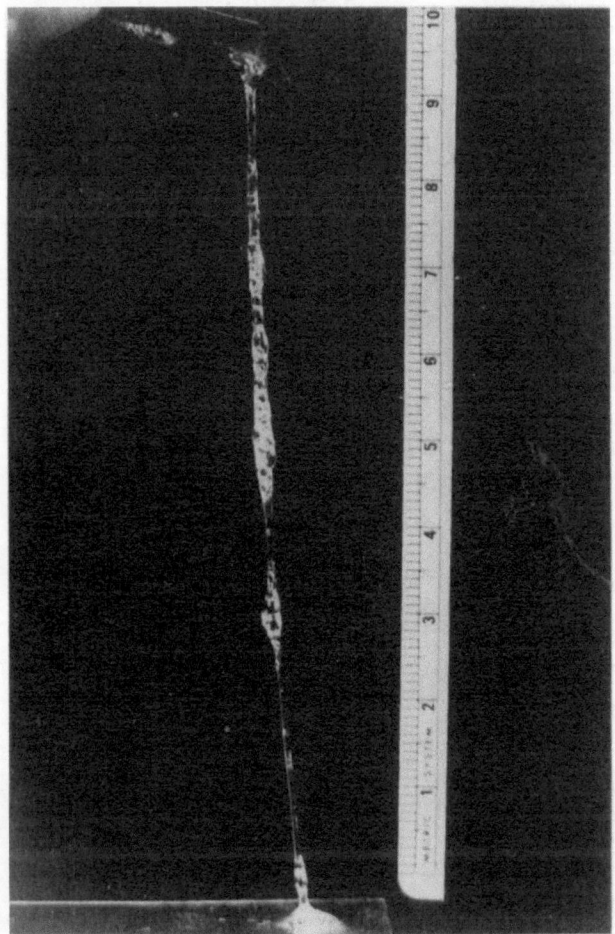

Figure 9-1. Elasticity (spinnbarkeit) of preovulatory cervical mucus.

was good ferning of cervical mucus (evidence of adequate estrogen secretion), in over 50% of the samples there was viable sperm 5 days after coitus.[19] Animal studies have demonstrated the continuous passage of sperm from the cervical mucus into the uterus.[20]

THE POSTCOITAL TEST

Spermatozoa will survive best in cervical mucus during the preovulatory phase, at which time, under the influence of high levels of estrogen, the cervical

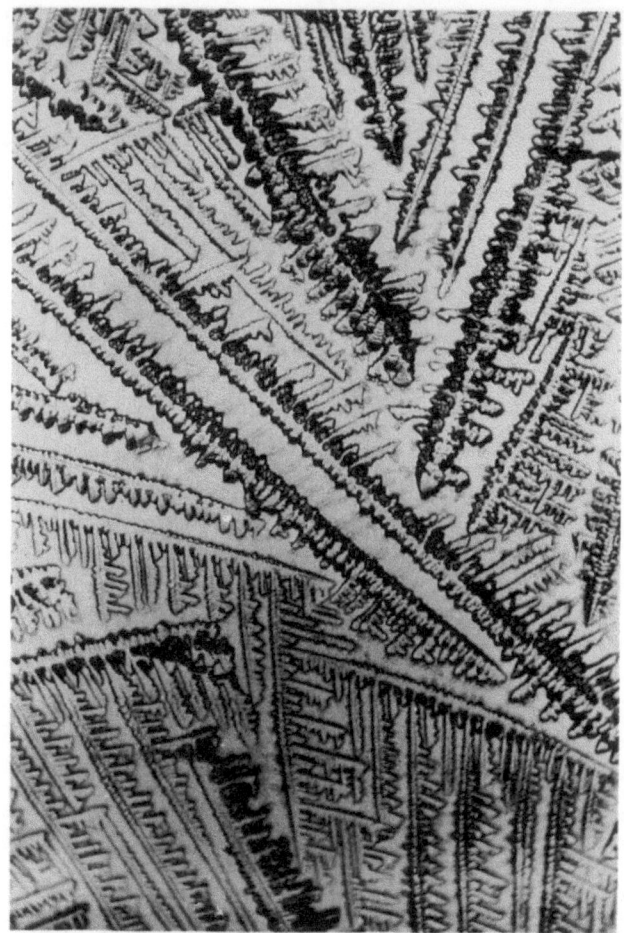

Figure 9-2. Full ferning of preovulatory cervical mucus.

mucus is thin, watery, and relatively acellular. Therefore, the test should be carried out as close to the preovulatory period as possible. During a 28-day cycle, this means the 14th or 15th day of the cycle. In women with irregular or prolonged cycles, it may be necessary to carry out many postcoital tests.

In my experience, many physicians carry out the tests 2 to 8 hours after coitus, and often at 2 hours or less. There is little biologic justification for this approach. Huhner stated that the test that bears his name should be performed as soon as possible after coitus.[21] He gave no reason. Southam and Buxton wrote that "perhaps the spermatozoa in the cervical mucus at the time of the postcoital test are those without enough strength to progress further, while

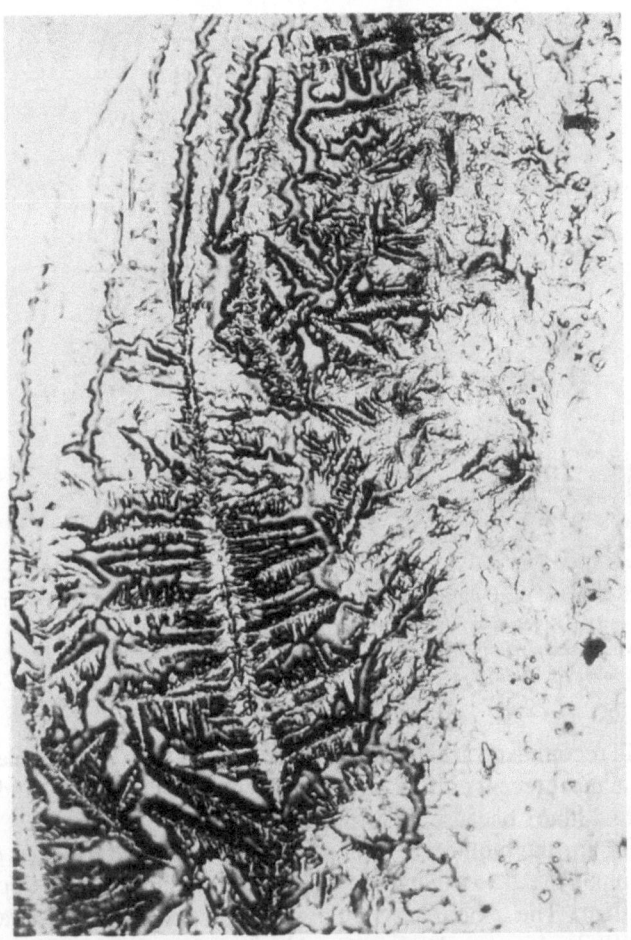

Figure 9-3. Partial ferning of cervical mucus indicative of only low estrogen activity or the addition of progesterone.

those with high velocity had progressed beyond the cervix."[22] But they offered no proof for this statement. Treadway suggested that the postcoital test be performed 2½ hours after coitus because he found this to be the time when most sperm were found.[23]

Most of the current, authoritative reviews of infertility continue to beg the question. In the latest (1988) edition of *Progress in Infertility*, there is no chapter on the cervical factor. In a chapter reviewing infertility, the postcoital test is mentioned, but the time after coitus when the test is performed is not specified. On the other hand, in the second edition of *Progress in Infertility*,

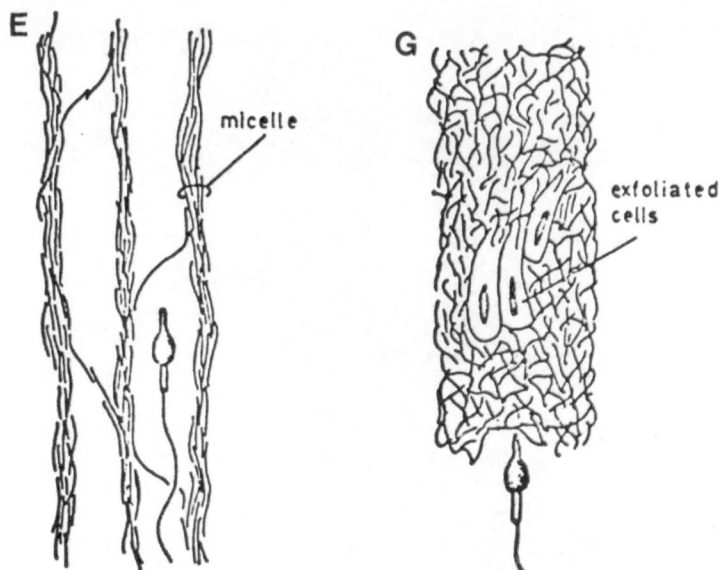

Figure 9-4. Schematic three-dimensional view of the structure of estrogenic (E) cervical mucus and postovulatory (G) cervical mucus with sperm moving inside the cervical plasma between the micelles of type E and a noninvading sperm outside type G (from Odebad E: *Acta Obstet Gynecol Scand* 47 (Suppl 1):61, 1968).

Davajan did recommend a 2-hour interval because it was "reasonable."[24] Similarly, in the most recent edition of *Gynecologic Endocrinology*, Andrews also advises 2 to 4 hours because it has proved "practical."[25]

Leaving for the moment the question of physiologic rationale, one could ask for whom is the 2- to 4-hour test "reasonable and practical." Certainly not for the patient. The 2-hour test requires that intercourse take place in the morning. While this may be a reasonable time for some couples to "make love," under these circumstances it is a time when they must perform the act according to a precise schedule that may conflict with daily routines and professional commitments of one or both partners. If a time interval for this test is being chosen solely on the basis of reasonableness and practicality, it certainly would be more comfortable for the couple to have intercourse "at bedtime," but not at a prescribed hour, on the evening prior to the day of testing. The appointment for the postcoital test could be made for any time in the working day that is mutually convenient for the physician and patient. We suspect that greater flexibility in timing the postcoital test (i.e., 10 to 16 hours after coitus) will lead to wider application of the test as well as more informative test results.

However, beyond reasonableness and practicality, there are also physiologic reasons for delaying the postcoital test. There is good evidence that the human cervical mucus serves as a reservoir for sperm. There is a significant relationship between sperm survival for 48 hours in cervical mucus and conception in donor artificial insemination cycles.[26] There is little change in motility of normal sperm after 48 hours in cervical mucus,[27] and sperm recovered from the mucus at this time can penetrate the human zona pellucida and fuse with zona-free hamster oocytes.[28] It is likely that conception depends in part on the ability of sperm to survive in cervical mucus and maintain function there. The oocyte is probably fertilizable for less than 24 hours. Most couples attempting to conceive are advised to have intercourse every other day in the periovulatory period. When sperm are able to survive in the cervical mucus for 24 hours or longer, it is logical that the chances of conception will be greater. As Treadway pointed out, most postcoital tests will be positive at 2½ hours.[23] But significant information may be lost when sperm survival at longer intervals is not observed. We have seen numerous cases in which the postcoital test is adequate at 2 hours, but unsatisfactory after a longer interval. These include cases of male and female factor infertility, some related to antisperm antibodies and some to nonimmunologic causes. In his excellent review, Moghissi emphasizes the importance of sperm longevity for fertility.[29] We are missing the opportunity to identify potentially treatable causes of infertility when we limit the interval of postcoital testing.

Both for physiologic reasons and for the emotional comfort of our patients, Overstreet and I have urged that physicians adopt a more rational and flexible approach to postcoital testing and take advantage of the clinical information that may be gained from observations of sperm longevity in the cervix.[30]

Procedure

With the patient in the lithotomy position and a bivalve speculum in place, the vaginal secretions are wiped from the cervix. The pH of the cervical mucus is tested. A large dressing forceps or a special mucus forceps (Fig. 9-5) is inserted about 1 cm into the cervical canal, opened, rotated, closed tightly, and then withdrawn. The mucus is placed on a microscope slide.

The *amount* is classified as scant, moderate, or profuse. The *degree of clarity is noted*. The sample is tested for a *spinnbarkeit* by placing a cover slip on the mucus and slowly drawing the cover slip from the slide, noting the amount in centimeters that the mucus will stretch. Under the microscope the degree of *cellularity* is noted, and the number of sperm is evaluated. It is best to scan the slide under low power, and once a representative field has been found, switch to high power and count the *number* of active, the number of sluggishly motile, and the number of nonmotile sperm per high-power field. The slide is then dried for *fern* formation evaluation.

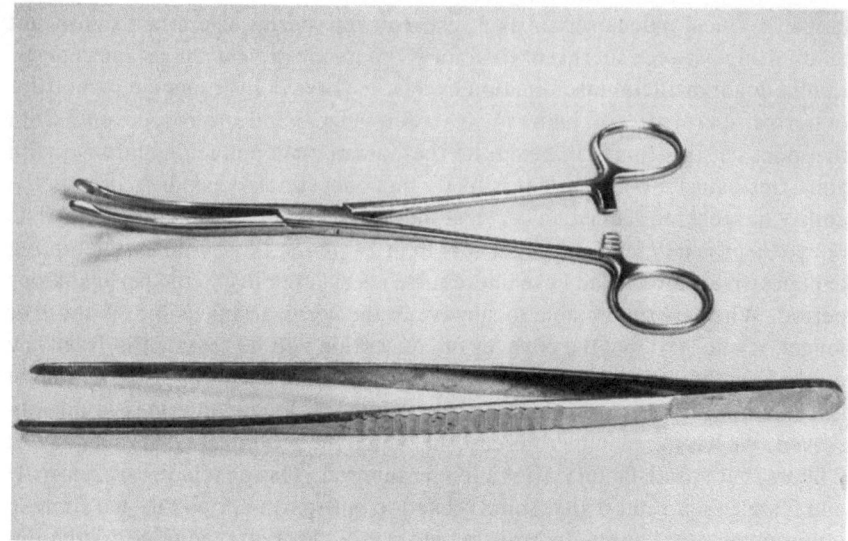

Figure 9-5. Instruments for obtaining a sample of cervical mucus.

Significance of the Postcoital Test

Because of the lack of a universal standard applied to the postcoital test in terms of timing the test and the number of active sperm that are meaningful, it has been difficult to evaluate the true significance of the postcoital test. In a recent symposium on cervical mucus, no attempts were made to demonstrate a correlation between the results of the postcoital test and pregnancy rates.[30]

Early enthusiasm for the postcoital test was dampened by reports indicating a lack of correlation between the findings and the pregnancy outcome. Other researchers have found that, if there are more than 20 active sperm per high-power field, there is a good correlation with pregnancy outcome,[3,8,31] but there is no statistical difference among groups with fewer numbers of active sperm.[32,33] On the other hand, others have shown that although pregnancies do occur when the postcoital test has shown less than five active sperm per high-power field and even when there have been no sperm, in general the higher the cervical mucus sperm count, the higher the conception rate.[33–35]

I am in agreement with those who believe that the findings of ten or more active sperm per high-power field is evidence of adequate insemination.[36] If there are less than five, this is a poor postcoital test. The findings between five and ten are considered fair or indeterminant.

Table 9-1 presents a correlation between the postcoital findings and pregnancy rate in 569 patients. Sperm counts less than 40 million, as well as tests associated with inadequate cervical mucus, have been excluded. When there

Table 9-1. Relationship of Postcoital Test to Pregnancy

Postcoital test	Number	Number pregnant	Percent
Excellent (>10)	168	79	47
Equivocal (5–9)	233	77	33
Poor (<5)	168	47	28
Total	569	203	36

was good insemination, the conception rate was 47% as compared with 28% for a poor postcoital test. These differences are statistically significant and lend some validity to the significance of the postcoital test. Jehe and Glass also found a positive correlation between a good postcoital test and pregnancy outcome.[32] As in our study, the length of time after coitus was 10 to 16 hours. In conclusion, it appears to be reasonable to treat the patient for whom the postcoital test consistently shows less than five active sperm per high-powered field.

Special Tests

Fractional postcoital tests have been described in which samples are taken at three levels of the endocervical canal by means of a special polyethylene catheter.[37] A significant correlation with the sperm count can be found among the number of motile sperm at various levels,[38] but correlation with conception has not been made.[31] Another study suggested that this was a more reliable method than the Sims-Huhner test.[39]

In vitro sperm migration tests are recommended when the postcoital test is poor but there is normal semen analysis.[40–42] Cervical mucus and seminal fluid are placed in apposition. Spermatozoa will make their way into the cervical mucus with varying degrees of efficiency. The Miller-Kurzrok test, described in 1928,[43] is performed by placing a small drop of cervical mucus on a slide. The drop is flattened to a diameter of 5 to 6 mm by a cover slip, and the corners of the cover slip are supported by small petroleum jelly pillars. Semen is applied to the edge of the cover slip and is allowed to flow around the cervical mucus. The slide is placed in a moist chamber at room temperature and read after 3 to 4 hours as follows: degree 0, sperm found only in peripheral part of the mucus; degree 1, the majority of the sperm have invaded the periphery, but some are present in the center of the cervical mucus; degree 2, sperm are equally distributed throughout the mucus.

The capillary tube cervical mucus penetration test described by Kremer in 1965 is probably the best in vitro test available.[44] It is a simple test that can be performed in the office. The distance that the spermatozoa travel can be measured, the density of the spermatozoa can be noted, the degree and character of motility can be determined, and the viability of the spermatozoa and the cervical mucus can be evaluated. One can compare sperm penetration by cross-matching with other mucus and semen samples.

To perform this test, a column of cervical mucus about 40 cm long is drawn up into a flattened capillary tube (Vitro Dynamic, Rockaway, NJ) with an inner diameter of 0.7 ml. The end of the tube is sealed with modeling clay. The sealed tube can be stored at 4 degrees centigrade until used (a few days to 1 week later). With the use of fresh cervical mucus, only one end need be sealed. If the frozen cervical mucus specimen is used, it should defrost at room temperature. One of the seals is removed, and the tube is immersed into a semen reservoir containing fresh semen. After 1 hour in a moist chamber, the extent of penetration by the spermatozoa into the cervical mucus is read as follows: degree 0, the foremost spermatozoa are within the 5 mm of the immersed end of the tube; degree 1, the foremost spermatozoa are beyond the 30-mm mark. Reichman and co-workers and Mahler have described other approaches to cervical mucus sperm penetration.[45,46]

Endometrial aspiration has been recommended by some as further means of assaying sperm migration.[47,48] The test is often difficult to perform, and usually the sample is heavily contaminated with blood. The significance is yet to be shown. Some have failed to find active sperm in the uterus despite good cervical insemination.[49] On the other hand, Grant reported a 10% incidence of positive fundal tests where the cervical secretions contained no sperm.[50] This is an area that requires further investigation.

Coital Positions

There is extensive literature on the significance of coital position in insemination. It is logical to assume that having the female in the recumbent position would be the most conducive position for having the cervical os rest in the seminal pool. However, with retroverted uterus, the cervix may point away from the pool, and prone or lateral positions might be better. If the postcoital test is adequate, there is little to be gained by interfering with coital position. But, if with repeated postcoital tests there is no explanation in terms of semen, cervical mucus, and antibodies, this possibility should be considered and discussed with the couple.

CAUSES OF POOR POSTCOITAL TESTS

Male Factor

One of the most obvious causes of a poor postcoital test is oligospermia. Occasionally, a relatively good test can be found despite significant oligospermia. This most likely is a chance occurrence, and its presence should not be taken as evidence of a lack of correlation between the postcoital test and semen analysis. It is indicative, however, that both tests should be performed for a thorough assessment of the fertility potential of the couple.

Infection

It is my opinion that the role of cervical infection in sperm survival has been overemphasized, a view forcefully expounded by Buxton and his co-workers in 1954.[51] Controlled studies indicate no difference in pregnancy rates between those who did and those who did not have antibiotic therapy. In most instances, the thick, tenacious, cellular mucus observed is due either to poor timing of the test, or to inadequate estrogen stimulation of the glands. What many consider evidence of infection is actually erosion of the portio vaginalis, usually caused by a congenital lesion, or is due to the alkaline secretion of the endocervical glands spilling over the squamous epithelium. Little is gained by antibiotics, much is lost by cautery.

Although infection with *Chlamydia trachomatis* has been shown to be a significant cause of tube infertility, there is no evidence that such an infection adversely affects the postcoital test.[52] On the other hand, the role of mycoplasma in affecting tests remains inconclusive (see chapter 17).

Inadequate Mucus—Cervical Stenosis

Despite good timing of the test, the cervical mucus can be found on occasion to be scant, and tenacious. Occasionally, this may be related to inadequate secretion that can be stimulated by estrogen- or iodine-containing preparations, but more often it is associated with a cervix that has been previously cauterized or infected, and in which the glands have been destroyed. The cervical canal itself is rigidly replaced by scar tissue.

The Immune Factor

Antibodies of sperm, probably residing in cervical mucus, are a significant cause of a poor postcoital test. If the timing of the test is correct and there is good cervical mucus and a normal semen analysis, there is a good correlation between the finding of a poor postcoital test and the presence of an immune factor.[53-55] Where the presence of antibodies has been shown to prevent mucus penetration, it is important to keep in mind that this is not an all-or-none phenomenon. There is often not a good correlation between cervical antibodies and sperm antibodies.[56] This is one of the reasons for the confusion about the importance of the sperm antibodies in the past.

REFERENCES

1. Sims JM: Sterility and value of the microscope in diagnosis and treatment. *Trans Am Gynecol Soc* 13:291, 1888
2. Huhner M: *Sterility in the Female, and its Treatment.* New York, Rebman, 1913
3. Giner J, Merino G, Luna J, Aznor R: Evaluation of the Sims-Huhner post-coital test on the fertile couples. *Fertil Steril* 25:145, 1974
4. Bergman P: Uterine cervical factors in the causation of infertility. *Acta Obstet Gynecol Scand* 28:172, 1948
5. Marcus S: The cervical factor in infertility. *J Reprod Med* 3:138, 1971
6. Davajan V, Nakamura M, Khrum L: Spermatozoan transport in cervical mucus. *Obstet Gynecol Survey* 25:1, 1970
7. Rubenstein BB, Strauss H, Lazarus M, Hankin H: Sperm survival in women. *Fertil Steril* 2:15, 1951
8. Cohen WR, Stein IF: Sperm survival at estimated ovulation time. *Fertil Steril* 2:20, 1951
9. Clift AF: Observations on certain rheological properties of human cervical secretion. *Pro R Soc Med* 39:1, 1945
10. Rydburg E: Observations on the crystallization of cervical mucus. *Acta Obstet Gynecol Scand* 28:172, 1948
11. Bennett JT, Vickery BH: Hormonal influence of the cervical factor in relation to fertility. *J Reprod Med* 3:123, 1971
12. Odebad E: Biophysical techniques of assessing cervical mucus and microstructure of cervical epithelium on cervical mucus. In Elstein M, Moghissi KS, Barth R (eds): *Human Reproduction.* Copenhagen, Scriptor, 1973, pp 58–74
13. Moghissi KS, Syner FN: The effect of seminal protease and sperm migration through the cervical mucus. *J Fertil* 15:43, 1970
14. Moghissi KS, Dabich D, Levine J, et al: Mechanism of sperm migration. *Fertil Steril* 5;15, 1964
15. MacDonald RR, Lumley IB: Endocervical pH measured in vivo throughout the normal menstrual cycle. *Obstet Gynecol* 35:202, 1970
16. Moyer DL, Rimdusit SL, Mishell DR: Sperm distribution and degradation in the human female reproductive tract. *Obstet Gynecol* 35:831, 1970
17. Perloff WH, Steinberger E: In vivo survival of spermatozoa in cervical mucus. *Obstet Gynecol* 88:439, 1964
18. Fraenkel L: Sterilisierung und konzeptionsverhutung. *Arch Gynaekol* 144:86, 1936
19. Nicholson R: Vitality of spermatozoa in the cervical canal. *Fertil Steril* 16:758, 1965
20. Mattner P: Spermatozoa in the genital tract of the ewe: 2. Distribution after coitus. *Aust J Biol Sci* 16:688, 1963
21. Huhner M: The Huhner test. *J Mt Sinai Hospital* 14:388, 1947
22. Southam AL, Buxton L: Seventy post-coital tests made during the conception cycle *Fertil Steril* 7:133, 1956
23. Tredway DT, Settlage DF, Nabamara RM, Motoshima M, Umezaki CA, Mishell DR: Significance of timing for post-coital evaluation of cervical mucus. *Am J Obstet Gynecol* 121:387, 1975
24. Davajan V, Nabamura RM: The cervical factor. In Kistner RW, Behrman, SJ (eds): *Progress in Infertility*, 2nd ed. Boston, Little, Brown, 1975, p 17
25. Andrews W: Investigation of the infertile couple. In Gold JJ, Josimovich JB (eds): *Gynecologic Endocrinology*, New York, Plenum Press, p 543, 1987.
26. Jonssen B, Eneroth R, Langdren B, Wilkborn C: Evaluation of in-vitro sperm penetration testing of 176 couples with the use of ejaculates and cervical mucus from donors. *Fertil Steril* 45:353, 1986

27. Hanson FW, Overstreet JW: The interaction of human spermatozoa with cervical mucus in vivo. *Am J Obstet Gynecol* 140:173, 1981
28. Gould JS, Overstreet JW, Hanson FW: Assessment of human sperm after recovery from the female reproductive tract. *Biol Reprod* 31:888, 1984
29. Moghissi KS: Cervical factor in infertility. *J Reprod Med* 3;142, 1971
30. Taymor ML, Overstreet JW: Some thoughts on the post-coital test. *Fertil Steril* 50:702, 1988
31. Stein I, Cohen M: Survival at estimated ovulation time: Prognostic significance. *Fertil Steril* 25:2, 1974
32. Jehe NT, Glass RH: Prognostic value of the post-coital test. *Fertil Steril* 23:29, 1972
33. Danezis J, Sujan S, Sobrero A: Evaluation of the post-coital test. *Fertil Steril* 13:559, 1962
34. Kovacs GT, Newman GB, Henson GL: The first post-coital test: What is normal? *Br Med J* 1:818, 1978
35. Grant N: Cervical hostility. *Fertil Steril* 9:321, 1958
36. Moghissi KS: Post-coital test: Physiologic basis, technique and interpretation. *Fertil Steril* 27:117, 1976
37. Davajan V, Kunitake GM: Fractional in vivo and in vitro examination of post-coital cervical mucus in the human. *Fertil Steril* 20:197, 1969
38. Tredway DR: The interpretation and significance of the fractional post-coital test. *Am J Obstet Gynecol* 124:352, 1976
39. Moran J, Davajan V, Nakamaura R: Comparison of fractional post-coital test with Sims-Huhner post-coital test. *Int J Fertil* 19:93, 1974
40. Moghissi KS: The function of the cervix in fertility. *Fertil Steril* 23:295, 1972
41. Perloff W, Steinberger E: In vitro penetration of cervical mucus by spermatozoa. *Fertil Steril* 14:231, 1963
42. Kesseru E: In vivo sperm penetration and in vitro sperm migration tests. *Fertil Steril* 24:584, 1973
43. Kurzrok R, Miller E: Biochemical studies of human and its relation to mucus of the cervix uteri. *Am J Obstet Gynecol* 15:56, 1928
44. Kremer J: A simple sperm penetration test. *Int J Fertil* 10:209, 1965
45. Reichman J, Insler V, Serr D: A modified in vitro spermatozoal penetration test. *Int J Fertil* 18:241, 1973
46. Mahler A: A new method for evaluation of cervical penetrability using daily aspirated and stored cervical mucus. *Fertil Steril* 27:533, 1976
47. Frankel DA: Sperm migration and survival in the endometrial cavity. *Int J Fertil* 6:285, 1961
48. Kleegman SJ: *Infertility in Women.* Philadelphia, FA Davis, 1966, p 84
49. Moghissi K: Human and bovine sperm migration. *Fertil Steril* 19:118, 1968
50. Grant A: Cervical hostility. *Fertil Steril* 9:321, 1958
51. Buxton L, Southam A, Herrmann W, et al: Bacteriology of the cervix in human sterility. *Fertil Steril* 5:493, 1954
52. Battin DA, Barnes RB, Hoffman DL, Shaater J, diZerega GS, Yonebura MC: *Chlamydia trachomatis* is not an important cause of abnormal post-coital tests in ovulatory patients. *Fertil Steril* 42:233, 1984
53. Kremer J, Jaeger S, Van Slochteren-Drasisma T: The "unexplained" poor post-coital test. *Int J Fertil* 23:277, 1988
54. Telang M, Rayniak JV, Shulman S: Antibodies to spermatozoa: VIII. Correlations of sperm antibody activity with post-coital tests in infertile couples. *Int J Fertil* 23:200, 1978
55. Wang C, Baker HWG, Jennings MG, Bunger HG, Lutjen P: Interaction between human cervical mucus and sperm surface antibodies. *Fertil Steril* 44:484, 1981
56. Friber J: Post-coital testing in relation to circulating sperm-agglutinating antibodies in women. *Am J Obstet Gynecol* 139:587, 1981

CHAPTER 10

Evaluation of the Tubal Factor

FUNCTIONS OF THE FALLOPIAN TUBES

When the physician understands the functions of the fallopian tubes, he or she is better able to evaluate the tubal factor in infertility.

Between the wide expanse of the endometrial cavity and the open spaces of the peritoneal cavity, the fallopian tube, with its diameter at some portion as small as 1 mm, provides a necessary conduit for both spermatozoa and the fertilized gamete. The tube does not function just as a passive channel; the fimbria are involved in ovum pickup, its ciliary and muscular movements are involved in sperm and ovum transport, and its secretions are vital to the nourishment and maturation of the zygote.

Sperm Transport

Spermatozoa, deposited and stored in the cervix, make their way rapidly to the fallopian tubes. Indeed, spermatozoa have been found at the fimbriated end of the tube as early as 5 minutes after cervical insemination. Little is known of their passage through the uterus.

Passage through the fallopian tubes is achieved mainly by the flagellate action of the sperm itself, since the action of the cilia sends a current of fluid toward the uterus. The current itself apparently serves as a counterforce against which the sperm swim in a relatively straight line. It has been theorized that, although the beat of the cilia in the ampullary portion of the tube creates a current of flow toward the uterus, this flow is reserved, particularly in the narrow isthmus portion of the tube. There, in addition, muscular contractions aid in transporting the sperm from one mucosal compartment to another.[1] The uterotubal junction probably acts as a barrier to prevent too many sperm from reaching the oocyte and reduces the danger of polyspermy. It is thought that the high incidence of abortion after tubal implantation for obliterated uterotubal junction occlusion may be due to polyspermy.[2]

Ovum Pickup

The concept that the tube serves merely as a conduit for the fertilized egg has given way to knowledge of the many functions of the tube in relation to the ovum: ovum pickup, site of fertilization, nourishment, maturation of the zygote, and precise time transport to the uterine cavity.

The ovum reaches the tube by a combination of the sweeping movements of the fimbria over the surface of the ovary and the flow of current toward the lumen created by the cilia of the fimbria and the ampullary portion of the tube. Doyle verified this grasping action of the fimbria by endoscopy.[3]

Ciliary action has been observed mainly in animals, but cilia are also seen in the human fallopian tube. In animals, progesterone increases the rate of beating of the cilia, and the progesterone level rises in association with the ovulatory peak of luteinizing hormone prior to ovulation.[4] It has been shown that the smooth muscle of the meso-ovarium and ovarian ligament intermittently contract and relax. Thus, when the ovary is fixed to the side wall of the pelvis or broad ligament by endometriosis or pelvic adhesions, there is a diminished chance of ovum pickup, even though the tube and fimbria are normal.

Ovum Transport

Our knowledge of the muscular and secretory functions of the fallopian tube, in relation to ovum transport, is also based primarily on animal experiments, with but few observations in humans. Therefore, our conclusions in relation to human infertility must be speculative.

The ovum is moved from the fimbriated end of the tube toward the uterus by a combination of cilia and muscular activity. The beat of the cilia is toward the uterus, and a current flow is established. Under the influence of progesterone, the rate of ciliary beat increases. In addition to the action of cilia, the movement of the ovum through the ampullary portion of the tube is aided by peristaltic-like contractions of the tube. This muscular activity is also increased at the time of ovulation and is also accelerated by progesterone. There is evidence, from animal experiments that a degree of retention of the ovum in the infundibulum is required to prevent premature entry into the uterus. Passage through the isthmus is primarily by muscular contraction. In experimental animals, this is fairly rapid and is aided by progesterone.

The fallopian tube then is not just a conduit; it plays a dynamic role in both sperm and ovum transport. Thus, diseases interfering with the action of cilia or the musculature of the tubal wall will have permanent effects upon fertility, even though surgical measures are taken to restore tubal patency.

EVALUATION OF TUBAL PATENCY

Unfortunately, despite our knowledge that the fallopian tube plays an important role in sperm and ovum development, and that cilia and muscular activity are important elements in ovum transport, our diagnostic evaluation is now limited to the determination of the patency or nonpatency of the tubes. Two methods are currently utilized: (1) hysterosalpingography and (2) direct observation at endoscopy. In the past, tubal insufflation with carbon dioxide, originally described by Rubin in 1920,[5] was solely used as an initial screening procedure, but this procedure has been virtually discarded. Because tubal disease is more common than it used to be a generation ago, and because hysterosalpingography is more accurate than tubal insufflation, hysterosalpingography is now the initial procedure for confirming tubal disease.

The accuracy of the x ray is in question in contrast to direct visualization with laparoscopy. One study reveals that, in 17% of the patients, abnormalities diagnosed by hysterosalpingogram could not be confirmed by laparoscopy.[6] In another study, 19% of patients with a normal hysterosalpingogram had pathology discovered by endoscopy.[7] Other studies show the variability to range from 37% to 40%.[7,8] However, in many instances the discrepancy was because hysterosalpingography revealed uterine lesions not demonstrable by endoscopy, and endoscopy revealed problems such as endometriosis and adhesions not discernible by x ray. The physician should not think that this discrepancy between hysterosalpingogram and endoscopy justifies performing laparoscopy as part of the initial tubal evaluation. The fact that the hysterosalpingogram may suggest problems (in actuality, one of the tubes might be normal) only dictates that endoscopy should be performed as a final evaluation *before* subjecting a patient to a laparotomy or tubal surgery. Conversely, because one tubogram out of six fails to reveal pathology (later to be uncovered by endoscopy), this does not justify subjecting the remaining five women to the expense, risk, and inconvenience of endoscopy without first trying more conservative therapy. Hysterosalpingography and endoscopic evaluation of the fallopian tube should not be considered competitive approaches, but as part of a progressive evaluation of the tubal factor in the total management of the infertile couple.

TECHNIQUES FOR EVALUATION OF TUBAL PATENCY

Hysterosalpingography

Hysterosalpingography should be performed in the follicular phase, in the window between the end of menses and a few days before anticipated ovulation. The purpose for this timing is to avoid radiation during the early stages of the fertilized oocyte development.

An antiprostaglandin given by mouth 30 to 60 minutes before the procedure reduces uterine contractibility and often diminishes much of the discomfort. Pain is also reduced if the cervical tenaculum is put into position slowly, and if the tip of the acorn is only between one-half and three-quarter inches in length so that it does not pass through the internal os. Once the tenaculum and cannula with its acorn tip are in place, the speculum can be removed, and the patient slides up under the fluoroscopic screen. With the fluoroscope on, dye is slowly injected and one watches the filling of the uterus, the flow through each tube, and spill from the tubes. Spot films are taken at various intervals. Usually 5 to 8 ml of dye and three spot films are sufficient. The instruments are removed and, if water-soluble material has been used, the patient takes a 360 degree roll on the table. An additional film to delineate the spread of media within the pelvis is taken.

If the patient has a history of pelvic infection, she should be given a prophylactic antibiotic before, during, and after the procedure. If dilated tubes are found, she should be placed on antibiotics after the procedure.

Two general types of contrast media are used: water soluble and oily media. The chief advantage of water-soluble media is that it is completely absorbed within 30 minutes. Other possible advantages are the rapid and easy flow through the syringe and tubes.

The rapidity of the absorption of water-soluble media is considered by many to be a disadvantage. The original oily media (i.e., Lipiodol®) remained in the peritoneal cavity for years after the test, and was believed to be responsible for adhesions. Newer oily media (Ethiodol®) are absorbed in approximately 30 days, and the physician has the advantage of observing whether the contrast media spills easily through the peritoneal cavity (Fig. 10-1) or remains loculated as by pelvis adhesions (Fig. 10-2), or within the fallopian tube. (Fig. 10-3) However, if hydrosalpinges are present, even Ethiodol may precipitate an inflammatory action, either acute or subacute. An experienced radiologist can usually differentiate between dye trapped in the tube or dye lying between adhesive bands. Furthermore, if the patient takes a 360 degree turn on the table

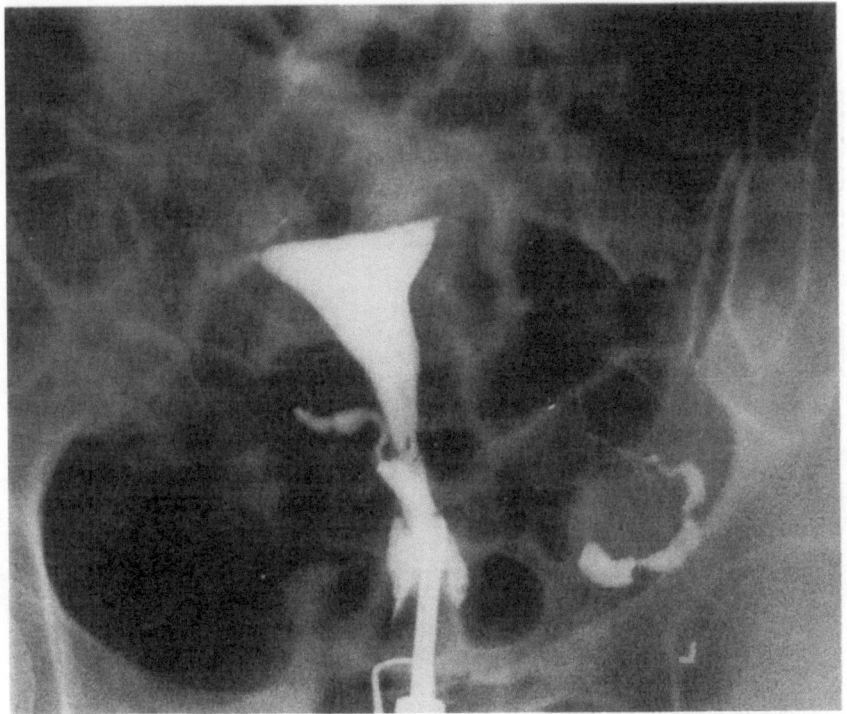

Figure 10-1. Normal hysterosalpingogram.

immediately after the procedure, the entrapment of dye by adhesions can be evaluated even if water-soluble media is used. For these reasons, water-soluble is the procedure of choice for more and more physicians.

Fluoroscopy with an image intensifier is the recommended radiologic equipment. An experienced radiologist, using a spot film system, can often differentiate between accumulation of the medium in the tubo-ovarian gutter and that trapped by peritubal adhesions. If fluoroscopy is not available, three or four films are taken after the fractional instillation of 1, 3, and 5 ml of medium. A follow-up film is taken a few minutes later after the patient has moved about. The amount of radiation should be kept at a minimum so that the average dose per examination is less than 500 mR.

The greatest error in hysterosalpingography is the failure of one or both tubes to fill, due to spasm of a relatively tight uterotubal junction. Surgery at the cornual end of the tube (Fig. 10-4) should not be contemplated without first rechecking a hysterosalpingogram and evaluating patency under endoscopy. A

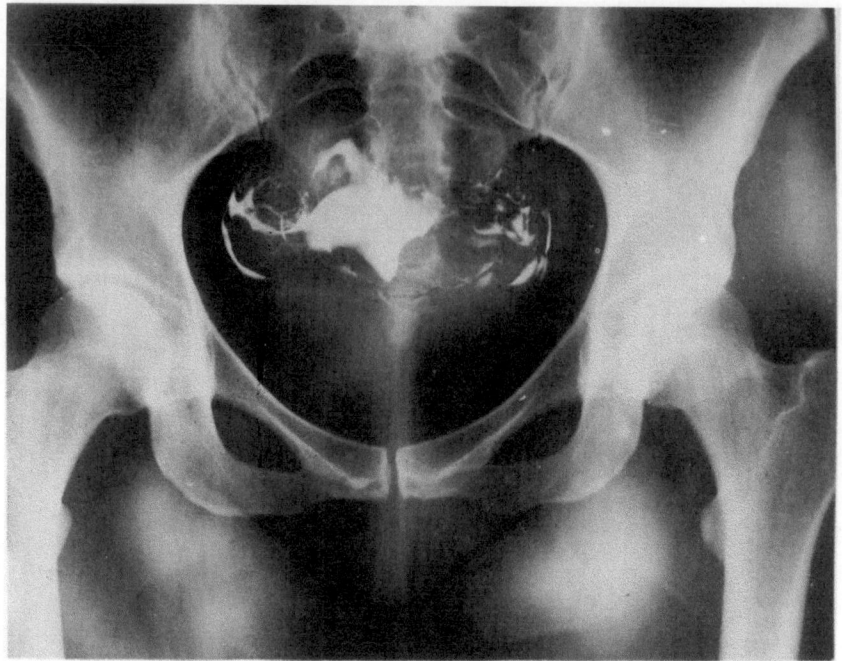

Figure 10-2. Loculation of dye in pelvis after 24 hours, resulting from pelvic adhesions.

final evaluation of patency or the lack of it should be made on laparotomy before dividing the tubes.

Endoscopic Evaluation

A critical part of diagnostic laparoscopy for infertility is the evaluation of tubal patency. The instrumentation is similar to that for tubal insufflation or hysterosalpingogram: a hollow cannula in the cervix and cervical tenaculum. Indigo-carmine dye is passed through this cannula into the uterus, and its exit through the tube is observed by direct vision. Obvious patency is demonstrated by observing the dye escape from the fimbriated end of the tube. A temporary occlusion of the escape of dye, followed by a dripping, of dye, suggests some degree of fimbrial adhesions or narrowing. Endoscopy is the final evaluation of tubal blockade or patency before surgery.

OTHER APPROACHES

Tubal irrigation with saline containing antibiotics has been recommended.[9] The rationale is that it provides better evaluation of "tight tubes."

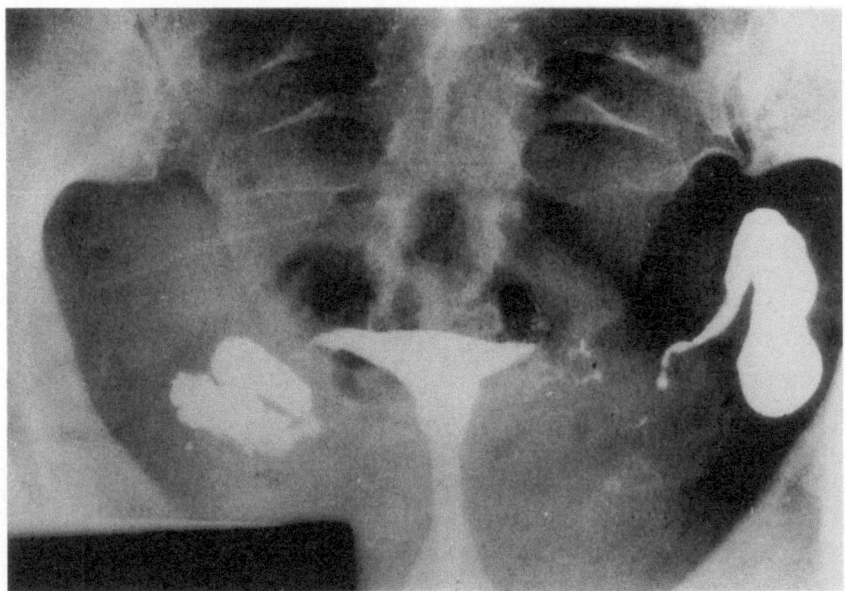

Figure 10-3. Bilateral hydrosalpinx.

Actually "tight tubes" can be evaluated by the reading of carbon dioxide passage as well. A combination of water-soluble dye, followed by insufflation, reportedly increases the accuracy of hysterosalpingography.[10]

The Speck test involves the injection of phenolsulfonphthalein through the cannula.[11–13] If this reaches the urine, tubal patency is expected. The test is simple, economical, and safe, but it cannot supplant x-ray or endoscopic confirmation.

SUMMARY

The tubal factor is one of the important factors in infertility. Tests are available to determine patency, although other tubal functions are not yet within our diagnostic reach. The two main approaches to the diagnosis of tubal patency, hysterosalpingography and endoscopy, should not be considered competitive; each has its distinctive role. Indeed, one additional reason for proceeding in a step-by-step manner is the reports of pregnancies that follow each step.[14,15] At this time, whether these resulting pregnancies are due solely to the procedure or to time alone, it is impossible to know.

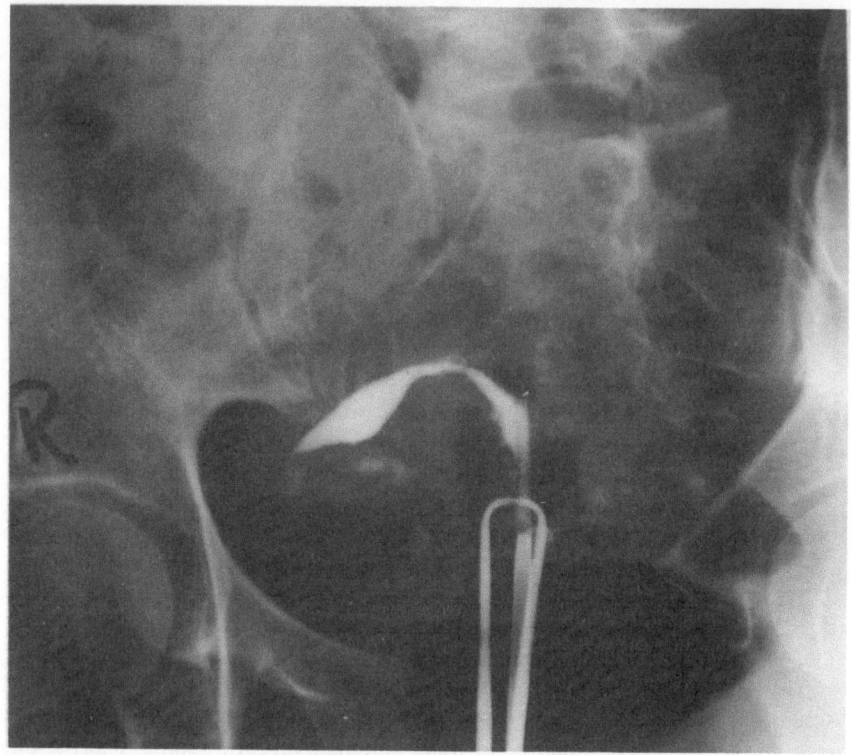

Figure 10-4. Cornual blockage.

REFERENCES

1. Settlage D, Fordney S, Motoshima M, Tredway D: Sperm transport from the external os to the fallopian tubes in women: A time and quantitative study. *Fertil Steril* 24:655, 1973
2. Hafez ESE: Sperm transport. In Behrman SJ, Kistner RW (eds): *Progress in Infertility*, 2nd ed. Boston, Little, Brown, 1975, p 151
3. Doyle JG: Tubo-ovarian mechanisms, observation at laparotomy. *Obstet Gynecol* 8:696, 1965
4. Yussman MA, Taymor ML: Serum levels of follicle stimulating hormone and luteinizing hormone and of plasma progesterone related to ovulation by corpus luteum biopsy. *J Clin Endocrinol Metab* 30:396, 1976
5. Rubin IC: Non-operative determination of patency of fallopian tubes in sterility: A preliminary report. *JAMA* 74:1017, 1920
6. Maathius JB, Horbach JGM, Van Hall EV: A comparison of the results of hysterosalpingography and laparoscopy in the diagnosis of fallopian tube dysfunction. *Fertil Steril* 23:428, 1972
7. Moghissi KS, Sim GS: Correlation between hysterosalpingography and pelvic endoscopy for the evaluation of tubal factor. *Fertil Steril* 26:1178, 1975
8. Swolin K, Rosenkrantz M: Laparoscopy vs. hysterosalpingography in sterility investigations. A comparative study. *Fertil Steril* 23:270, 1972

9. Horne HW, Kosasa T: Quantitative method of evaluating the functional patency of human uterine tubes: Correlation with 61 laparotomy cases. *Obstet Gynecol* 39:3, 1972

10. Roland M, Clyman A: Further studies on the value of water-soluble media in hysterosalpingography. *Fertil Steril* 17:605, 1966

11. Davis ME, Ward ME, King AG: An evaluation of the PSP (Speck) test for tubal patency. *Fertil Steril* 3:217, 1962

12. Speck G: Revision of the PSP (Speck) test for tubal patency. *Fertil Steril* 1:328, 1950

13. Israel S, Freed C: The PSP (Speck) test for tubal patency. *Fertil Steril* 1:328, 1950

14. Wahby O: Hysterosalpingography in relation to pregnancy and its outcome in infertile women. *Fertil Steril* 17:520, 1966

15. Horbach JGM, Maathius JB, Van Hall EV: Factors influencing the pregnancy rate following hysterosalpingography and their prognostic significance. *Fertil Steril* 24:15, 1973

CHAPTER 11

Evaluation of the Ovulatory Factor

The presence or absence of ovulation and the quality of the corpus luteum function, both important factors in infertility, are evaluated initially by three approaches: (1) basal body temperature chart, (2) endometrial biopsy, and (3) the determination of progesterone levels in the blood. It should be emphasized that these three approaches are only presumptive evidence of ovulation, all dependent on the secretion of progesterone by the corpus luteum. Occasionally, a luteinized follicle can secrete progesterone and imitate the hormonal features of ovulation.

BASAL BODY TEMPERATURE CHART

The basal body temperature chart was first described in 1904,[1] and for over fifty years has been widely used to assess the presence or absence of ovulation.[2] Progesterone causes an increase in the basal body temperature level, the waking temperature, before any physical activity occurs. The basal temperature generally is well below 98°F before ovulation, and around or above 98°F after ovulation. A biphasic chart, in which the basal temperature of the last 13 to 15 days of the cycle demonstrates a sustained rise of 0.3 to 1.0 degrees higher than the follicular phase, is almost certain evidence of ovulation. A classic chart is shown in Fig. 11-1. A fairly recent study, on the other hand, indicated that some women with nonphasic charts also may be ovulating.[3]

It is widely accepted that ovulation actually occurs on the day of the low point that is followed by a sustained rise that lasts for 13 to 15 days. This can be

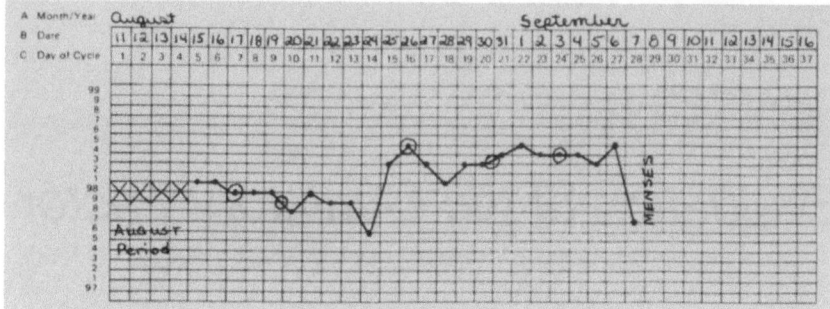

Figure 11-1. Basal body temperature chart. Classical biphasic chart of normal ovulation.

determined only retrospectively, after the entire cycle is completed. Furthermore, studies in which the temperature chart was correlated with corpus luteum biopsy demonstrated that ovulation could occur anywhere from 24 to 28 hours after the temperature shift, and in some cases even greater discrepancies between ovulation and temperature rise were noted.[4–6] It requires a certain amount of progesterone, approximately 0.4 ng/ml, to cause the temperature increase. Since there is a variable amount of progesterone production even before ovulation, it is not surprising that this lack of correlation exists.[7] More current studies utilizing luteinizing hormone (LH) levels indicate that the basal body temperature increase is usually on the onset of LH surge and the first high point occurs 8 hours after ovulation.[8]

For this reason, the use of the temperature chart to time intercourse must be condemned. One cannot predict in advance the day of ovulation. Prolonged reliance on the temperature chart for this purpose does harm to the psychosexual adjustment of the couple. If sperm count and motility are normal, sperm will remain viable in the uterus and tubes for at least 48 hours.[9] Thus, if a couple has a routine of coitus two to three times a week, there will be many times during a year or two in which sperm will be waiting for the ovum to be released. This cannot be improved upon by putting off intercourse for a number of days and waiting for the so-called crucial dip. It is impossible to know in advance which dip is the crucial one, even then, ovulation may occur before this event.

Unfortunately, a large number of patients have been advised to wait for the dip in the temperature charts. Sometimes there is no dip. The temperature rises and ovulation is past. At other times, the dip occurs on the 9th or 10th day, followed by a rise and a number of alternating dips and rises. Coitus occurs on each dip but, by the time ovulation does occur, the husband is physiologically and psychologically exhausted. An act of love becomes duty. One can imagine the tensions and hostilities that build up as a wife urges her husband on because of her physician's orders. In situations of borderline semen quality, often more than 48 hours are required for the quality to rebound. Therefore, by the time that ovulation does occur, the chances for conception are considerably decreased. No wonder many patients are hostile to using the temperature chart; no wonder many physicians have developed a nihilistic attitude toward the thermometer.

The physician should exercise a moderate and rational approach toward the chart. The chart is necessary during the initial workup to retrospectively note that the postcoital test was performed in the preovulatory period. The temperature chart should not be used to time intercourse in an ongoing cycle. However, 3 or 4 months of recording the temperature gives the physician proof of ovulation, as well as information concerning the quality of ovulation and an average estimation of when the cycle ovulation does occur. Some couples can then be told to concentrate coitus during this time period. Then, unless there are further reasons for the temperature chart, taking temperatures can be stopped. Additional charting aids the physician in roughly estimating the timing of ovulation for insemination therapy, in the evaluation of the effectiveness of ovulation-inducing compounds, and in the evaluation of therapy for luteal phase deficiency.

The basal temperature chart can be of diagnostic help in luteal phase deficiency. In this condition ovulation occurs, but because of deficient function or shortened life of the corpus luteum, there is a deficiency of progesterone. A concomitant deficiency in the development of the endometrium results so that, even if fertilization does take place, implantation does not occur. Three different patterns are seen in the basal body temperature chart that suggest the presence of a luteal phase deficiency: first, the length of the luteal phase may be a normal 13 to 15 days, but the temperature rise may be a gradual one that is not well maintained (Fig. 11-2); or it may contain many dips; or it may be a short luteal phase lasting anywhere from 5 to 12 days. However, confirmation of these changes in the temperature pattern is required by endometrial biopsy or progesterone assay.

ENDOMETRIAL BIOPSY

Sampling of the endometrium for assessing progesterone production by the corpus luteum is another method giving indirect evidence of the presence or absence of ovulation. The cyclic changes in the endometrial glands and stroma, corresponding to the days of the menstrual cycle, were classically described by Noyes and his co-workers.[10] They concluded that, more than any other method available at that time, examination of the endometrium during the secretory phase gave more information regarding ovulation and the degree of progestational change, normality, and abnormality of the endometrium.

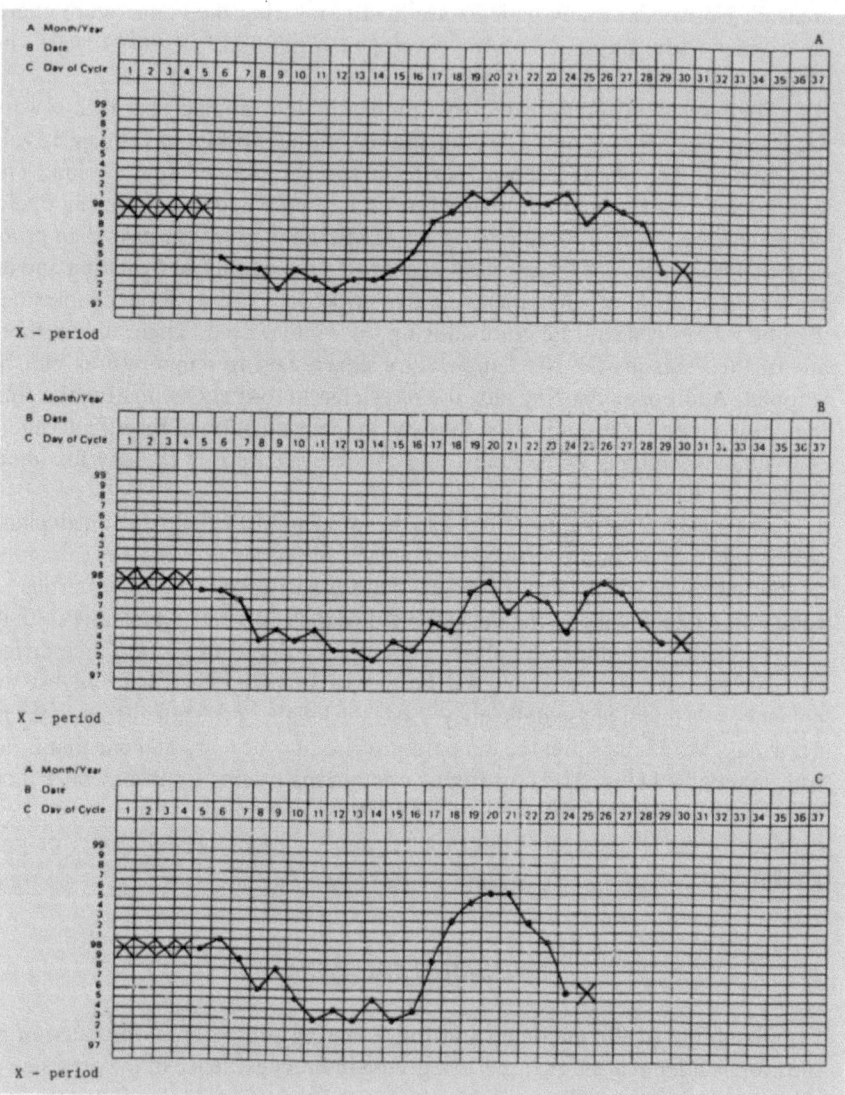

Figure 11-2. Basal temperature charts associated with progesterone deficiency.

If one is interested in only the presence or absence of ovulation, either the basal body temperature chart or the endometrial biopsy, alone, will usually give that information. On rare occasions, however, the temperature rise is so minimal or so questionable that it is difficult to interpret, and the addition of the endometrial biopsy gives needed verification. Moghissi, in a recent study, reported that in approximately 20% of ovulatory cycles proven by progesterone levels, the basal body temperature failed to demonstrate ovulation.[11]

More important information than just noting the absence or presence of ovulation is often needed. An assessment of the *quality* of the corpus luteum function, as manifested by the endometrial response to estrogen and progesterone, is an important part of the infertility workup. Since neither approach is consistently accurate, an evaluation of both basal body temperature and endometrial biopsy is helpful; the more information the better.

There is controversy as to when in the cycle is the best time to take the endometrial biopsy. For the simple yes or no diagnosis of ovulation, any time in the luteal phase is satisfactory, but to evaluate better the full ripening of the endometrium, the closer to the onset of the menses the better. Many recommend that the biopsy be performed within 12 to 18 hours after the start of the menstrual flow. It has been claimed that at this time the endometrium is difficult to read, but most pathologists have no difficulty. Figure 11-3 shows the fully developed picture of menstrual endometrium in a specimen taken 16 hours after the onset of menses: we see exhausted secretory glands, compact stroma, and polymorphonuclear leucocytes. Figure 11-4 is from another biopsy taken shortly after the onset of menses. Here, despite the fact that it was taken at the onset of menses, the findings are consistent with midsecretory endometrium. This is clear evidence of diminished progesterone effect from inadequate corpus luteum function.

The time disadvantage of such a biopsy is that the physician must be available 7 days a week. In an effort to get around this inconvenience, some physicians recommend performing the biopsy routinely on the 1st day of flow (except weekends). For those patients whose menses begin on a weekend, a biopsy can be scheduled the following month for menses day -1, or -2.

Furthermore the need to wait for the onset of menses has been obviated by the availability of sensitive urine pregnancy tests. These can be performed in the office within 2 or 3 minutes, and can detect a pregnancy 4 or 5 days before the expected onset of menses. Taking all these facts into consideration, it would seem that a biopsy taken on day 25 to 27 would be the most convenient, give the most information, and still be safe for pregnancy. In any event, a biopsy taken during a conception cycles does not invariably interrupt pregnancy. A review of the literature revealed a 0% to 22% chance of such an interruption, which compares favorably with the incidence of spontaneous abortion.[12]

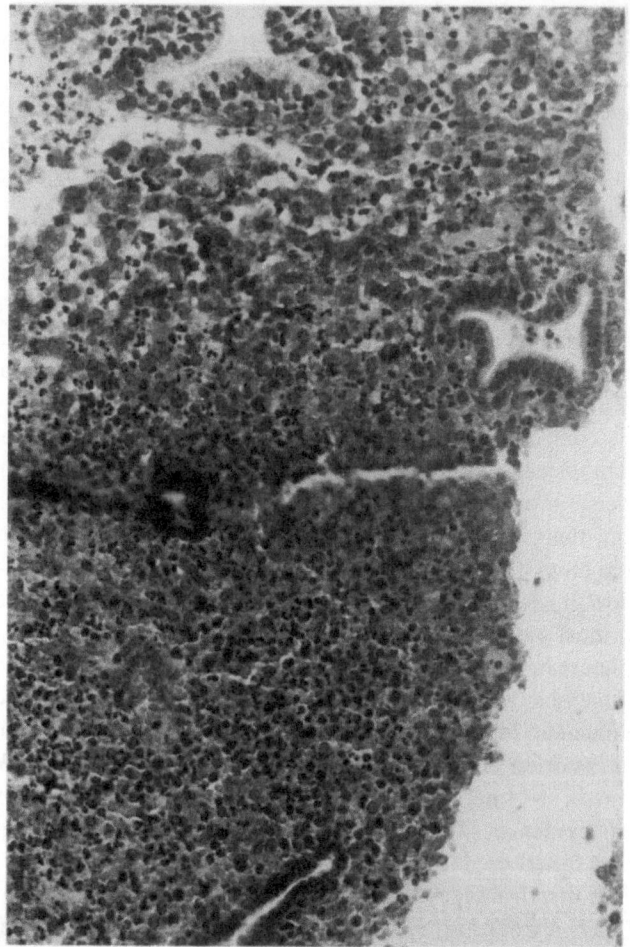

Figure 11-3. Normal endometrial histology 16 hours after onset of menstrual flow.

Other infertility therapists recommend that the biopsy be performed on approximately the 19th day of the cycle. This avoids injuring the fertilized ovum because implantation has not yet occurred. The dating of the endometrium is then correlated by subtracting from 28 the number of days until menses. While this appears to be a logical approach, it is possible that the corpus luteum may function normally for the first part of its life span, and then produce a deficient amount of progesterone in the latter half. The 20-day secretory endometrium may be normal for its time, but the deficiency would not be seen as it developed later in the cycle. The availability of a sensitive pregnancy test makes this approach unnecessary.

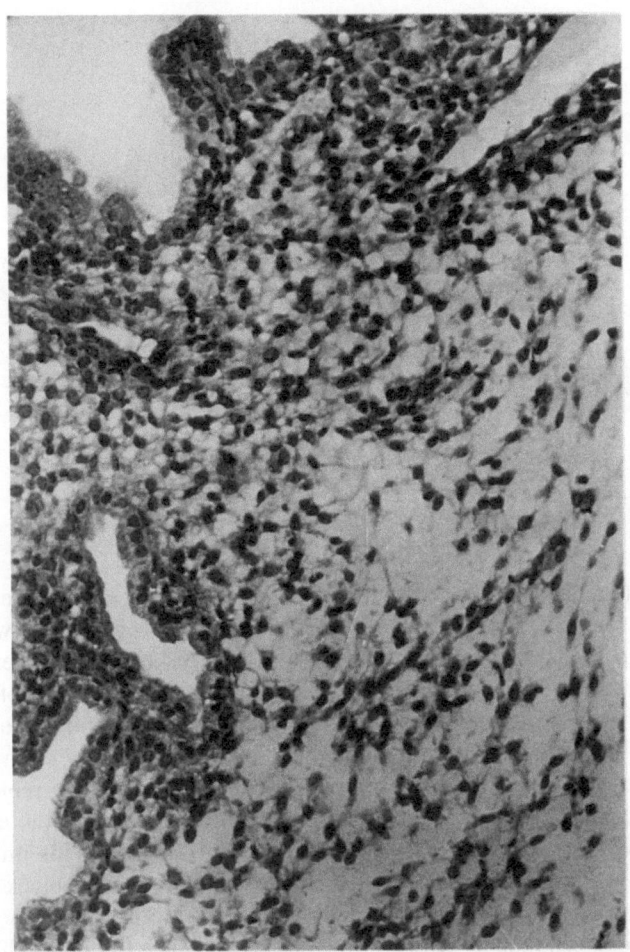

Figure 11-4. Midsecretory endometrium obtained by endometrial biopsy at onset of menstrual flow.

Technique of Endometrial Biopsy

In the past, endometrial biopsies were performed with metal instruments, either a ridged suction tip curette (Novak) or a malleable one (Meigs) (Fig. 11-5). This was an invariably painful procedure. A less traumatic instrument now available is a thin disposable plastic suction curette that is relatively easy to insert and causes relatively little discomfort (Fig. 11-6). If one must resort to the metal biopsy curette, a paracervical block should be performed.

A preliminary pelvic examination should be carried out to determine the

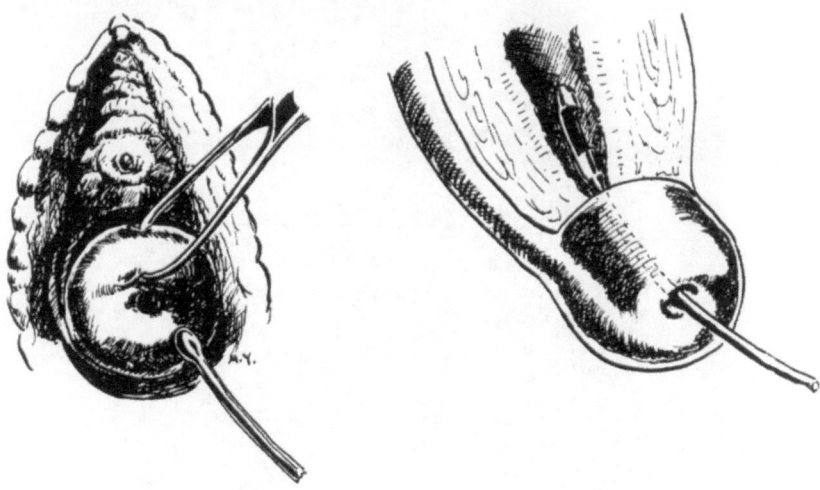

Figure 11-5. Older technique of endometrial biopsy.

position of the uterus. The cervix is exposed, and the exocervix and external os are wiped with an antiseptic. The plastic suction tube is bent in its wrapper to conform to the approximate position of the uterus and then inserted. The insertions can be accomplished without a cervical tenaculum 80% of the time. With a sharply angulated uterus, a tenaculum may be required to partially straighten the canal. When the cannula is in place, a plunger is withdrawn rapidly, the cannula is partially rotated a few times, the cannula is removed, and the procedure is complete. In approximately 10% of the time, the angulation may be too great or there is a degree of cervical stenosis. This impedes the entrance of the pliable cannula. In that situation, a paracervical block should be given and the uterine cavity sounded to confirm the direction. A Meigs or Novak curette can then be utilized. Specimens are taken from both the anterior and posterior walls. In either instance, the tissue taken from the curette is quickly placed in formalin for transfer to the pathology laboratory.

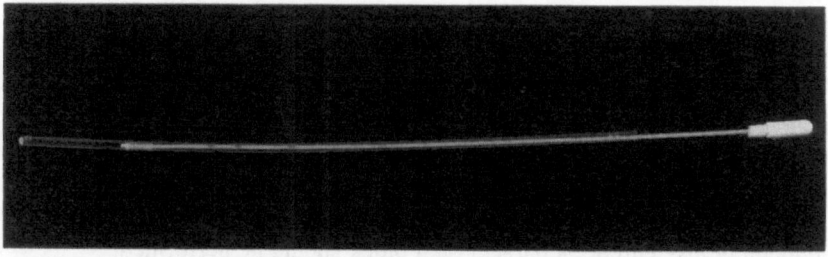

Figure 11-6. Plastic suction cannula for endometrial biopsy.

PROGESTERONE LEVELS

Some physicians utilize a particular level of progesterone both to determine the presence or absence of ovulation, and to assess the quality of corpus luteum function. As with the endometrial biopsy taken at any time in the luteal phase, a single level of progesterone in the blood of 5 to 20 ng/ml is presumptive evidence of ovulation, and has been recommended by some as a replacement for biopsy.[13] The chief advantage is that the procedure is less painful than the biopsy.

Once again, however, the proper assessment of the endocrine factor means more than just the simple determination of the presence or absence of ovulation; it also means an assessment of the degree and quality of corpus luteum function. This latter evaluation is more difficult. On average, there is a distinctive pattern to progesterone level in the secretory phase of the cycle (Fig. 11-7). The levels of progesterone usually lie between 10 and 20 ng/ml 5 to 10 days after the luteinizing hormone peak. There is, however, considerable variation, with no sharp demarcation of what is normal or abnormal on a given day. In addition, the day of ovulation cannot always be selected in advance. Therefore, to assess the function of the corpus luteum, it is necessary to carry out a minimum of two or more progesterone determinations, and even these are not always adequate. At this point, the expense and time involved become a consideration. With the newer instrumentation available for biopsy, and use of local anesthesia in par-

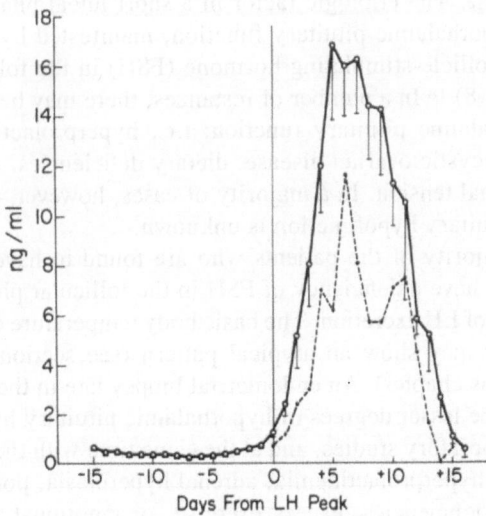

Figure 11-7. Serum progesterone levels during the normal menstrual flow. ○—○, Mean; ●--●, lowest range.

ticularly difficult situations, a well-timed biopsy can provide more accurate information.

Other physicians have reported considerable variation in progesterone levels in relation to endometrial histology, and they believe that both endometrial biopsy and serum progesterone are required for the diagnosis of the inadequate luteal phase.[14]

LUTEAL PHASE DEFICIENCY

Luteal phase deficiency, or corpus luteum insufficiency, results from inadequate progesterone secretion by the corpus luteum and inadequate maturation of the endometrium. This is more likely to result in chronic first-trimester abortion, but primary infertility also occurs. Jones reported a 35% incidence in chronic abortion, but only a 3.5% incidence in infertility.[15] Others have reported an incidence as high as 10%.[16] This discrepancy comes about because of the difficulties in diagnoses and evaluation of therapy. Wentz gives a figure of 5%.[17]

Etiology

There are two major types of luteal phase defects, the one with a short luteal phase (11 days or less in length) and one with an essentially normal-length luteal phase. The etiologic factor in a short luteal phase is found in a deficiency of hypothalamic pituitary function, manifested by a deficiency of serum levels of follicle-stimulating hormone (FSH) in the follicular phase of the cycle (Fig. 11-8).[18] In a number of instances, there may be specific factors affecting hypothalamic pituitary function; i.e., hyperprolactinemia, adrenal hyperplasia, polycystic ovarian disease, dietary deficiencies, excess exercise, or severe emotional tension. In a majority of cases, however, the cause of the hypothalamic pituitary hypofunction is unknown.

The vast majority of the patients who are found to have a luteal phase deficiency do not have a deficiency of FSH in the follicular phase nor do they have a deficiency of LH excretion. The basic body temperature chart either is of normal length or may show an atypical pattern (see section on basal body temperature in this chapter). An endometrial biopsy late in the cycle is abnormal. There may be lesser degrees of hypothalamic pituitary hypofunction not discernible by laboratory studies, and at the same time with the same pituitary etiologic factors: hyperprolactinemia, adrenal hyperplasia, polycystic ovarian disease, dietary deficiencies, excess exercise, or emotional tension. A rare cause is a deficiency of progesterone receptors in the endometrium.[19]

Severe organic disease such as endometriosis[20] or severe scarring from

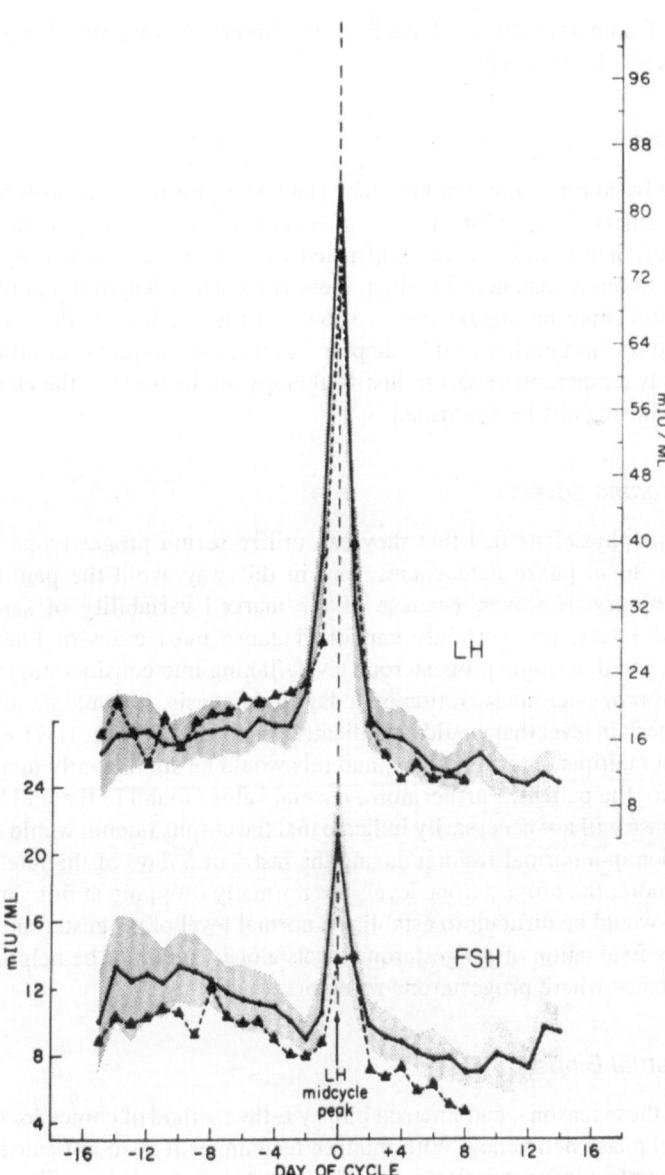

Figure 11-8. Mean daily LH and FSH levels (solid lines) in 16 cycles with 13 or more days post LH peak intervals compared to mean daily LH and FSH levels (dotted lines, solid triangles) in 7 cycles with post LH intervals of 8 days or less (reprinted with permission from Ross *et al.*[18]).

pelvic inflammatory disease have been incriminated as causes of luteal phase deficiencies of either type.

Diagnosis

The basal body temperature chart can be helpful in some cases and of no value in others. A short luteal phase of less than 11 days is diagnostic of luteal phase deficiency and can be confirmed by biopsy or serum progesterone levels.[21] In many instances in which there is a normal-length luteal phase, the temperature may be suggestive as shown in the section on the basal body temperature chart earlier in this chapter, but there is too much variation in the basal body temperature chart to justify therapy on the basis of the chart alone. The diagnosis must be confirmed.

Progesterone Levels

Some physicians feel that they can utilize serum progesterone levels to diagnose luteal phase deficiencies, and in this way avoid the painful endometrial biopsy. However, because of the marked variability of serum progesterone levels, one certainly cannot diagnose most cases of luteal phase deficiency with a single progesterone level. Taking into consideration the variability of progesterone secretion on a day-to-day basis, it would be difficult to select a certain level that would be indicative of normality (Fig. 11-7). One must carry out multiple determinations, and this would be significantly more inconvenient for the patient. Furthermore, normal values found in the middle of the luteal phase will not necessarily indicate that the corpus luteum would continue to function in a normal fashion during the last 4 or 5 days of the luteal phase. Furthermore, the progesterone levels are normally dropping at this time. Once again, it would be difficult to establish a normal level of progesterone for days 24 to 28. Evaluation of progesterone levels alone would not be helpful in this circumstance where progesterone receptors are low.

Endometrial Biopsy

For these reasons, endometrial biopsy is the method of choice for diagnosing luteal phase deficiency. With modern techniques it need not cause significant discomfort in most patients. Serum progesterone levels can still be utilized for those who cannot tolerate even that degree of discomfort. The biopsy need only be taken once during the cycle. A further advantage of the biopsy is that it can be performed a day or two before expected menses, and the full effect of ripening or nonripening of the endometrium can be evaluated. A biopsy performed in the midluteal phase does not always indicate what may happen to the development of the endometrium over the next 4 to 5 days, and also can precipitate an early menses that would contribute to a false-positive diagnosis. The biopsy taken on day 26 or 27 of the cycle is also easier to read.

The endometrium may be read as 11 days post ovulation. If menses occurs the next day, the endometrium is only 2 days out of phase. If the biopsy read as ovulation plus 8 days and menses occurs on the next day, the biopsy is 5 days out of phase. Because of the inability to pinpoint endometrium timing with less than a 48-hour error, luteal phase deficiency should only be diagnosed if there is more than a 2-day lag in the endometrium.[22] Diagnoses made on the basis of a 2-day deficiency only lead to an abnormally high incidence of luteal phase deficiency and extreme difficulty in evaluating therapy.

Another problem is that luteal phase deficiency often does not occur in every cycle in a patient.[21] It may be present one month and not a second.[23,24] This is more likely to occur in the milder degrees of inadequacy. For that reason, before starting therapy in a patient with only a 3-day lag, two consecutive biopsies should ideally be carried out.

Other Diagnostic Aids

It is probably wise to draw prolactin and dehydroepiandrosterone-sulfate levels on patients with luteal phase deficiency before starting therapy, as these may point to a primary cause of the condition. Vaginal smears have also been used to identify the condition.[25,26]

REFERENCES

1. Van der Velde TA: *On the Connections Between Ovarian Activity Cyclical Periodicity and the Menstrual Flow*. Haarlem, R. Bohm's successors, 1904
2. Rubenstein BB: The relation of cyclic changes in human vaginal smears to body temperature and basal metabolic rates. *Am J Physiol* 119:635, 1937
3. Bauman JE: Basal body temperature: Unreliable method of ovulation detection. *Fertil Steril* 36:729, 1981
4. Buxton CL, Engel ET: Times of ovulation. *Am J Obstet Gynecol* 60:539, 1950
5. Kalant N, Pattee C, Simpson G, et al: Timing of ovulation. *Fertil Steril* 7:57, 1966
6. Moghissi VS, Syner FN, Evans TN: A composite picture of the menstrual cycle. *Am J Obstet Gynecol* 114:405, 1972
7. Yussman MA, Taymor ML: Serum levels of follicle stimulating hormone and luteinizing hormone and of plasma progesterone related to ovulation by corpus luteum biopsy. *J Clin Endocrinol Metab* 30:396, 1970
8. De Mouzon J, Testart J, Lefevre B, Pouly JL, Frydman T: Time relationship between basal body temperature and ovulation or plasma progesterone. *Fertil Steril* 41:254, 1984
9. Tyler ET: The vagina and fertility. *NY Acad Sci* 83(Annual):294, 1959
10. Noyes RW, Hertig AT, Rock J: Dating the endometrial biopsy. *Fertil Steril* 1:3, 1950
11. Moghissi K: Accuracy of basal body temperature for ovulation detection. *Fertil Steril* 27:207, 1976

12. Wentz AC, Herbert CM III, Maxson WS, Hill GA, Pittaway DL: Cycle of conception: Endometrial biopsy. *Fertil Steril* 46:196, 1980

13. Israel R, Mishell DR, Stone SC, et al: Single luteal phase serum progesterone assay as an indicator of ovulation. *Am J Obstet Gynecol* 112:1043, 1972

14. Sprong JW, Archer DF, Salazar H: Relationship of serum progesterone and endometrial histology in infertile women. *Fertil Steril* 27:205, 1976

15. Jones GSJ: The luteal phase defect. *Fertil Steril* 27:351, 1976

16. Murphy YS, Arronet GH, Parek MC: Luteal phase inadequacy, its significance in infertility. *Obstet Gynec* 36:758, 1970

17. Wentz AC: Luteal phase inadequacy. In Behrman SJ, Kistner RW, Patton GW Jr (eds): *Progress in Infertility*, 3rd ed. Boston, Little, Brown, 1988, p 405

18. Ross GT, Cargille CM, Lipsett MB, et al: Pituitary and gonadal hormones in women during spontaneous and induced cycles. *Recent Prog Horm Res* 26:1, 1970

19. Laatikainen T, Andersson B, Karkkbainen J, Wahlstrom T: Progesterone receptor level in endometria with delayed or incomplete secretory change. *Obstet Gynecol* 62:592, 1983

20. Naples JD, Batt RE, Sadigh A: Spontaneous abortion rate in patients with endometriosis. *Obstet Gynecol* 57:509, 1981

21. Downs KA, Gibson M: Basal body temperature graph and the luteal phase defect. *Fertil Steril* 40:466, 1983

22. Annos T, Thompson IE, Taymor ML: Luteal phase deficiency and infertility: Difficulties encountered in diagnosis and treatment. *Obstet Gynecol* 55:705, 1980

23. Israel SL: *Diagnosis and Treatment of Menstrual Disorders and Sterility*, 5th ed. New York, Harper and Row, 1967

24. Jones GES, Pourmand K: An evaluation of etiologic factor and therapy in 555 private patients with primary infertility. *Fertil Steril* 13:398, 1962

25. Vorys N, Neri AS, Boutselis JG: Menstrual dysfunction. In Gold, JJ (ed): *Gynecologic Endocrinology*, 2nd ed. Hagerstown, MD, Harper and Row, 1975, p 227

26. Hammond DO: Colpocytologic evidence of progesterone production. *Obstet Gynecol* 21:308, 1963

CHAPTER 12

Semen Analysis

Perhaps no other aspect of infertility is more controversial than the evaluation of the male factor and, in particular, the evaluation of semen quality. Not only is this evaluation difficult, but somehow an adequate investigation of the male role in the infertile couple is often neglected. Such negligence is surprising, especially when one considers that, in approximately 40% of the infertile couples, relative deficiencies in the male partner play at least a partial role and in 20% of the couples, a fairly absolute role in infertility.

WHO SEES THE MALE?

The reason for this neglect often comes down to either geography or responsibility. If the couple lives in an area where there is a fertility specialist, or fertility clinic, the male is more likely to be seen. Usually, however, it is the gynecologist who first sees the female partner, and it is his or her responsibility to ensure that the male factor is properly evaluated and treated. If the gynecologist is untrained in this area, he or she should refer the husband to a urologist with whom he can maintain a close contact. Too many gynecologists, unfortunately, rely solely on the results of a postcoital test or a semen analysis carried out in either their office or a clinical laboratory. Evaluating the male factor only by results of a single postcoital test can be misleading. Occasionally, even when sperm counts are less than 20 million ml, and when the percentage of motile forms is less than 35%, a reasonably good postcoital test will be found. Therefore, one good postcoital test does not necessarily mean that the overall fertility of the couple is not reduced, nor that the male is not still a contributing factor. Only by investigating the male directly can this information be obtained. Other characteristics of the semen—its volume, motility, and morphology—cannot be analyzed by the postcoital test, and it is imperative that motility and morphology be analyzed in assessing the fertility potential of a semen sample.

HISTORY AND PHYSICAL EXAMINATION

To diagnose accurately and correlate abnormal findings of the male with those in the female, it is vital to take a history and do a physical examination. All factors that produce relative deficiencies of sperm count and motility can only be uncovered by such a thorough procedure. Semen analysis, alone, is insufficient. For example, in the occasional case of hypospadias, which results in faulty deposition of the semen at the cervical os, semen analysis is normal.

Moreover, the gynecologist or fertility specialist can take this opportunity to establish a firm relationship with the husband, to provide him with an understanding of the problem, and to tell him what the couple may expect in terms of time, effort, and financial involvement. Such a discussion, giving the husband insight into the reasons for the course of treatment, will often result in the whole-hearted cooperation of the couple as they proceed through the labyrinth of the tests and therapy. Some husbands, however, are reluctant to be seen by a physician; a rare husband is reluctant even to have a semen analysis.

The physician should attempt to explain the importance of these examinations in the context of the problem of infertility and urge his cooperation. This is not to say the investigation of the infertile couple cannot continue even without the husband's full cooperation. Semen analysis without a history and examination is better than nothing.

STANDARDS OF INFERTILITY

The lack of absolute standards of fertility or infertility in terms of sperm count, motility, and morphology have caused additional controversy in evaluation of the male factor. This is particularly true as far as sperm density is concerned. MacLeod suggested that only when sperm count was less than 20 million/ml was there a significant drop in fertility,[1] and the majority of physicians and particularly urologists now agree with this tightening of criteria. These observations have been recently extended by David and co-workers (Table 12-1). Men with sperm counts less than 10 million/ml were ten times more likely to consult for infertility. Men with sperm counts of 40 million/ml

Table 12-1. Relative Risk of Infertility
According to Sperm Count[a]

Sperm count millions/ml	Relative risk	Significance
<10	10.3	$P<10^{-9}$
10–19	5.2	$P<10^{-3}$
20–39	3.1	$P<0.001$
40–59	1.7	$P<0.02$
60–159	1.0	
160–199	1.3	NS
200+	1.5	NS

[a]Unit risk is taken as that obtained for counts of 60 to 159×10^6/ml; NS = not significant; from David et al.[2]

were 1.7 times more likely to be infertile than those men with sperm counts of 60 million/ml or greater. Therefore, there are still many who believe that counts between 20 and 40 million represent at least diminished fertility. The acceptable range of values among various authors is shown in Table 12-2.

There is no doubt that pregnancies occur in the 20 to 40 million range (Table 12-3). They occur at counts less than 20 million,[1,7,8] and have been reported with counts as low as 1 million.[9] Tyler believed that some of the pregnancies occurring with low sperm counts were due to spontaneous variations in sperm count.[10] I believe that fertility of the wife is a decisive factor as to whether or not a 20 to 40 million sperm count will be significant in the overall fertility of the couple. Pregnancies occurring at low levels of sperm density may be due in a large measure to highly fertile females. The failure to take into account the relative fertility of the female partners may be a pitfall in attempting to set up isolated standards of fertility for the male.

That there is a difference in fertility potential between 20 and 40 million counts is suggested by the results shown in Table 12-4. The relation of count to fertility is remarkably similar to that found by Nelson and Bunge (Table 12-3) if one adds all percentages above 40 million together (49%). Accepting that a count of more than 40 million does not increase fertility, the data suggest that

Table 12-2. Variability in Standards for "Normal" Semen Quality

Reference	Year	Count in millions	Motility 2 hr (%)	Motility 6 hr (%)	Normal morphology (%)
MacLeod[1]	1951	20	50	35	70
Simmons and Taymor[3]	1955	60	40	—	70
Amelar[4]	1966	40	60	—	70
Speroff et al.[5]	1973	20	50	—	60
American Fertility Society[6]	1971	40	60	25	80

Table 12-3. Frequency Distribution of Sperm Counts from Allegedly Fertile Men Requesting Vasectomy Compared to MacLeod's Report

Sperm count (millions/ml)	MacLeod[1] (%)	Nelson and Bunge[7] (%)	Rehan et al.[8] (%)
10.1	2	4.7	2
10.1–20.0	3	15.5	5
20.1–40.0	12	30.8	16
40.1–60.0	12	21.0	18
60.1–80.0	14	14.3	21
80.1–100.0	13	6.7	13
100.0	44	7.0	24
Number of subjects	1000	386	1300

there is indeed decreased fertility with a count of less than 40 million. The significance in pregnancy outcome is greater if one considers that the individuals with infertile specimens (less than 20 million) receive treatment, as well, to achieve conception. Conversely, in addition to pointing out the significance of sperm counts less than 40 million, the data indicate that pregnancies are possible with treatment at the lower levels, and undue pessimism about the physician's ability to help the male in infertility is unwarranted.

Despite the above figures, it is generally agreed that sperm motility is a more important parameter than sperm density,[11–13] although this does not completely negate the role of sperm density. It is not as well known that considerable variation in sperm counts occurs on a day-to-day and week-to-week basis. MacLeod has shown that, when semen quality is graded on a 1 to 3 + basis, the variability is usually to the next grade.[14] Rarely does the quality go from 1 to 3 or vice versa. Another feature that has been reported is the usually good correlation between the various factors, i.e., density, motility, and morphology.[15] This is not to say that sufficient disagreement does not occasionally occur, and, therefore, all parameters must be investigated.

Table 12-4. Pregnancy Percentages Associated with Infertile, Subfertile, and Fertile Sperm Counts from 734 Infertile Males

	Number of cases	Number of pregnancies	Percent
A. Infertile (<20 million)	253	44	17
B. Subfertile (20–40 million)	147	48	33[a]
C. Fertile (>40 million)	334	143	43

[a]The difference between B and C is statistically significant to .05.

TECHNIQUE OF SEMEN EVALUATION

Collection of Semen

Semen should be collected in a small, clean, wide-mouthed jar of 1 or 2 oz. Using a larger jar will often result in the drying of the semen specimen along the sides while being transported to the office or laboratory. The preferred method of semen collection is masturbation, but if this is objectionable to the male, coitus withdrawal may be used without affecting the results.[16,17] If there is a loss of a portion of the semen by coitus withdrawal, it should be noted. A rubber condom should never be used, as it will kill the sperm. A plastic pouch can be used, but it makes the collecting and the analysis of the semen more difficult.

For the initial evaluations, there should be a minimum of 3 days, and no more than 5 days, of abstinence prior to collection. A minimum of two specimens, 1 to 2 weeks apart, should be part of the basic workup. Later, to assess more accurately the sperm being delivered to the cervix, the physician might want to collect specimens to coincide with the coital pattern of the couple.

The specimen should reach the laboratory within 2 or 3 hours. There is no need for examination in less than 2 hours. During transportation it should be kept at as near to room temperature as possible, and during cold weather it can be held close to the body in transit.

Preliminary Evaluation

After delivery to the laboratory, the specimen is evaluated for viscosity and volume. Normally, semen is ejaculated as a coagulum, but it will liquefy in 5 to 20 minutes, after which it flows easily and freely. Retention of a viscous state is one abnormality that may be associated with reduced fertility.

Volume between 2.5 and 8.0 ml is considered normal. Less than 2.5 ml often results in poor cervical insemination. A volume greater than 8 ml is usually accompanied by diminished density. This is an indication for the use of homologous insemination with a split ejaculate.

Motility

After thorough mixing, a drop of semen is placed on a microscopic slide. The overall density of the sperm is noted, as well as the number of leukocytes and the presence of autoagglutination. The percentage of motility is determined by judging the number of active forms versus inactive forms in four or five estimations, and a mean is then taken. Although this form of measurement is relatively inaccurate, this is the one used by most experts and seems to serve well in the usual clinical situation. More accurate but more expensive methods

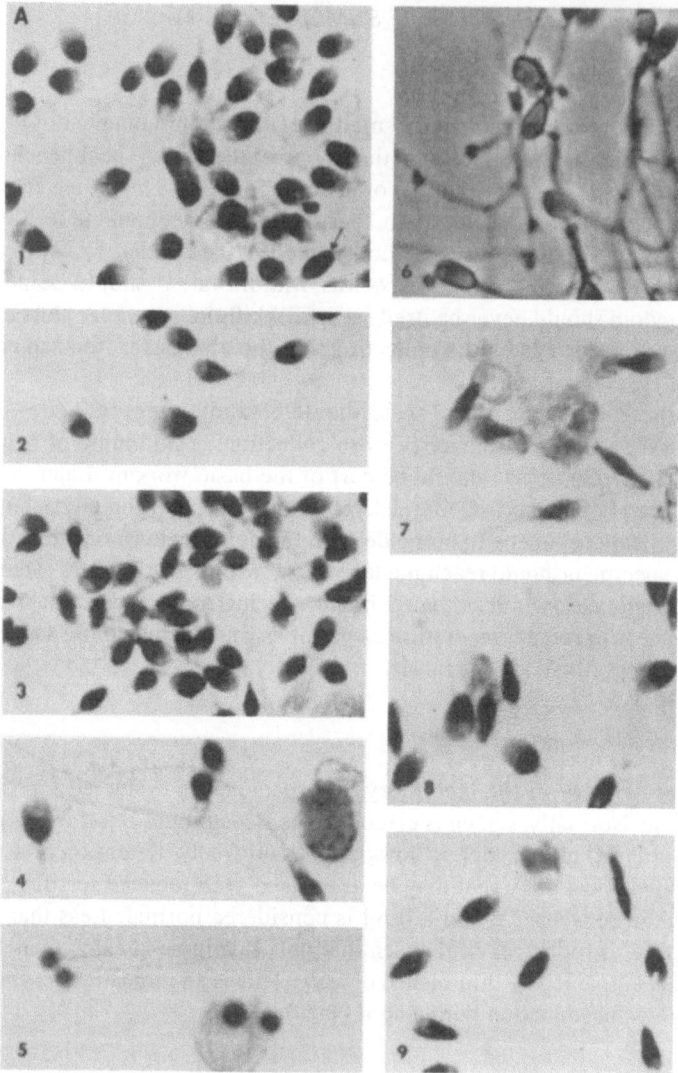

Figure 12-1. (A) (1) Normal specimen. Oval shaped, little variation in size. Vacuoles in the sperm head are without significance. (2) One extra-large sperm head is seen among normal ones. (3) Variations in size of sperm heads. A half-dozen sperm heads are seen in side view and thus appear "arrow head" shaped. (4) Two small-headed sperms, one normal (oval) and one moderately tapering. At right, an extraneous cell, and above this is a coiled sperm tail that has detached itself from the head. (5) Only small round-headed sperms were produced by this patient. At right, a spermatid. (6) This specimen contains several pin-headed sperms. (7) Tapering sperm heads. (8) Tapering forms. (9) One linear tapering head, with coiled tail. The latter condition is also a sign of abnormality. (B) (1,2) Duplicate heads, very common throughout the semen sample of this

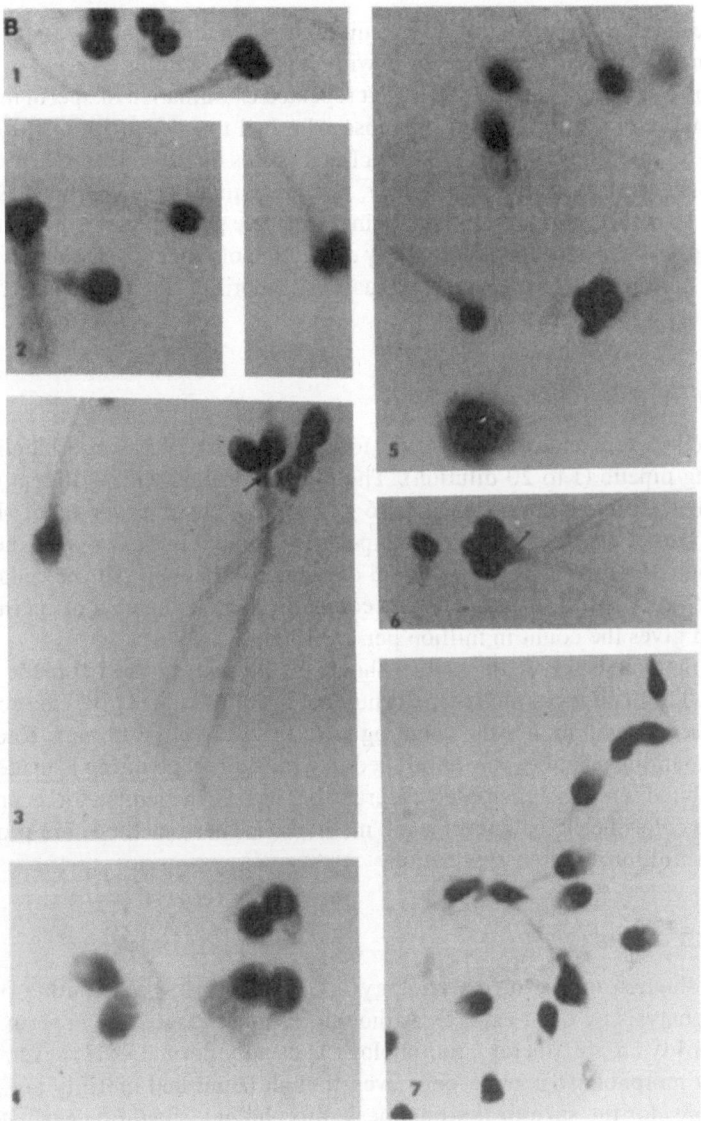

patient. (3) Double-headed sperm, with common cytoplasmic droplet (arrow). Also, a single sperm with very large cytoplasmic droplet. The presence of the droplet is evidence of immaturity of the sperm, for normally the droplet is shed in the epididymis. (4) Two spermatids, possible precursors of two-headed sperm. (5) At right, a four-headed sperm. (6) Four-headed sperm, with common cytoplasmic droplet (indicated by line), which stains red with eosin in Papanicolaou's stain. (7) Sperm heads of various sizes, several in silhouette. Note: The apparent doubling of tails in some photographs is due to double refraction of the portions of the specimens slightly out of focus. (From Amelar R: *Infertility in Man*. Philadelphia, FA Davis, 1966, p 41).

have been developed utilizing video micrography and computerization.[18] Another more accurate measurement is with supravital staining.[19]

Some fertility experts believe that repeated examination of sperm motility is not necessary.[20,21] I am among those who feel that longevity of the sperm may be an important parameter.[22] MacLeod points out that since sperm reaching the cervix leave the seminal fluid, residence in a bottle of semen is not a natural state for sperm. Yet longevity in the female genital tract is important to enhance chances of conception, so any evaluation of longevity should be meaningful. For this reason, a second evaluation of motility should be carried out 5 to 6 hours after ejaculation.

Sperm Concentration

Well-mixed semen is drawn up to the 0.5 mark of a white blood cell–counting pipette (1 to 20 dilution). The pipette is filled with a diluent of 4% sodium bicarbonate and 1% phenol (16 g of sodium bicarbonate, 4 g of phenol, and 400 ml of distilled water). The pipette is thoroughly shaken, and the cells are counted in the red blood cell field of a hemocytometer. All the cells lying within 5 blocks of 16 squares each are counted. The total number of sperm cells counted gives the count in million per milliliter.

If the count is low, the semen should be brought to the 1.0 mark of the pipette (1 to 10 dilution), and then the number of cells doubled gives the count in millions. This will reduce the counting error in severe oligospermia. Recently, a new counting chamber was developed in which direct counting is made from an undiluted sample.[23] Increased accuracy has also been claimed for techniques that use colorimetric or fluorometric methods.[24] These methods are probably more useful for research application.

Sperm Morphology

Evaluation of sperm morphology is considered to be a routine part of semen analysis by most experts. Although, in most cases, when sperm count and motility are satisfactory, morphology is usually normal.[25] However, occasionally morphology may be poor even though count and motility are good. Therefore, for the sake of thoroughness, morphology should be evaluated. A relatively simple method involves preparing a smear on a slide for a blood smear and allowing partial fixing by drying. Additional fixation with 10% formalin for 1 minute is carried out. The slide is first rinsed in water, stained in Meyer's hematoxylin for 2 minutes, rinsed again in water, and allowed to dry. It is examined under an oil immersion lens. A more complicated but better stain is the Papanicolaou stain.

The major classes of sperm morphology are shown in Figure 12-1. There is

Table 12-5. Standards of Semen Quality

	Fertile	Subfertile	Infertile
Count	>40 million	20–40 million	<20 million
Percent motile (6 hr)	>50%	40–50%	<40%
Percent normal	>70%	60–70%	<60%

little unanimity about the significance of abnormal forms and the number of normal forms. Some experts set the fertile level at 60%, some 70%, and others 80%. Although such variability makes one wonder about the significance of morphology, sperm morphology is most helpful for establishing a diagnosis of severe impairment of fertility. The presence of more than 1 million immature forms per milliliter has been reported to give a universally bad prognosis.[26] A high percentage of tapering forms has been seen in association with varicocele.[27]

SUMMARY

There is no sharp line of demarcation between fertility and infertility based on available evidence so far as the parameters of semen quality are concerned. Taking into account the variable role of the female partner, the role of motility as opposed to count, and the role of disturbed morphology, it may be best to group semen analyses into fertile, subfertile, and infertile as outlined in Table 12-5. Therapy in the subfertile and infertile groups is dependent on the evaluation of the couple as a unit.

REFERENCES

1. MacLeod J: Semen quality in 1,000 men of known fertility and in 800 cases of infertile marriages. *Fertil Steril* 2:15, 1951
2. David G, Jouanuet P, Martin-Boyce A, Smira M, Schwartz D: Sperm counts in fertile and infertile men. *Fertil Steril* 31:413, 1979
3. Simmons FA, Taymor ML: Failure of conception in 100 completely studied couples. *Fertil Steril* 6:32, 1955
4. Amelar RI: *Infertility in Men*. Philadelphia, FA Davis, 1966, p 38
5. Speroff L, Glass RH, Kase N: *Clinical Gynecologic Endocrinology and Infertility*. Baltimore, Williams and Wilkins, 1973, p 204
6. American Fertility Society: *Minimal Standards for Evaluation of Infertile Couples*. Birmingham, 1971
7. Nelson CM, Bunge R: Semen analysis: Evidence for changing parameters of male fertility potential. *Fertil Steril* 25:503, 1974
8. Rehan NE, Sobrero A, Fertig JW: The semen of fertile men: Statistical analysis of 1300 men. *Fertil Steril* 26:492, 1975

9. Murphy D, Torrano E: Male fertility in 3620 childless couples. *Fertil Steril* 16:337, 1965
10. Tyler ET: Male infertility: Status of treatment, prevention and research. *JAMA* 169:91, 1956
11. Rutherford R, Banks A, Coburn W, et al: Sperm evaluation as it relates to normal, unplanned parenthood. *Fertil Steril* 14:521, 1963
12. MacLeod J, Gold RZ: The male factor in fertility and infertility: VI. Semen quality and certain other factors in relation to ease of conception. *Fertil Steril* 4:10, 1953
13. Santonauro A, Sciarra J, Varna A: A clinical investigation of the semen analysis and postcoital test in the evaluation of male infertility. *Fertil Steril* 24:245, 1973
14. MacLeod J, Gold R: The male factor in fertility and infertility: VIII. A study of variations in semen quality. *Fertil Steril* 7:387, 1966
15. Sobrero A. Rehan N: Semen of fertile men: II. Semen characteristics of 100 fertile men. *Fertil Steril* 26:11, 1975
16. Hotchkiss RS, Brunner EK, Grenlay P: Semen analysis of 2001 fertile men. *Am J Med Sci* 196:362, 1938
17. Freund M: Interrelationships among the characteristics of human semen and factors affecting semen specimen quality. *J Reprod Fertil* 4:143, 1962
18. Makler A: A new chamber for rapid sperm count and motility estimation. *Fertil Steril* 30:313, 1978
19. Eliasson R, Triechl L: Supravital staining of human spermatozoa. *Fertil Steril* 23:134, 1971
20. MacLeod J: The semen examination. *Clin Obstet Gynecol* 8:115, 1965
21. Amelar RI: *Infertility in Men*. Philadelphia, FA Davis, 1966, p 37
22. Eliasson R: Analysis of semen. In Behrman SJ, Kistner RN (eds): *Progress in Infertility*, 2nd ed. Boston, Little, Brown, 1975, p 697
23. Makler A: Use of a microcomputer in combination with the MEP technique for human sperm motility determination. *J Urol* 124:372, 1980
24. Paz G, Homonai ZT, Korenblum H, Kracier PF: Comparison of colormetric and fluorometric methods for estimation of sperm concentration in human ejaculates and not epididymal sperm. *Int J Androl* 1:570, 1978
25. MacLeod J, Gold RZ: The male factor in infertility and fertility: IV. Sperm morphology in fertile and infertile marriage. *Fertil Steril* 2:394, 1951
26. Frank IN, Benjamin JA, Sergerson JE: Cytologic examination of semen. *Fertil Steril* 5:217, 1954
27. MacLeod J: Seminal cytology in the presence of varicocele. *Fertil Steril* 16:735, 1965

PART IV

Management of the Infertile Couple

CHAPTER 13

A Timetable of Management

The foregoing section has covered the basic workup of the infertile couple. In virtually all instances, before embarking on more intensive therapy, the physician should first complete the basic workup with the couple. The workup may reveal that infertility may be caused by a number of minor factors in both the husband and the wife, each of which alone, would not cause infertility; added together they significantly decrease the couple's fertility potential. For example, time and energy might be wasted treating a husband with moderate oligospermia when a luteal phase deficiency in his wife has not been diagnosed and simultaneously treated.

The basic workup should uncover approximately 90% of the obvious factors involved in infertility. Often, these will lead directly to the next investigative step. For example, the absence of tubal patency by hysterosalpingogram should be followed fairly promptly by laparoscopy. The presence of anovulation indicates the need for hormonal studies, and then specific therapy for the induction of ovulation. Complete azoospermia means that a testicular biopsy should be considered.

At the same time, a number of minor factors also will be uncovered. Therapy for all of these factors should be instituted simultaneously: progesterone suppositories, when indicated, or improvement of environmental factors for the husband. It is important that physicians allow an interval of time to pass so that they can evaluate the results of correcting these minor factors.

Where only factors of minor significance, or where no factors whatsoever, have been uncovered during the basic workup, the therapist should allow time, itself, to play a beneficial role. The reassurance to the couple of their basic normality provided by the workup, in addition to the salutary effects of minor therapeutic maneuvers and the therapeutic potentialities of the tests themselves, may combine to produce the desired results. There are many patients with borderline situations who after 4 to 6 months begin to be concerned about their fertility. Rather than being reassured at this early time by the physician, they are immediately put on the temperature chart (for timing coitus) by either a physician, a nurse, or advice from a friend. The vicious cycle of infertility–emotional tension–infertility begins. It is this couple who responds well to the positive reassurance of a negative basic workup.

For this reason, the practice of admitting patients to the hospital for a 2- to 3-day crash program, including uterotubogram, D&C, culdoscopy or laparoscopy, and a complete endocrine survey, is to be condemned. There are many objections to this crash program. Endoscopy, particularly laparoscopy, is not a completely benign procedure. It involves considerable expense to the patient and can be a waste of medical energy. Each procedure carries with it the slight chance of infection, even at a subclinical level. There should be a specific indication for each procedure to justify any risk whatsoever.

A number of patients may conceive after the basic workup. Whether this is due to the workup, alone, or to the role of time combined with reassurance is an impossible question to answer.

Additional reasons for spacing the total diagnostic possibilities over a 6- to 8-month period are (1) each diagnostic maneuver may have a therapeutic benefit and (2) a sufficient number of opportunities must be allowed for the union of the egg and sperm to test the value of each test and each new therapeutic approach. During this time the physician should maintain a reassuring manner that keeps the couple's anxiety at a minimum. If all the tests were completed within a month or two and if conception did not occur within a few short months, a couple might become frustrated and move on to another physician. If the physician involved is a capable, conscientious practitioner with special training in infertility, the patient has nothing to gain by establishing a relationship with one physician after another. A painful and distressing workup would have to be repeated with an accumulation of anxiety and frustration. Spacing the workup over a period of a year is thus not so that the physician can hold on to his patient for material benefits, although the physician will indeed benefit because more pregnancies will occur while the patients are "under his care."

With this philosophy in mind, the following timetable for the workup is recommended: (1) one should allow a period of observation for 3 to 4 months following the basic workup of the couple with essentially negative findings; (2) if indicated, special tests as outlined in part 5 should be carried out; (3) for those with a negative basic workup at the end of 4 months a laparoscopy should be performed; if positive, infertility surgery or assistant reproductive technology will be considered.

These procedures should consume about 6 to 8 months. At the initial visit or at the end of the basic workup, it would be wise for the physician to discuss this timetable with the couple. The timetable may have to be modified, from time to time, to fit an individual couple's needs, but this approach will allow the maximum opportunity for the cumulative effect of therapy, diagnostic tests, and time itself. Even if the result is unsuccessful, the physician and the couple have a greater chance of feeling that a thorough job has been accomplished. The couple will be emotionally more amenable to accepting the reality of childlessness or the move to adoption, whichever their choice may be.

CHAPTER 14

Infertility Counseling

With Ellen Bresnick, MSW

To reproduce and rear offspring must be one of the most powerful human instincts, an integral part of our ancestral heritage. Millions of years of biological shaping supported by social rituals favoring reproduction and fecundity make infertility "antibiological, unnatural, and antisocial" to many people in our culture. It should also be said that while fewer women choose to bear children in present day society, and the childless parent is more socially acceptable, there are, nevertheless, a core of couples seen in practice who feel what they consider to be the social pressures to become parents.

The social and psychological preparation for parenthood in these individuals begins in childhood where, in role-modeling, the child relates the parent to younger children, dolls, or small animals. This role-playing is a normal growth and crisis experience; young fantasies of future parenthood are constructed, broken, and reformed. As the realistic possibility of parenthood approaches with physical maturation, the psychological investment appreciably intensifies. As concrete plans for pregnancy and parenthood are made, usually in young adulthood, even more emotional energy becomes invested in the goal of childbearing. If that goal is frustrated, delayed, or interrupted, this emotional investment is left in limbo. As a woman and her partner begin to realize that she may never bear a child, an emotional state develops that can be called the "crisis of infertility," affecting all areas of their life together, social, psychological, moral, and religious. In the glaring reality of failure to reproduce, the complacency of a young marriage may gradually be shattered by the recognition of an intense problem. This crisis exacts an emotional toll that manifests itself in various forms of anxiety, depression, frustration, guilt, isolation, and obsession. It is imperative that all those who deal with infertile couples understand their already intense emotional distress, and realize that infertility, itself, may exacerbate existing biological, emotional, or social problems. The couple's emotional tensions can also affect their biological processes so that a vicious cycle of failure to conceive is established. Emotional trauma and its effects, then, are clearly a part of the entire problem of infertility. The physician should recognize and treat the *total* problem of infertility to minimize the overall emotional devastation.

When an individual approaches the physician regarding the failure to reproduce, she or he has already experienced many losses: the loss of a sense of well-being, the loss of self-image, and the loss of achievement of goals. The patient may view himself or herself as "not whole," as defective or diseased. During the infertility workup, the patient's self-image may be further threatened as his or her personal health, sexual identity, sexual activity, and ideas of parenthood are carefully scrutinized. Someone else, the therapist, is now involved, scanning the most intimate private aspect of the young couple's life. The more one invests emotionally in efforts to reproduce, the more vulnerable it seems one becomes to the ensuing disappointment. The very goal the couple is attempting to achieve gradually becomes the source of intense pain.

"We had a very good sexual relationship," one patient explained, "until we realized we had a problem. Then it got horrendous. My body and desires did not always match my temperature chart."

Another patient states, "For years it went on. I dreaded the endless, seemingly futile visits to the doctors. I felt like an outcast as I eyed the successfully pregnant women. I often hoped that they would find something wrong with me, for the words 'relax,' 'keep trying,' only served to drive on my already frustrated, confused guilty self."

Couples must "perform" sexually so that someone else can medically evaluate the results. One young man with a low sperm count became increasingly anxious as yet another test needed to be done. He wondered if his physical well-being contributed to his low count. He had to work the night before the test and thought that because he might be tired it would affect the results. He debated taking sick leave. "It is like a report card to tell you how you did. If you are not feeling well you are afraid your sperm count will be off."

The above feelings become compounded by an increasing sense of guilt and isolation. Infertile couples report feeling uncomfortable in their neighborhood because all their neighbors have children; they do not feel that they belong. Friends may not tell them of their own pregnancies for fear of upsetting them. Holidays, especially, find the childless couple feeling alone. One couple frequently talked of wanting to entertain family and friends at home on holidays, but because they had no children they always felt it was easier for them to travel. They never encouraged visits to their home, and found themselves left out of gatherings where children were involved. Normal social questions became guilt-arousing interrogations; "Do you have any children?" always aroused uncomfortable feelings. The isolation is reinforced; as a chronic aborter stated,

> I was numbed by my first miscarriage. I grabbed every book on pregnancy I could find, desperately trying to find a fitting description of my plight. I felt isolated and lonely as I seemed unable to find anything to hang on to. My second and third miscarriages left me feeling different and alone. I felt like a beetle on its back, desperately fighting for something to help change this cruel pattern. I began to blame myself, feeling I am paying for some unknown sins in my life.

The tests involved in the infertility workup are expensive, often painful, and usually inconvenient. Young working couples, frequently required to take time off from their jobs, feel unable to explain the reasons to their employers. Their feeling that the truth must be hidden, encourages isolation and feelings of inadequacy. Tests, such as the postcoital test and semen analysis, and treatment, such as homologous insemination, interfere with the normal sexual patterns of the couple. Infertile couples must reexamine their sexual feelings as three kinds of sex now confront them regularly: sex for love, sex for the physician, and sex for reproduction. Unfortunately, this pattern can continue for years. As pressures mount, husbands and wives find their ability to perform sexually becomes increasingly unsatisfactory. Temporary premature ejaculation or impotence may result, further compounding feelings of frustration and inadequacy. Suddenly there becomes a right and wrong way to perform the sex act! Many couples' most bitter arguments occur around the time of necessary sex. They resent one another. They fear another failure. They resent the intrusion. They resent the "command performance." They resent their vulnerable positions. Couples may survive all this for a while, but eventually, this produces disastrous results in their sex life and in their whole marriage.

Another source of emotional tension may arise when it is apparent that the couple must accept their life together without a child. Couples must then begin to evaluate their original goals for a family and consider alternatives. Adoption, once a ready alternative, is much more difficult and uncertain today. Not only do couples have to deal with the reality of what they consider their own biological failures, but also with the possibility of childlessness. Added to those psychological burdens with which the couple is already struggling are the realities of adoption if they decide to pursue it. The adoptive channels through which they must work, the time expended, the types of children available, all pose complicated and emotionally demanding problems.

Another resolution that can stimulate emotional tensions and problems is the decision to use donor insemination (AID), an area that today involves complicated legal issues, as well as the obvious psychological ones. How do couples reach this decision confidently, with full awareness of the implications? How do they handle this privately and socially? Today, AID is not discussed, and many consider it "secret." AID remains a promising realistic solution to many infertile couples, but it is not without its emotional consequences.

In vitro fertilization and gamete intrafallopian tube transfer present special problems. The intense involvement in this form of therapy that sometimes requires up to a 2-week period magnifies the anxieties and problems previously outlined: the sense of inadequacy, the interference with natural lovemaking, the interference with job responsibilities, the fear of the medication and the procedure, and the financial sacrifice that has to be made by most couples. Finally, the failure to achieve pregnancy after all of the above becomes another bitter pill to swallow.

COUNSELING

The importance of the emotional concomitants of infertility is undoubtedly recognized by many physicians, but through either lack of time or perhaps the disinclination to involve themselves personally in their patients' emotional trauma, this treatable symptom of infertility is often neglected.

Each couple undergoing the basic workup for infertility should have the option of meeting with an infertility counselor who, ideally, should be a trained psychiatric interviewer, well acquainted in the field of obstetrics, gynecology, and infertility. As a rule it is difficult and often time consuming for the physician to obtain and fully assess the couple's sexual and emotional history, so the counselor's help may be especially important for both the physician and the couple. The interviewer may well be in a better position to elicit this detailed, guarded, and often painful information. In front of the physician, couples prefer to present a "good" picture and may withhold information and deny feelings. Their intense sense of helplessness compounds the denial and serves to conceal the profound emotional effects of infertility. Nevertheless, gathering such information is necessary to evaluate thoroughly the general life-style of the couple, the degree of marital stress, and to estimate the couple's ability to deal with their plight.

The history taking also involves a review of the couple's understanding of their particular medical problems, tests, and possible therapeutic interventions. Questions are encouraged. Emotional support is offered. Follow-up counseling is offered to any couples who may desire it.

During the next 2 to 3 months, coinciding with the basic workup, the couple is urged to attend a series of orientation conferences. Four to six couples in similar situations meet together with both the physician and the counselor. The sessions deal with the facts of reproduction, the infertility tests, and the treatment. Emotional and sexual problems that frequently emerge during this period are explained to the couples. The course is viewed as part of the total treatment plan. The greater the patient's understanding of his or her body, of the reasons for certain tests and therapies, the more responsibility he or she may assume in sharing the information with the physician, and the more capable he or she may become in understanding and coping. Through ongoing discussions, the fertility patient's sense of helplessness and feelings of being victimized can be reduced. Explanations of tests and treatments help allay fears engendered by misinformation and ignorance. The patient may assume a more active, less helpless role. He or she can begin to feel involved in the treatment rather than its victims. The general effects of the tests and therapies on the couple's sexual enjoyment and adjustment are discussed, and they are prepared to expect some problems. Anticipating effects often minimizes their severity. Finally, the effect of the infertility problem on the marriage as a whole, one's feeling of self-worth, the ultimate possibility of adoption, AID, or childlessness are discussed.

Many couples report that before counseling they did not verbalize their concerns sufficiently because each feared "upsetting" the other. For the majority of couples, insight into their current and future problems prepares them to work out their problems together. Many find this new understanding of their present crisis enough to sustain them. For other couples, particularly those with long-standing infertility or those who face prolonged therapeutic regimens, such as homologous insemination, treatment of inadequate luteal phase, induction of ovulation, or who are chronic aborters, more sustained ongoing recourse to emotional support and general information may be needed. This can be in the form of individual counseling or group sessions. Aside from the economic benefit, group sessions offer peer support that ameliorates the loneliness and the isolation that these people are already experiencing. One woman, who had been part of a group, expressed great relief; she felt strong enough to deal with questions of infertility at a party. Having shared with others in a similar situation, she knew she was no longer alone with her problem: she felt less isolated and inadequate as she dealt with a social situation. "I actually smiled inwardly when my friend suggested that once we adopt, I could become pregnant. I remembered our discussion and knew I wasn't alone. I didn't feel so vulnerable." This opportunity to share, to give and take is very salutary.

While counseling of the couple as a unit is the ideal, in our culture it is the woman who makes the greatest apparent emotional investment in handling an infertility problem. If her husband refuses to participate, she, herself, should not be denied an opportunity for counseling. Some physicians are surprised that more and more husbands are not only participating, but seeking out ongoing help. As the expression of feeling becomes more acceptable for men, their emotional involvement and responsibility appear to be increasing.

Counseling should not be viewed as the final method of resolving infertility problems when all other medical resources have failed, but rather as a prescription to alleviate an intense, often overwhelming symptom: emotional turmoil. The additional benefits of counseling can be viewed as part of the physician's concern for maintaining, encouraging, and enhancing the well-being of his or her patients.

PART V

Special Areas and Special Diagnostic Tests

CHAPTER 15

Laparoscopy and Operative Laparoscopy

The widespread use of laparoscopy in infertility diagnosis and treatment represents one of the most significant advances in the management of the infertile couple.

LAPAROSCOPY

Historical Background

Endoscopy of the abdominal contents, including the pelvis, dates back to the early 20th century. It was at times called celioscopy, or laparoscopy. Because the procedure was accompanied by a significant degree of complications, it never was widely used in the management of infertility.

In 1944, Decker described the use of the culdoscope in infertility diagnosis. For the next 20 years, this became a well-accepted and valuable tool in infertility management.[1] Culdoscopy, however, never achieved the widespread use and popularity now enjoyed by laparoscopy because of the relatively high percentage of failures. These failures were mainly caused by improper positioning of the patient, or by delegating the positioning to someone without experience, or by failure to pay attention to the details of technique that would ensure a successful puncture. During the days when culdoscopy alone was available, another drawback was often the relatively faulty equipment available,

113

which was prone to fail during the procedure. Finally, when compared to modern laparoscopy, the visualization was relatively limited.

Technologic improvements, such as a better lens system and the use of fiber optics, coincided with the reintroduction of the improved laparoscope in the mid-1960s. Thus laparoscopy never suffered the problems that harassed culdoscopy and grew in popularity because of its improved instrumentation, excellent visualization, and increased potential for therapeutic use. Since most gynecologists use laparoscopy for purposes other than infertility diagnosis and treatment, such as routine gynecologic diagnosis and tubal ligation, an increasing number of gynecologists maintain constant familiarity with the techniques involved in the use of the laparoscope.

These advantages appear to far outweigh the disadvantages of general anesthesia and the slightly increased risks of laparoscopy as opposed to culdoscopy. At this time very few gynecologists still use culdoscopy.

Procedure

Since the laparoscope is now a basic diagnostic tool in general gynecology, virtually all gynecologists have become familiar with the techniques involved in its use. In the past, many authors have described clearly the indications, contraindications, and hazards, and how the pitfalls may best be avoided.

In mastering the technique, as it pertains to infertility diagnosis, it is not sufficient to establish only the normal appearance of the uterus, ovaries, and tubes, as well as freedom from obvious adhesions or endometrial implants. Free mobility of the tubes and ovaries must also be noted. This can sometimes be accomplished first by pulling the uterus down and into the pelvis and then lifting the ovary out of the pelvis with the fundus of the uterus. Even though the presenting surfaces appear normal, however, a second puncture is usually required to demonstrate that the ovaries are not adhering to the broad ligaments by adhesions or by endometriosis. Without a double puncture, it is also often difficult to examine adequately the fimbriated ends of the tubes. It is not enough to see that dye has entered the pelvic cavity when instilled through the uterine cannula. The character of flow through the fimbriated ends of the tubes, free or impeded, should be evaluated. The blunt probe is the best instrument for lifting the ovaries or ends of the tubes into view. Sharp forceps should be avoided. For infertility diagnosis with laparoscopy, then, a second puncture is almost always indicated.

Indications for Laparoscopy in Infertility

Tubal Pathology. When blocked tubes have been demonstrated by uterotubogram, a laparoscopy should precede the planned tuboplasty. When the x ray has shown blocked tubes at the cornual ends, Peterson and Behrman have noted adequate patency with laparoscopy in as high as 25% of their patients.[2] Spasm or faulty x-ray procedure in these cases produced the blockage. Of equal importance is evaluation of the tubes for distal obstruction before surgery. At preliminary laparoscopy, too much disease in the pelvis or tubes too distorted by disease might be found, and tuboplasty would not be justified. Thus an unnecessary laparotomy is avoided. This too, has been reported at an incidence of upwards of 25%.[2]

Endometriosis. Most patients suspected of having minimal endometriosis, where fertility is not in question, can be observed or treated medically for pain. While minimal endometriosis is not a serious hazard, endometriosis, particularly when there is fixation of the ovaries, can diminish fertility. Medical treatment of endometriosis will not dissolve adhesions; lysis by surgery is required. Therefore, when the gynecologist suspects endometriosis by history or by pelvic examination in an infertile woman, laparoscopy should be planned relatively early in the workup. An enlarged ovary with suspected endometriosis also requires early intervention; not because of infertility alone, but to prevent further progressive destruction of ovarian tissue. The physician, by undertaking proper therapy at the earliest possible date, will avoid losing valuable time.

Suspected Pelvic Disease. A history of ruptured appendix, previous surgery, or pelvic inflammatory disease also suggests the need for early laparoscopy. Pelvic adhesions, diagnosed by uterotubogram, can be confirmed by laparoscopy. Laparotomy should not be carried out solely on the basis of x-ray findings.

Ovulation Disorders. Laparoscopy can occasionally help in the differential diagnosis of ovulation disorders. When there is a problem of hirsutism associated with an ovulatory disturbance, it is sometimes difficult to differentiate between adrenal disease, idiopathic hirsutism, and polycystic ovarian disease. The laboratory findings are often not clear-cut. The demonstration by endoscopy of enlarged, pale, smooth ovaries can sometimes be a diagnostic aid. On the other hand, when the laboratory findings are fairly indicative of a specific disorder, the risks of laparoscopy should be weighed against the good obtained by a mere visual inspection of the ovaries. The decision, in such cases, often should be against laparoscopy. Furthermore, ovarian biopsy usually adds little to the diagnosis, since in most cases only a portion of the capsule is obtained. It is, of course, possible to obtain deeper biopsies, but here too, one must weigh the advantages against the risk of bleeding and the additional danger of producing adhesions by extensive biopsy and cauterization.

When, however, there is a significantly elevated plasma-testosterone level, accompanied by studies that rule out an adrenal problem, then laparoscopy is indicated to differentiate between polycystic ovarian disease and a masculinizing ovarian tumor.

In the differential diagnosis of amenorrhea, laparoscopy can supplement hormone assays in firmly establishing the diagnosis of ovarian agenesis or dysgenesis, particularly in some of its atypical forms. When hormone studies are equivocal, it is also helpful in establishing whether there is primary ovarian failure. Once again, I would caution that laparoscopy should not be considered as a routine procedure; the physician must constantly weigh the advantages to be gained against the risks.

Routine Infertility Diagnosis. The preceding sections have described specific conditions where prior findings indicated the need for early laparoscopy. In addition, laparoscopy can be a vital tool in the management of the infertile couple, even when no specific pathology is suspected. The incidence of unsuspected lesions, such as pelvic adhesions or unexpected endometriosis, found at laparoscopy ranges as high as 60%.[2,3] Occasionally, despite a normal hysterosalpingogram, narrowing of the tubes will be noted; therefore, despite normal x-ray findings, tubal lavage is indicated in all infertility laparoscopies.

The majority of the lesions found are treatable and lead to a higher success rate in infertility management, but even a negative laparoscopy finding provides important information. The significance of borderline disturbances discovered during the basic workup, such as a borderline postcoital test or questionable luteal phase efficiency, is reenforced when the pelvis and pelvic organs are found to be completely normal. Thereafter, the physician can direct his or her attention to the correction of these minor factors, with the wholehearted cooperation of the patient. Furthermore, a negative laparoscopy finding can sometimes be considered as the final test in the infertility workup. When infertility persists, despite negative findings, the time to end further testing has arrived.

I reemphasize that the advantages of a routine laparoscopy in infertility diagnosis must be weighed against its potential dangers. The following serious complications, although rare, can occur: bowel perforation, bleeding from a major vessel in the abdominal wall, and retroperitoneal hematoma from injury to the vena cava. Although in only 0.1% of cases is a laparotomy required to repair these complications, laparoscopy must not be thought of as a benign procedure.

Other serious complications include the subfascial injection of gas, omental emphysema, and pelvic infection. Since most laparoscopies are performed under anesthesia, we must not forget the significant number of complications secondary to endotracheal pneumoperitoneum, such as cardiac irregularities and carbon dioxide embolus.

Therefore, when deciding to use endoscopy in infertility management as a routine diagnostic step, the physician must first determine that sufficient information will result that is not obtainable by other methods that will outweigh the possibility of complications. Some therapists use laparoscopy as one of the first steps in infertility workup and management. The main objection to such routine use is that only a small percentage of laparoscopies result in positive findings. Among many patients being needlessly laparoscoped, attention to minor factors, or time alone, would bring about the desired result. In still other patients, a serious cause of infertility, treatable but as yet undiscovered, would preclude the ultimate need for laparoscopy. Aside from the unnecessary expense, the risks of the procedure are not yet balanced out by the potential benefits.

On the other hand, if laparoscopy is deferred until after the basic workup is completed, if a trial of therapy has been instituted for factors already uncovered, and if time itself has been given a chance to play a therapeutic role, then the yield of positive laparoscopies increases to 50% or 60%; here the benefits significantly outweigh the dangers. In most cases, a laparoscopy is indicated 3 to 6 months *after* completing the basic diagnostic workup provided that no factors have been uncovered indicating an earlier endoscopic investigation. When factors indicating the need for laparoscopy are found, the advantages even for early laparoscopy outweigh the disadvantages.

Screening for In Vitro Fertilization (IVF) and Gamete Intrafallopian Tube Transfer (GIFT). When IVF was first performed and the retrieval of oocytes was carried out primarily by laparoscopy, it was vital to perform a screening laparoscopy to evaluate ovarian accessibility. With the use of vaginal ultrasound retrieval, such a step is now not routinely required unless one suspects complete obliteration of the cul-de-sac by adhesions or endometriosis. Diagnostic laparoscopy still plays a role in the evaluation of the extent and prognosis of distal tubal disease. Whereas surgery for some lesser degrees of hydrosalpinges can be followed by 30% to 40% pregnancy rates, more extensive tubal disease only yields results that can be approximated by the much less invasive procedure, IVF. Thus the physician and patient are greatly aided in their decision making by the laparoscopic findings.

Evaluation of a patient for GIFT however, does require a screening laparoscopy. This is necessary to evaluate not only ovarian accessibility, but also the accessibility of the distal ends of the fallopian tubes. It is not sufficient to simply determine tubal patency by hysterosalpingogram.

Technique of Laparoscopy

With the patient in lithotomy position prepped and draped, the bladder is emptied, the uterus examined for position, and a tenaculum is placed on the cervix; a hollow cannula is inserted to both manipulate the uterus during the procedure and to allow for hydrotubation. With the table flat or in Trendelenburg position, a small puncture stab is made with a scalpel at the inferior margin of the umbilicus. If the Verres needle is inserted in the direction of the hollow of the sacrum, an extremely safe approach is provided. However, there is an increased chance that the diagonally traveling needle will push the peritoneum away rather than pierce it, and one finds lack of entry into the peritoneum cavity more common when the needle is inserted in this direction. Inserting the needle perpendicularly through the peritoneum provides a more certain entry into the peritoneum cavity. By lifting up on the skin, the needle is taken well away from the vital structures overlaying the vertebrae, and this also further tenses the peritoneum. The needle is inserted under careful control. Under an ideal situation, the hub of the needle will rise as the needle pierces the rectus sheath, and it will drop as it goes through the muscle. It will rise again as it goes through the posterior sheath and peritoneum and drop again as it enters the peritoneum. Familiarity with a particular insufflation machine allows the operator to be confident that he is in the peritoneum cavity after watching that the pressure develops when flow into the cavity has begun. An average of 3.5 L is required to adequately fill the peritoneum cavity. When an adequate pneumoperitoneum has been obtained, the intraumbilical incision is enlarged to accommodate the size laparoscope that is to be used. For observation laparoscopy a 5-mm scope is adequate. It is much easier to insert, and it is less likely to cause severe damage if there is a problem with insertion. For operative laparoscopy or documentation by photography or video, a 10-mm scope is usually required.

The patient is placed in fairly steep Trendelenburg, the trocar is inserted through the incision in the abdominal wall through the corium and then advanced a one-half inch or so to produce a z-like incision through the abdominal wall. Once again, the abdominal wall is lifted up and held firmly by the operator and the assistant, and now the trocar is inserted in the direction of the hollow of the sacrum with a firm, steady, screwing motion. After noting that the laparoscope is in position, a double puncture is made approximately three-finger breadths above the top of the symphysis pubis. This puncture should be made under direct vision, with the operator using one hand to push the second trocar through a small incision in the abdominal wall while observing the advancement of the trocar through the peritoneum and its avoidance of pelvic structures.

Complications of Laparoscopy

Although complications from laparoscopy are rare, they do occur. They seem to decline with the increasing experience of the surgeon. A report by the

American Association of Gynecologic Laparoscopists, analyzing 125,566 laparoscopies, reveals complications rates of .45% for hemorrhage, 0.42% for bowel injury, 0.42% for infections, and 0.16% for anesthetic complications.[4]

Operative Laparoscopy

An advantage of laparoscopy over culdoscopy is the number of surgical procedures that can be carried out without resorting to full laparotomy. Although Clyman had described a number of such procedures in association with culdoscopy, there has not been widespread use of his approach.[5] Because of better visibility, the ability to use two and even three puncture sites and because more versatile instruments have been designed, the potential for surgery through the laparoscope has always been present and continues to grow. Lysis of minor adhesions with a cautery scissors is a relatively simple and worthwhile maneuver. With better instruments, the experienced surgical gynecologist can safely divide and cauterize even dense adhesions between the ovary and adjoining structures or between the omentum and pelvic organ.[5] Aspiration of simple ovarian cysts is possible and reasonable. Gomel has described dilatation of phimotic tubal ostia.[6] More extensive surgery to the tubes, where precise dissection with fine instruments and hemostasis with microcautery are important, should be carried out by individuals with specialized training or be reserved for laparotomy.

If minor surgical procedures can be carried out successfully through the laparoscope, the patient experiences less risk, less discomfort, less expense, and a shorter hospital stay and convalescence than with a laparotomy and is still provided with a satisfactory approach to her problem. If extensive bleeding and cauterization are to be encountered, the surgeon should then consider the better results obtained by open laparotomy and that careful microsurgical techniques can outweigh the advantages of operative laparoscopy.

Minimal lesions of endometriosis can be coagulated with a unipolar cautery[6] although the significance of this maneuver in the correction of infertility remains open to question.

PELVISCOPIC SURGERY

Semm has been an advocate of more extensive surgery under laparoscopic visualization, a procedure also called pelviscopic surgery.[7] Multiple punctures, specialized instruments, and extensive experience and training are required to carry out this surgery successfully and safely. The main goal is to reduce the length of hospital stay and complications from those associated with laparotomy. There is also a feeling that less adhesions form, but this has not been well documented.

For procedures that are not necessarily associated with infertility, such as myomectomy, removal of ovarian cysts, salpingostomy or salpingectomy for ectopic pregnancy, and thermocoagulation of extensive endometriosis, pelviscopic surgery in experienced hands can be successfully carried out with marked gain to the patient.

On the other hand, the role of extensive pelviscopic surgery in infertility therapy remains to be determined. Minor adhesions and minor degrees of endometriosis can be handled equally well through the laparoscope or laparotomy, and no doubt there is an advantage here. However, lysis of thick extensive adhesions, the removal of large chocolate cysts from the ovary, primary neosalpingostomy for blocked fallopian tubes, or ovarian wedge require extensive handling of tissues, extensive coagulation for hemostasis, and often suture placement. If we accept that microsurgery techniques are important, if we accept that the first surgical approach to these problems has the best chance of success, an approach designed primarily to save the hospital stay can be questioned. Until large control studies are demonstrated, and at least an equality in results shown, final judgment should be withheld.

So far, the evidence for better results has yet to be shown. In surgery for distal disease of the tube, the laparoscopic approach is usually performed in conditions with less severe degrees of tubal damage. Leventhal has described six pregnancies in 18 patients (30%) treated laparoscopically, but only three came to term (16.5%). All were noted to have apparently undamaged tubal fimbria that were released at the time of surgery.[8]

LASER LAPAROSCOPY

A further extension of the therapeutic use of laparoscopy is to use a carbon dioxide laser at the time of laparoscopy, laser laparoscopy. As with any new procedure, its early advocates were enthusiastic about the indications, potential, and successes.[9–11] However, because of the need for expensive equipment and specialized training and possible significant complications, it has taken time to have extensive studies reported. As time passes, more individuals will have had an opportunity to assess this approach, and this should result in more balanced conclusions about the procedure.[10]

The laser provides a rapid method of cutting tissue with minimal damage, and it provides an excellent method of destroying implants of endometriosis and cysts of endometriosis with minimal damage to healthy tissue. For these reasons, it is a significant aid in the lysis of pelvic adhesions and the treatment of moderate to severe endometriosis at open laparoscopy. Whereas in open pelvic surgery, the vaporizing effects of laser have significant advantages over other methods of cutting tissue, in a laparoscopic approach these advantages are somewhat offset by the inability to reach all areas of the pelvis with equal safety. Some surgeons are becoming exceedingly expert with this technique, but many will find their range limited and only carry out the amount of incision or vaporization that could be as easily taken care of with the endoscopic cautery. Both the expense of the equipment and the extra time needed to set up the instrument come into play in the determination of whether or not to use the laser in association with laparoscopy.

Instrumentation

The instrumentation has been thoroughly described by Daniel.[11] The carbon dioxide laser is ideal for use in the pelvis because with its low level of penetration, it can perform its mission with minimal damage to surrounding tissues and organs. A number of excellent carbon dioxide machines are on the market. One most important part of the instrumentation is the articulating joint between the laser and laparoscope, or between the laser and the double puncture tube that will carry the beam to the pelvis. The articulating arm must be so constructed that the beam from the laser will be centered after traveling through the scope or accessory tube. If the beam is not centered, there should be a mechanism for easy correction of this problem.

The single puncture method utilizes a somewhat enlarged single puncture laparoscope with a 5-mm operating channel through which the laser tube carrying the beam passes. The double puncture technique uses the usual observation laparoscope for viewing, and 250- or 350-mm-long tubes that carry the laser beam through a third incision made between the umbilicus and pubis. The usual second incision at the pubis allows for the installation of fluid and for the evacuation of smoke indications.

Indications in Infertility Treatment

At the present time, laser laparoscopy provides a significant advantage for infertility therapy when used to lyse fairly extensive pubic adhesions and in the treatment of some cases of moderate endometriosis.

Endometriosis. To my mind its use in minimal and mild endometriosis is still open to question, chiefly because there is no clear evidence that the treatment of minimal or mild endometriosis leads to increased pregnancy rates.[12] However, there is evidence that if one sees endometrial implants there are probably many areas of endometriosis that are not visible through the laparoscope. If one feels that mild and minimal endometriosis is to be treated, medical treatment would reach lesions not seen through the scope. Use of the laser in such cases could lead to a false sense of security about the elimination of all endometriosis. Furthermore, the procedure is not without significant risk.

On the other hand, the ability to vaporize chocolate cysts of the ovaries is a very distinct advantage. Since the ovaries can be brought into view, fairly good-sized cysts can be unroofed and vaporized with minimal damage to a normal ovary and can thus eliminate endometriosis that medical therapy could not reach.

Lysis of Adhesions. Adhesions are very amenable to laser surgery. The lysis is usually bloodless and causes minimal tissue damage. A backstop behind the laser beam lends safety to the procedure. If the problem in infertility is the presence of peritubular or periovarian adhesions, an adequate lysis can usually be carried out with a laser through the scope without significant risk.

Salpingostomy. Salpingostomy has been successfully performed with a laser through the laparoscope and pregnancies do occur. However, the series reported have been small. Furthermore, the less severe are usually selected for laser laparoscopy therapy, and even then the results of term pregnancy are not spectacular.[7] It is difficult to utilize truly meticulous, microsurgical techniques through the laparoscope. The first attempt at salpingostomy is the one most likely to succeed. Until better results are demonstrated, then, salpingostomy with a laser through the laparoscope is not justified.

REFERENCES

1. Decker A, Cherry TH: Culdoscopy, new methods in diagnosis for pelvic disease. *Am J Surg* 64:40, 1944
2. Peterson EP, Behrman SJ: Laparoscopy and hysteroscopy. In Behrman SJ, Kistner RW (eds): *Progress in Infertility*, 2nd ed. Boston, Little, Brown, 1975, pp 865–887
3. Israel R, March C: Diagnostic laparoscopy: A prognostic aid in the surgical management of infertility. *Am J Obstet Gynecol* 125:7, 1976
4. Phillips JM, Halka J, Peterson HB: American Association of Gynecologic Laparoscopists, 1982 Membership Survey. *J Reprod Med* 29:592, 1984
4a. Sulewski JM, Carcio EJ, Bronlsky C, Stengen VG: The treatment of endometriosis at laparoscopy for infertility. *Am J Obstet Gynecol* 138:128, 1980
5. Clyman M: Endoscopy: A new panculdoscope: Diagnostic, photographic and operative aspects. *Obstet Gynecol* 21:343, 1963
6. Gomel V: Laparoscopic tubal surgery in infertility. *Obstet Gynecol* 46:47, 1975
7. Semm K: Advances in pelviscopic surgery: Current problems. *Obstet Gynecol* 5:1, 1982
8. Leventhal JM: Laparoscopy in female infertility. In Hunt R (ed): *Atlas of Female Infertility Surgery*. Chicago, Year Book Publishers, 1986, p 189
9. Baggish MS: Status of carbon dioxide laser in infertility surgery. *Fertil Steril* 40:442, 1983
10. Adamson GD, LU J, Subak LL: Laparoscopic Co_2 laser vaporization of endometriosis compared with traditional treatments. *Fertil Steril* 50:764, 1988
11. Daniel JF: Laser laparoscopy. In Baggish MS (ed): *Basic and Advanced Laser Surgery in Gynecology*. East Norwalk, CT, Appleton-Century-Crofts, 1985, p 343
12. Bayer SR, Seibel MM, Saffan DS, Berger MJ, Taymor ML: Efficacy of Danazol treatment for minimal endometriosis in women. *J Reprod Med* 33:179, 1988

CHAPTER 16

The Prediction of Ovulation

The ability to predetermine the arrival of ovulation can obviously enhance the chances of conception, and this is a subject that has intrigued fertility clinicians and researchers for many years. To the time honored methods of charting the basal body temperature and of examination of cervical mucus have now been added new information and new approaches that improve the accuracy of this aid to infertility treatment.

THE BASAL BODY TEMPERATURE CHART

The basal body temperature chart is a useful, inexpensive method for *retrospectively* determining the approximate timing of ovulation. It is the general consensus that ovulation occurs around a thermal nadir that is followed by a sustained rise in temperature lasting from 12 to 15 days (see Fig. 11-1). In a recent report utilizing urinary luteinizing hormone (LH) kits, the LH surge was found to begin on the day of the thermal nadir.[1] It was further suggested that ovulation occurred sometime during the 24 hours after the thermal nadir. However, other studies have shown that a thermal nadir in relation to ovulation can vary as much as 2 or 3 days in each direction. Furthermore, often there is no clear nadir. Finally, there is much less cycle regularity than patients believe. In a study of basal body temperature charts, 49% of women with 12 graphs had a cycle variability of more than 5 days.[2] Accepting this variability then, it would appear that if charts are going to be used for coital timing even in future cycles, one should select only women with fairly regular cycles, average a relatively large number of cycles, and provide a fairly wide window for coital activities such as the 11th, 13th, 15th, and 17th day or the 10th, 12th, 14th, and 16th day of the cycle. Even with this advice, patients should be told that it is not a strict rule but just a guideline.

It is well recognized that one cannot utilize the charts to predict the coming of ovulation in an ongoing cycle, and fortunately its use for this purpose has been for the most part discarded. However, as indicated in chapter 11, there are other important uses for the basal body temperature chart.

CERVICAL MUCUS CHANGES

In the 1950s and 1960s much attention was directed to changes in cervical mucus, those brought about by the rising level of estrogen that peaks 1 to 3 days before ovulation. There are changes in the physical characteristics of the mucus, including ferning and spinnbarkeit, that together have been characterized as a cervical score.[3] Peaks in concentration of sodium chloride[4] or glucose[5] were also used to predict the coming of ovulation. Although these changes were helpful in a few cases, in many others, particularly in women with markedly irregular cycles, the changes were not distinct enough nor consistent enough to be of real value.

LUTEINIZING HORMONE: RELATIONSHIP OF THE SURGE TO OVULATION

The pioneering work of Zondek and Ascheim demonstrated a direct relationship between pituitary gonadotropin secretion and ovarian function.[6] Fevold and co-workers were the first to separate follicle-stimulating hormone (FSH) and LH.[7] McArthur was the first to show a consistent midcycle surge in LH by means of the rat ventral prostate assay.[8] Since that time, many investigators, using a variety of assays, have sought to use assays for LH as a marker of ovulation and have done so with varying accuracy as time has progressed.

In 1959, our first study was reported in which corpus luteum biopsy was correlated with LH assays to relate in a temporal way the peak of LH excretion to ovulation in humans.[9] A subsequent study using radioimmunoassay for LH and corpus luteum biopsies showed the mean time of ovulation to be 28 (24 to 40) hours after the surge and 22 (20 to 30) hours after the peak of plasma LH.[10] Later, a collaborative study was reported by the World Health Organization that involved 107 patients subjected to ovarian inspection or corpus luteum biopsy associated with indicated laparotomy.[11] LH determinations were limited, however, to 8-hour intervals. The mean result was remarkably close to the previous observations performed 10 years before, but there was no further narrowing of the range. Ovulation occurred 32.0 (23.6 to 38.2) hours after the onset of the LH peak. The relatively large variation in this latter series, even with a large number of cases, was because the LH determinations were made at 8-hour intervals and the patients were observed over a long time span both before and after ovulation.

A study involving a combination of rapid LH assay at 4-hour intervals with laparoscopic removal and examination of the maturing oocyte or visualization of an early corpus luteum put ovulation as occurring 36 to 38 hours after the onset of the LH surge and 22 to 26 hours after the occurrence of the LH peak.[12] Testart also showed that by 37 hours after the onset of the LH surge, almost all subjects had ovulated.[13] A summary of these studies relating the time of ovulation to the onset of the LH surge and occurrence of the LH peak is shown in Table 16-1.

The time interval of 36 to 38 hours between the onset of the LH surge and ovulation is for plasma levels of LH. In clinical practice, the urinary determination is often more practical. The onset of ovulation after the onset of the surge is earlier in urine, closer to 28 hours.

Urinary LH Kits for Home Detection

A number of kits for the home assay of urinary LH are available. In general, they have been found to be quite reliable in predicting ovulation within the next 24 hours. According to one report, Ovutest® is 87.5% accurate and First Response®, 53.7%.[14] However, others have questioned the reliability of these tests.[15]

Accepting a degree of accuracy for the tests, the major question is which patients can benefit from the knowledge that their ovulation will occur in the

Table 16-1. Studies Relating Time of Ovulation to Onset of LH Surge and LH Peak (Serum)

Study	Year	Onset of surge (hr)	Peak (hr)
Taymor[9]	1959	—	26 (12–48)
Yussman and Taymor[10]	1970	32.8[a] (28–44)[b]	17.6 (16–24)
Ferin et al.	1973	21–36	—
Croxatto et al.	1974	—	14–?
Pauerstein et al.	1978	—	9 ± 2
WHO[1]	1980	32 (23.6–38.2)	16.5 (9.5–23.0)
Garcia et al.	1981	27.3	17.5
Testart[13]	1982	37	—
Taymor et al.	1983	36–38	22–26

[a]Hours before ovulation.
[b]Range.

next 24 hours. If the cervical mucus is normal and receptive to sperm, if the sperm count is within normal limits, and if the couple regularly engages in coitus, approximately every other day, there is little to be gained by knowing when ovulation will occur. There will be sperm waiting for the egg most of the time. The cause of the infertility is undoubtedly elsewhere. The LH kit is a relatively costly one that often does not help solve the problem, and indeed may do harm by producing frustration engendered by high expectations, by the pressure of dictating "love making" according to the test, and by a delay in the resolution of the real problem. In other words, the tests have been oversold.

This is not to say that there are no indications for the use of home LH kits. In patients whose natural sex drive calls for relatively infrequent intercourse, such information for timing may be helpful. When couples are geographically separated because of their jobs, they can be happily brought together at the appropriate time. In timing insemination treatments, whether with husband or donor sperm, a beneficial increment is added to the therapeutic maneuvers by the knowledge that ovulation is imminent.

One would hope that the test would be particularly helpful in pinpointing ovulation in grossly irregular cycles where the day of ovulation might vary over a 10- to 15-day period from month to month. Unfortunately, in such cases one does not know when to start testing, and often in such cases the end points are not sharp, and there are multiple minor surges of LH before the one that ends in ovulation.

THE ROLE OF ULTRASOUND

With the first descriptions of the use of ultrasound to scan the development of the ovarian follicle, it was hoped that a relatively simple method would be available to predict the coming of ovulation.[16] However, it soon became apparent that the variability in follicle size at the time of ovulation was too great, and that the ultrasonic changes from follicle to corpus luteum were too subtle to allow for accurate timing of ovulation in advance of the event.

The scanners have improved through the years and, particularly, the use of vaginal transducers provides a clearer delineation of the ovarian structures. Although most authors believe that 20 mm is the usual size of the preovulatory follicle, there is a marked degree of variability. The size of the preovulatory follicle has been recorded as being from 20 mm[17] to 27 mm[18] (Fig. 16-1). Ultrasound scanning, therefore, cannot predict that ovulation is imminent or that it has occurred (Fig. 16-2). It can indicate that it will probably occur within the next few days. Its best use is in determining when a follicle or follicles are ready to receive the LH stimulation necessary to result in ovulation, and thus it provides invaluable information as to when to administer human chorionic gonadotropin (HCG) in induced cycles.

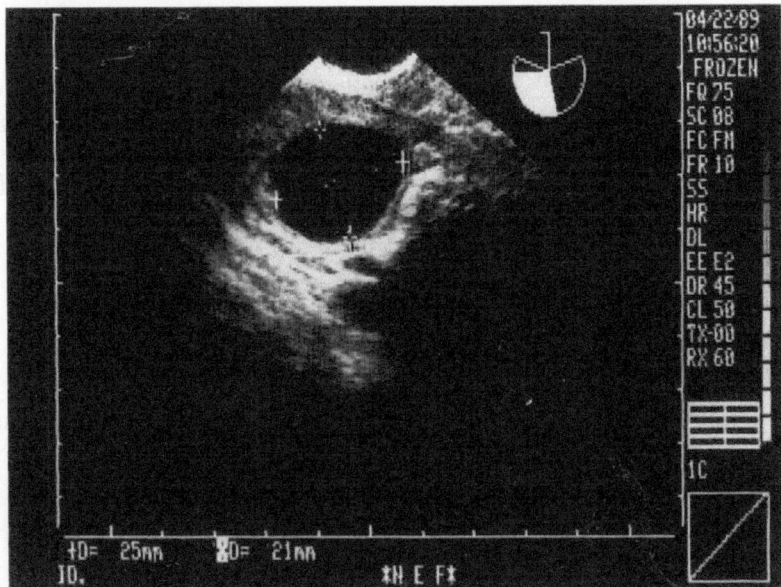

Figure 16-1. A preovulatory follicle by vaginal ultrasound.

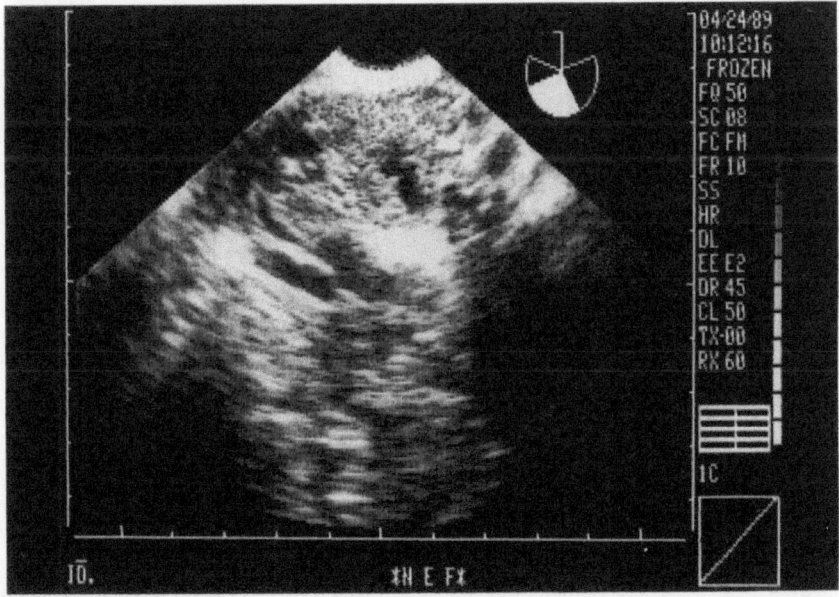

Figure 16-2. Disappearance of the preovulatory follicle indicating that ovulation has occurred.

ESTRADIOL LEVELS

Although rising levels of estradiol in the late follicular phase of the cycle plays a significant role in stimulating the onset of the preovulatory LH surge, the premenstrual increase is not distinct enough nor consistent enough to allow one to select a point where one could predict the coming of ovulation by this measurement alone[19] (Fig. 16-3).

OVULATION TIMING BY OVULATION INDUCTION

Clomiphene

Clomiphene acts by stimulating the release of FSH and LH. Follicular development occurs, and this may be multiple. The occurrence of ovulation,

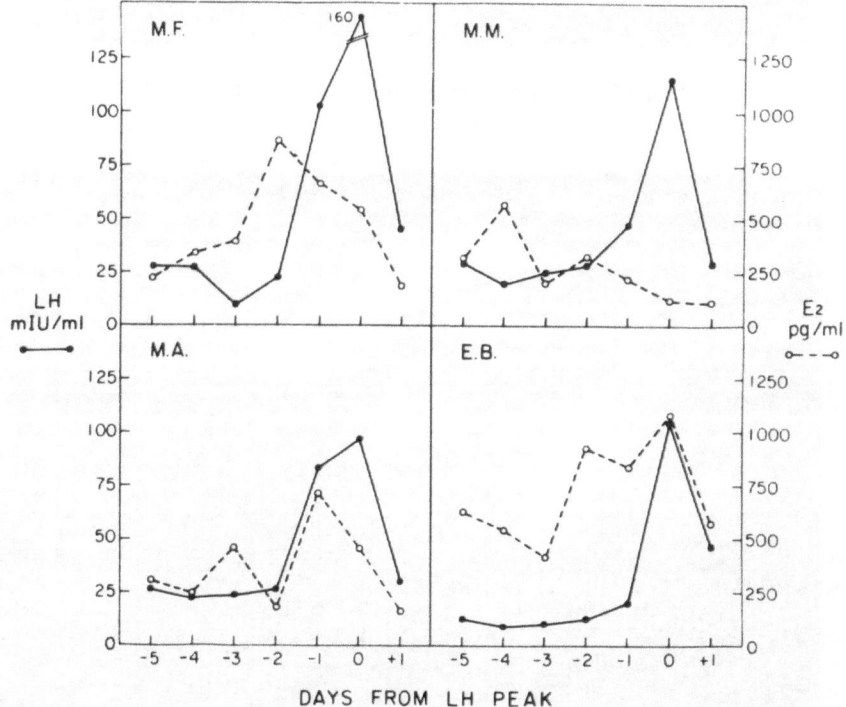

Figure 16-3. Variability of relationship of peak estradiol levels to peak LH levels in four normal subjects.

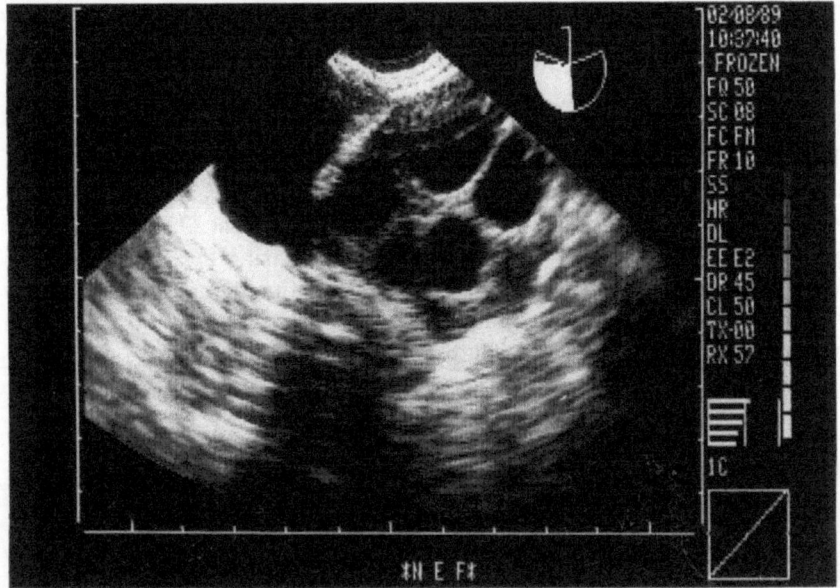

Figure 16-4. Multiple preovulatory follicles induced by gonadotropin therapy.

however, and the hormonal events surrounding ovulation are similar to that in the normal menstrual cycle. Measurement of the LH surge is the best indicator of the incipient ovulation, and the same indications for the use of the home LH kits prevail. However, ovulation can be triggered by the administration of HCG.

Gonadotropins

Under a variety of conditions it may be helpful to control the ovulatory process in ovulatory women by the use of gonadotropins administered during the follicular phase of the cycle. These indications are in vitro fertilization (IVF), gamete intrafallopian tube transfer (GIFT), and intrauterine insemination, conditions where one wants to retrieve oocytes or insert spermatozoa just prior to ovulation. The contributions of the gonadotropin therapy are twofold: (1) by starting the gonadotropin administration early in the follicular phase, days 2 to 4, multiple follicles can be brought to the preovulatory phase and the ovulation of a number of oocytes can theoretically enhance fertility (Fig. 16-4); (2) the use of HCG to trigger ovulation once mature follicular development has been reached means that the therapy planned can be carried out at the appropriate time, i.e., just before ovulation.

The Use of HCG

Where HCG is used, following either clomiphene or gonadotropins, the endogenous LH surge is no longer in control of ovulation (unless the LH surge has begun prior to the administration of the HCG), but is under the control of the HCG. From the work of Edwards, it has been shown that in a manner very similar to endogenous LH, ovulation occurs 36 to 38 hours after the administration of HCG if adequate follicular development is present.[20] This knowledge gives the therapist an enormous advantage in advising the time for coitus following ovulation induction, for timing insemination therapy when it is carried out in combination with clomiphene HCG or gonadotropin therapy, and in performing IVF and GIFT procedures.

REFERENCES

1. Corson SL: Self-prediction of ovulation using a urinary luteinizing hormone test. *J Reprod Med* 31(Suppl 8):761, 1986
2. McCarthy JJ, Rockette HE: Prediction of ovulation with basal body temperature. *J Reprod Med* 31(Suppl 8):743, 1986
3. Insler V, Melamed H, Eichenbrenner I, et al: The cervical score: A simple semi-quantitative method for monitoring of the menstrual cycle. *Int J Fertil* 10:223, 1972
4. McSweeney DJ, Sbarra AJ: A new cervical mucus test for hormone appraisal. *Am J Obstet Gynecol* 88:705, 1964
5. Birnberg CH, Kurzrock R, Laufer A: Simple test for determining ovulation time. *JAMA* 166:1174, 1958
6. Zondek B, Ascheim S: Des hormone des hypophysen vor der lappens. *Klin Wochenschr* 6:248, 1927
7. Fevold HL, Hisaw FC, Leonard SL: The gonad stimulating and luteinizing hormones of the anterior lobe of the hypophysis. *Am J Physiol* 97:291, 1931
8. McArthur JW: Midcycle changes in urinary gonadotropin excretion. In Lloyd CW (ed): *Recent Progress in the Endocrinology of Reproduction*. New York, Academic Press, 1959, p 67
9. Taymor ML: Timing of ovulation by LH assay. *Fertil Steril* 10:212, 1959
10. Yussman MA, Taymor ML: Serum levels of follicle-stimulating hormone and luteinizing hormone and of plasma progesterone related to ovulation by corpus luteum biopsy. *J Clin Endocrinol* 30:396, 1970
11. World Health Organization: Task force on methods for determination of the fertile period. *Am J Obstet Gynecol* 138:838, 1980
12. Taymor ML, Seibel MM, Smith DM, Levesque L: Ovulation timing by luteinizing hormone assay and follicle puncture. *Obstet Gynecol* 62:191, 1983
13. Testart J, Frydman R: Minimum time lapse between luteinizing hormone surge or human chorionic gonadotropin administration and follicle rupture. *Fertil Steril* 37:50, 1982
14. Vermesh M, Kletzky OA, Davajan V, Israel R: Monitoring technique to predict and detect ovulation. *Fertil Steril* 47:259, 1987
15. Darcel JC Jr, Lonergan BB, Sullivan PK, Taylor SP: Evaluation of "Determine: The Ovutest" as a device for identifying optimal time for conception. *Fertil Steril* 47:590, 1987
16. Queenan, JT, O'Brien GD, Bains LM, Simpson J, Collins WP, Campbell S: Ultrasound scanning of ovaries to detect ovulation in women. *Fertil Steril* 34:99, 1980

17. O'Herlihy E, Pepperell RJ, Robinson HP: Ultrasound timing of human chorionic gonadotropin administration in clomiphene stimulated cycle. *Obstet Gynecol* 59:40, 1982
18. Renaud RL, Macier S, Dervain I, et al: Echographic study of follicle maturation and ovulation during the normal menstrual cycle. *Fertil Steril* 33:272, 1980
19. Taymor ML, Thompson IK, Arfania J, Kosasa TS: Studies on gonadotropin-steroid relationships in the menstrual cycle. In Crosignani PG, James VHT (eds): *Recent Progress in Reproductive Endocrinology*. New York, Academic Press, 1974, p 523
20. Edwards RG, Steptoe PC: Control of human ovulation, fertilization and implantation. *Proc Roy Soc Med* 67:932, 1974

CHAPTER 17

Immune Factors and Infections in Infertility

IMMUNE FACTORS

For many years the role of immune factors in infertility had been a subject of controversy. However, in the last few years, with the availability of more precise and more specific tests for sperm antibodies, this relationship has been placed on a much firmer basis, and few can now question the fact that such a relationship does exist.

Historical Background

Since Landsteiner[1] and Metchnikoff[2] independently described the presence of antibodies to sperm in 1899, numerous studies both in animals and in humans have confirmed their findings. These studies have been reviewed extensively by Behrman.[3] The relationship between immunology and human infertility was first suggested by Wilson in 1954 when he described the discovery of spermagglutins in human semen and blood.[4] The relationship of antibodies to semen or sperm has been extensively studied ever since Franklin and Dukes first reported spermagglutinating activity in the serum of 78% of women with unexplained infertility.[5] However, these results have not been subsequently confirmed. The reported incidence of spermagglutinating antibodies have ranged from a low 7% to a high 45%.[6,7] Such inconsistent findings have led many to doubt that immune factors in infertility are significant. A more balanced view might be that although immune factors may not always occur in the high incidence of 78% reported by Franklin and Duke's original article, there is ample evidence for the existence of such factors.

In the 1970s a variety of tests were developed for both spermagglutinating and sperm immobilizing antibodies: gelatin agglutination test, tube slide agglutination test, tray agglutination test, complement-dependent sperm immobilization test, and mixed agglutination reaction. These tests, reviewed by Ansbacher, all gave a relatively high incidence of false negatives and false positives, and as late as 1981 the exact significance of the immune factor remained open to question, particularly in relation to the presence of antibodies to sperm in the female.[8]

Recently, however, more precise methods of assessing antibodies have been developed. Now the evidence for the immune factor in infertility is quite convincing. Furthermore, in the early 1980s, Mather and her colleagues, utilizing an immunofluorescent cytotoxic method, showed convincing evidence that antibodies to sperm do exist in the cervical mucus of infertile women, and that the titer correlates with the results of the postcoital test and with pregnancy outcome.[9,10]

New approaches to therapy have developed along with these improved methods of diagnosis. However, the information being developed at this time is relatively new and as yet has not been tested with prospective control studies. Consequently, we still must have some reservation as to the true significance of the tests and the meaning of the outcome of the results. One fact that must be kept in mind is that immunity of the sperm is a relative phenomenon and is not an all-or-nothing situation. Some individuals can carry antibodies and still conceive.

Methods of Measuring Antibodies

The current methods of identifying and measuring antibodies have been reviewed by Bronson.[11] One of the current methods commonly used is that of immunobead binding.[12] This method uses commercially available micronsized polyacrylamide spheres to which isotope-specific rabbit antihuman antibodies are linked. This allows one to detect directly immunoglobulins on the surface of human sperm, serum, and cervical mucus. IgG, IgA, and IgM antibodies can be identified.

Antibodies in the Male

Antibodies in the male are caused by disruption of the barrier between sperm cells and the circulation. Trauma, infections, the presence of varicocele, or previous vasectomy can lead to the production of antibodies to sperm in the male. It has also been proposed that there are cases in which immunity to sperm rises spontaneously.[11] Males whose partners have unexplained poor postcoital tests should have their sperm and serum studied for the presence of antibodies. Because agglutination of the sperm in the semen sample is not always present, all cases with a poor postcoital test should be studied. It is important to differentiate between antibodies directed toward the tail and those toward the head.[13] Tail antibodies will more likely interfere with the postcoital test, and with a cervical mucus penetration test, but are treatable. Antibodies distributed to the head will probably interfere with zona pellucida penetration and fertilization; therefore, this problem is less amenable to treatment. The serum in the male is usually not affected or the titer is relatively low.

Antibodies in the Female

Immunity to sperm resides throughout the female reproductive tract: cervix, uterus, and fallopian tubes. The process of the immunologic response is complex and has recently been reviewed by Jones.[14] In simple terms, the tissues lining the reproductive tract have cells sufficiently competent to produce an immune response to the foreign protein of the sperm. The sperm protein need not necessarily pierce the tissue blood barrier so serum antibodies need not always be present. The antibodies of sperm may affect fertility by immobilizing sperm, by causing agglutination that prevents adequate penetration of cervical mucus, by interfering with sperm capacitation, or by directly blocking fertilization.[11] The uterine cervix and its mucus are most accessible to investigation, but the process does go on throughout the female reproductive tract.

Indications for Investigation

When the postcoital test contains less than five motile sperm with normal semen parameters in well-estrogenized cervical mucus and particularly if motile but vibrating and shaking sperm are noted, an immunologic investigation should be carried out. This involves measurement of sperm antibodies in cervical mucus to the sperm of the male, in the male and female serum, and of the sperm itself. A cervical mucus penetration test (see chapter 10) should also be carried out. Bronson has emphasized the qualitative nature of the immune response.[15] When less than 50% of sperm are bound, there is no impairment of mucus penetration. Sperm antibodies are not necessarily present in the serum even though there are potent antibodies in the cervical mucus.[16] An immunologic workup should also be carried out in couples with unexplained infertility.

In the male one need not limit immunologic investigation to the cases in which observation of clumping of sperm in semen analysis was made. Significant antibody reactions can be present without clumping. Furthermore, one might not necessarily see serum antibodies in the male even though significant sperm antibodies are present.[17]

Therapy

Condom therapy was first recommended by Franklin and Dukes.[5] Subsequent reports have not confirmed their encouraging results, and the benefit of this form of therapy remains questionable.

Considering all the confusing information on immune factors, it is not surprising that our experience with Franklin and Dukes' agglutinization method and condom therapy between the years 1970 and 1978 produced no definite conclusions. We selected 172 patients who had persistently poor postcoital tests, despite "normal" semen analysis and "good" cervical mucus. Of these, 63 (36.6%) were found to have positive sperm agglutination tests by the Franklin-Dukes method (Table 17-1). Contrary to the findings in their series, however, 23 of 79 patients (29.1%) with no organic cause for infertility (group A) exhibited agglutination, while 40 of 93 patients (43%) with known organic causes for infertility (group B) demonstrated agglutination. Despite our divergence from the Franklin and Dukes' report, the fact that none of the 15 control group subjects (group C, fertile women with three or more viable pregnancies) had positive sperm agglutination tests strongly suggests the existence of an immunologic factor in the other groups.

Condom therapy has been recommended by Franklin and Dukes.[5] Table 17-2 summarizes the results of such therapy in two groups from my practice. Patients with negative titers were used as controls. Of 23 patients with no organic cause for infertility other than a positive sperm agglutination test who were treated with condom therapy for 6 to 12 months, 12 (52.2%) conceived within 1 year of therapy. On the other hand, only 7 of 40 patients (17.5%) with known organic problems and positive sperm agglutination tests conceived with condom therapy. This difference is statistically significant.

Spontaneous pregnancy rate in the patients with negative agglutination test results served as control, and 35.7% of those without organic problems

Table 17-1. Incidence of Positive Immune Tests

	Total number	Number positive	Percent
Infertile patients	172	63	36.6
Group A Unexplained cause	79	23	29.1
Group B Explained cause	93	40	43
Group C Pregnant controls	15	0	0

(group A) conceived within 1 year. The difference between 52.2% and 35.7%, while highly suggestive, is unfortunately not statistically significant.

This "highly suggestive but not statistically significant" finding characterizes the problem with the immune factor. Other studies have failed to show a significant improvement with condom therapy.[16,17]

Corticosteroid therapy has been utilized based on the concept that such therapy reduces the immune response.[18] Fairly large dosages have been used, 96 mg of prednisolone daily for 7 days is administered beginning on the 21st day of the female partner's cycle. This therapy appears to be most effective for antibodies in the male.[19,20] These larger doses are not without some risks and the patients should be monitored carefully. Lower doses, 16 mg of prednisolone daily for 30 days, have also been used.[16,21] Most studies have failed to show a statistical improvement. Further adequately controlled studies are needed to ascertain the efficacy of this approach to the therapy for male antibodies.

The lower doses have been recommended particularly for the female in the presence of antibodies. Prednisolone, 15 mg/day, for 3 weeks to 6 months has been recommended.[10] However, good results have not always been noted.[22] Part of the discrepancy in results may be due to the inadequacy of immune testing in the past. With the improved methods now available and more rigidly controlled trials, a true, more accurate evaluation of the role of corticosteroids may be available in the future.

If one accepts that the immunologic factor is a relative one, there appears to be a place for artificial insemination in treatment, particularly utilizing the newer approaches to intrauterine insemination. In vitro fertilization has also been shown to be a successful approach to the treatment of the immune factor.[23]

INFECTIONS

Salpingitis and its sequelae are a well-established cause of severe impairment of fertility. Whereas in the past the Neisseria gonococcus was known to be

Table 17-2. Couples Achieving Pregnancy

	Number of patients	Pregnancies[a]
Condom therapy for patients with a positive immune test		
Group A No organic cause	23	12 (52.2%)
Group B Organic problems	40	7 (17.5%)
Patients with initial negative immune test (controls)		
Group A No organic cause	56	20 (35.7%)[b]
Group B Organic problems	53	16 (30%)

[a]Pregnancies 12 months after completion of condom therapy or no therapy in group A controls.
[b]Not statistically significant.

the prime etiologic agent, in the last decade other agents have played an increasing etiologic role: *Chlamydia trachomatis*, possibly T-mycoplasma, and the intrauterine device (IUD).

Gonococcal and Nongonococcal Infections

In the past, most salpingitis was considered to be caused either by the gonococcus or a mixture of aerobic and anaerobic bacteria. Gonococcal infections give the clinical picture of large retort-shaped hydrosalpinges with marked atrophy of the endosalpinx. On the other hand, infections with nongonococcal bacteria are more likely to produce a situation with thickened muscular walls, with less swelling and less damage to the tubal epithelium. Gonococcus is sexually transmitted. Bacterial infections are secondary to the introduction of bacteria into the reproductive tract by instrumentation or subsequent to an induced or even spontaneous abortion. The role of the gynecologist as far as infertility is concerned is early recognition, correct diagnosis of the infectious agent, and prompt, appropriate treatment.[24] It has been reported that if patients are treated within 2 days of the onset of symptoms, none will be subsequently infertile and all will have patent tubes as diagnosed by hysterosalpingography.[25]

Chlamydia

Chlamydia trachomatis has recently become another common sexually transmitted pathogen. Direct culture of chlamydia or increased antibodies have been found in patients with tubal disease in significantly higher number than in controls.[26–28] Infection with chlamydia often appears to give a mild salpingitis that cannot always be recognized clinically, but the degree of damage to the tubes can be extremely severe.[29] For that reason all patients with pelvic infection or who are asymptomatic but with a high risk of pelvic infection, i.e., those having frequent sexual contact and IUD users, should be routinely cultured for chlamydia. On the other hand, there is no evidence that *Chlamydia trachomatis* can cause infertility other than through damage to the fallopian tubes, so the necessity for routine culture of all infertility patients in the face of open fallopian tubes is questionable.

T-Mycoplasma

For many years, mycoplasmas and in particular T-mycoplasma have been isolated frequently in a number of genital disorders: (1) nongonococcal urethritis, (2) spontaneous abortion and stillbirth, (3) vaginitis, and (4) pelvic inflammatory disease. Because of the accompanying high incidence in asymptomatic controls, there is still no conclusive evidence to establish definitely mycoplasma's etiologic role.

In 1972, Gnarpe and Friberg first suggested that infection with T-mycoplasma plays an etiologic role in human infertility.[30] The high frequencies (85% and 95%) of T-strain mycoplasma isolated from their two patient groups, as compared with a control group of fertile females (23%), were statistically significant. It was subsequently reported that 25% of patients with more than 5 years of unexplained infertility conceived within 5 months following treatment with doxycycline, a pregnancy rate that is higher than expected in a group of untreated couples with a similar duration of infertility.[31]

Gnarpe and Friberg's studies have presented suggestive evidence, but their studies as well as those of others have not established definitely the relationship between T-mycoplasma and infertility. Kundsin described a very high pregnancy rate (84% within 1 year) in patients with unexplained infertility, positive T-mycoplasma culture, and treatment with Declomycin®.[32] In 1973, Horne and his co-workers demonstrated a positive correlation between T-mycoplasma and subacute endometritis in 63% of cases.[33] A possible mechanism of interference with fertility was suggested by studies that demonstrated that T-mycoplasma attaches to sperm cells.[34,35] Semen quality appeared diminished in infertile men with positive T-mycoplasma cultures, as compared with those with negative cultures.[36] Yet, no reports have confirmed the highly suggestive but statistically inconclusive studies of Gnarpe and Friberg.

It may be hazardous to bestow etiologic properties on T-mycoplasma because it occurs in a higher percentage in one small group of infertile women than in one small group of controls. In other studies, Adler found a 50% infection rate in infertile women,[37] and Dunlop found 37 T-mycoplasma cultures in 39 sexually active women with unspecified infertility.[38]

The etiologic role of T-mycoplasma in infertility has been challenged in studies by DeLouvois who found no significant differences in the occurrences of T-mycoplasma in infertile or fertile couples. No increase in conception rate was demonstrated after treatment with doxycycline.[39] Matthews, in an attempt to study the frequency of T-mycoplasma infection, isolated T-mycoplasma from 66% of fertile women as compared with 52% of infertile patients.[40] Schowb could not demonstrate any differences in prevalence of T-mycoplasma in seminal fluid with normal cytology compared with abnormal cytology.[41]

A Personal Study

We studied 161 infertility patients over a period of 3 years from January 1974 to January 1977. At the time of the initial postcoital test, an endocervical culture for T-mycoplasma was taken by using a sterile dry cotton swab to collect endocervical secretions. Specimens were cultured in a cell-free agar medium (Hayflick's medium without thallium acetate, which inhibits T-mycoplasma growth).[42] Inoculation was done under anaerobic conditions. Broth media containing urea and phenol were also used for detecting any pH changes caused by urease-positive T-mycoplasma.[43] Dienes stain, which stained mycoplasma blue, was used. Because of urease property, however, the T colonies appeared brown; thus two types of mycoplasma were easily demonstrable.

Incidence of T-mycoplasma Infection. The incidence of positive cultures for T-mycoplasma in infertility patients is shown in Table 17-3. As in previous studies, the 55% incidence of T-mycoplasma infections in cases of unexplained infertility was higher than the 41% incidence in explained infertility, but not statistically significant even in this large series. The control group, C, made up of pregnant women and women of known fertility seen in a family planning clinic and a private gynecologic office, showed an infection rate of 33%, significantly lower than group B (unexplained infertility) patients.

Results of Treatment. T-mycoplasma infection responds to double-dose tetracycline therapy in about 90% of cases. Both the man and woman should be treated with 500 mg four times a day for 10 days. About 10% of these patients are resistant to tetracycline and require doxycycline, clindamycin, or minocycline, which have more gastrointestinal side effects. The true indication of the effectiveness of therapy is the pregnancy rate. Seventeen of our 54 patients who developed a negative culture after appropriate antibiotics became pregnant within 6 months (Table 17-4, groups A and B). Group A comprises patients with other known causes for their infertility. Group B includes couples in whom the only finding was that of a positive culture for T-mycoplasma. In Group B, 42% of the patients with unexplained infertility conceived within 6 months, as opposed to 23% with other infertility factors in group A; this result is suggestive but not conclusive.

The records of 67 patients seen in the 3 years of the study whose infertility was unexplained and who had negative mycoplasma cultures (group D) were analyzed for control purposes. Without any treatment whatsoever, 25% of these

Table 17-3. Incidence of Positive Cultures for T-Mycoplasma

Group	Total	Number positive	Percent
A Explained infertility	121	50	41
B Unexplained infertility	40	22	55
C Controls[a]	67	22	33

[a]Difference between groups B and C statistically significant to .03.

Table 17-4. Six-Month Conception Rates after
Successful Treatment of T-Mycoplasma Infection

Group	Total number	Conception	Percent
A Explained infertility	30	7	23
B Unexplained infertility	24	10	42
D Unexplained infertility (negative culture)a	67	17	25

aDifference between groups B and D not statistically significant.

patients conceived within 6 months. The difference between pregnancy rates in group B and group C is not statistically significant.

The etiologic role of T-mycoplasma in infertility still remains an enigma. Until now no well-controlled studies have successfully demonstrated such a role. Our own studies and those of others failed to show a statistically significant relationship when controls are used.[44-46] Since the therapy is relatively innocuous in patients with persistent or unexplained infertility, the physician should proceed with the culture and carry out antibiotic treatment where indicated. Routine antibiotic treatment for all patients with unexplained infertility is not yet justified as there is no equivocal proof of a relationship between T-mycoplasma and infertility.

IUD

If a patient gives a history of having worn an IUD, the physician should be more alert for the possibility of a low-grade pelvic infection with resultant tubal damage. IUDs increase the chances of infection in a number of ways. First, the introduction of the IUD can introduce pathogenic bacteria. However, the more likely situation is that the foreign body effect of the IUD alters the host defensive mechanisms against infection at any time that the IUD is in place. This is more likely to occur with a large tight-fitting IUD such as the Dalkon Shield® that compresses the endometrium. A third avenue of infection is the IUD string, which allows bacteria to ascend into the uterus.

REFERENCES

1. Landsteiner K: Zur kenntnis der spezifisch auf blutorperchen wirkenden sera. *Zentralbl Bakteriol* 25:546, 1899
2. Metchnikoff S: Etudes sur la resorption des cellules. *Ann Inst Pasteur Lille*, 13:737, 1899
3. Behrman SJ: The immune response and infertility. In Behrman SJ, Kistner RW, Patton GW Jr (eds): *Progress in Infertility*, 2nd ed. Boston, Little, Brown, 1975, pp 793–815
4. Wilson L: Sperm agglutinins in human semen and blood. *Proc Soc Exp Biol Med* 85:652, 1954
5. Franklin RR, Dukes CI: Antispermatozoal antibody and unexplained infertility. *Am J Obstet Gynecol* 89:6, 1964

6. Tyler A, Tyler ET, Denny PC: Concepts and experiments in immunoreproduction. *Fertil Steril* 18:153, 1967
7. Shulman S, Jackson H, Stone ML: Antibodies to spermatozoa: VI. Comparative studies of sperm agglutinating activity in groups of infertile and fertile women. *Am J Obstet Gynecol* 123:139, 1975
8. Ansbacher R: Sperm antibodies and infertility. *Fertil Steril* 36:446, 1981
9. Mathur S, Williamson HO, Baker ME, et al: Sperm motility on postcoital testing correlates with male autoimmunity to sperm. *Fertil Steril* 41:81, 1984
10. Mathur S, Baker ER, Williamson HO, Derrick FC, Teague KS, Fudenberg HH: Clinical significance of sperm antibodies in infertility. *Fertil Steril* 33:239, 1980
11. Bronson R, Cooper G, Rosenfeld D: Sperm antibodies and their role in infertility. *Fertil Steril* 42:171, 1984
12. Mandelbaum S, Diamond M, DeCherney A: Relationship of antisperm antibodies to oocyte fertilization in in vitro fertilization and embryo transfer. *Fertil Steril* 47:644, 1987
13. Bronson RA, Cooper GW, Rosenfeld DC: Sperm-specific antibodies and autoantibodies inhibit the bonding of human sperm to the human zona pellucida. *Fertil Steril* 38:724, 1982
14. Jones WJ: Immunology and infertility. In Behrman SJ, Kistner RW, Patton GW Jr (eds): *Progress in Infertility*, 3rd ed. Boston, Little, Brown, 1988, p 751
15. Bronson RA, Cooper GW, Rosenfeld DC: Autoimmunity to spermatozoa: Effect in sperm penetration of cervical mucus as reflected by post-coital testing. *Fertil Steril* 41:609, 1984
16. Sudo N, Shulman S, Stone ML: Sperm agglutination phenomenon in cervical mucus in vitro: A possible cause of infertility. *Am J Obstet Gynecol* 129:360, 1977
17. Schumacher GFB: Immunologic factors in infertility: Antibodies against spermatozoa. *J Reprod Med* 23:272, 1979
18. Shreiber AD: Clinical immunology of corticosteroid. *Prog Clin Immunol* 3:103, 1977
19. Shulman JF, Shulman S: Methylprednisone treatment of immunologic infertility in the male. *Fertil Steril* 38:591, 1982
20. Hendry WF, Stedronska J, Parslow J, Hughes L: The results of intermittent high dose steroid therapy for male infertility due to antisperm antibodies. *Fertil Steril* 36:351, 1981
21. Hendry WF, Trechuba K, Hughes L, et al: Cyclic prednisolone therapy for male infertility associated with autoantibodies to spermatozoa. *Fertil Steril* 45:249, 1986
22. Smarr SC, Wing L, Hammond MG: Effect of therapy on infertile couples with antisperm antibodies. *Am J Obstet Gynecol* 158:969, 1988
23. Ackerman SB, Graff D, Van Clem J, Swanson RJ, Veeck LL, Acosta AA, Garcia JE: Immunologic infertility and in vitro fertilization. *Fertil Steril* 42:474, 1984
24. Sweet RC: Pelvic infections in infertility. In Behrman SJ, Kistner RW, Patton GW Jr (eds): *Progress in Infertility*, 3rd ed. Boston, Little, Brown, 1988, p 37
25. Viberg L: Acute inflammatory conditions of the uterus adnexa. *Acta Obstet Gynecol Scand* 43(Suppl 4):5, 1964
26. Kane JL, Woodland RM, Forsey T, Darougay, Elder MG: Evidence of chlamydial infection on infertile women and without fallopian tube obstruction. *Fertil Steril* 42:843, 1984
27. Moss TR, Hawkswell J: Evidence of infection with *Chlamydia trachomatis* in patients with pelvic inflammatory disease: Value of partner investigation. *Fertil Steril* 41:429, 1986
28. Hartford SL, Silva PS, diZerega GS, Yanekura ML: Serologic evidence of prior chlamydial infection in patients with tubal ectopic pregnancy and contralateral tubal disease. *Fertil Steril* 47:118, 1987
29. Svenson L, Westrom L, Ripa K, et al: Differences in some clinical and laboratory parameters in acute salpingitis related to culture and serologic findings. *Am J Obstet Gynecol* 138:1017, 1980
30. Gnarpe H, Friberg J: Mycoplasma and human reproductive failure: I. The occurrence of different mycoplasmas in couples with reproductive failure. *Obstet Gynecol* 114:727, 1972

31. Friberg J, Gnarpe H: Mycoplasma and human reproductive failure: III. Pregnancies in "infertile" couples treated with doxycyline for T-mycoplasma. *Am J Obstet Gynecol* 116:23, 1973

32. Kundsin RB: Mycoplasma infections of the female genital tract. In Taymor ML, Green TH (eds): *Progress in Gynecology*. New York, Grune and Stratton, 1976, p 291

33. Horne HW, Hertig AT, Kundsin RB, Kosasa TS: Subclinical endometrial inflammation and T-mycoplasma. *Int J Fertil* 18:226, 1973

34. Gnarpe H: T-mycoplasma on spermatozoa and infertility. *Nature* 245:97, 1973

35. Fowlkes DM, Dooher GB, O'Leary WM: T-mycoplasma and human infertility. Correlation of infection with alternatives in seminal parameters. *Fertil Steril* 26:1212, 1975

36. Fowlkes DM, Macleod J, O'Leary WM: Evidence by scanning electron microscopy for an association between spermatozoa and T-mycoplasmas in men of infertile marriage. *Fertil Steril* 26:1203, 1975

37. Adler HE: Mycoplasmosis in animals. *Adv Vet Sci Comp Med* 10:205, 1965

38. Dunlop EMC, Hare MJ, Jones BR, Robinson DT: Mycoplasmas and non-specific genital infection: II. Clinical aspects. *Br J Vener Dis* 45:274, 1969

39. DeLouvois J, Stanley VC, Leak BG: Ecological studies of the microbial flora of the female generative tract. *Proc Soc Med* 68:269, 1975

40. Matthews CD, Elmslie AR, Clapp, KH, Svigos JJ: Frequency of genital mycoplasma infection in human fertility. *Fertil Steril* 26:988, 1975

41. Schowb BC, Jacobs YR, Hylen E, Freedman R: The role of mycoplasma in human infertility. *S Am Med J* 50:445–447, 1976

42. Hayflick L: Tissue cultures and mycoplasmas. *Tex Rep Biol Med* 23 (Suppl 1): 285, 1965

43. Shepard MC, Luneford CD: Differential agar medium for identification of T-mycoplasma in primary cultures. *Bacteriol Proc* 83, 1970

44. Idriss WM, Patton WC, Taymor ML: On the etiologic role of *Ureaplasma urealyticum* (T-mycoplasma) infection in infertility. *Fertil Steril* 30:293, 1978

45. Nagata Y, Iwasaka T, Wada T: Mycoplasma infection and infertility. *Fertil Steril* 31:392, 1979

46. Robinson TD: Evaluation of role of *Ureaplasma urealyticum* in the female genital tract. *Pediatr Infect Dis J* 5:S262, 1986

CHAPTER 18

Uterine Factors

Problems with the uterus itself are not a common cause of infertility. However, since the cause still remains unknown in many cases and since new methods are being made available for both physiologic and endoscopic evaluation of the uterus, the physician should not rule out the uterine factor, at least in those cases that fail to resolve themselves with routine techniques. Two excellent reviews, by Wallach and Patton, have been published.[1,2]

EVALUATION OF THE UTERINE FACTOR

Hysterosalpingography and hysteroscopy are the diagnostic aids for evaluation of a uterine factor in infertility.

Hysterosalpingography, when used as a routine step in workup of the infertile couple, usually provides the first inkling that a uterine problem is present. The injection of dye into the uterine cavity will demonstrate abnormalities of the uterus caused by congenital anomalies, tumors, polyps, medications such as diethylstilbestrol (DES), and adhesions. Hysteroscopy is used to confirm the diagnosis and to distinguish between certain filling defects not clearly identified by a hysterosalpingogram such as endometrial polyps or small submucous fibroids. Hysteroscopy will occasionally pick up small lesions not seen on a hysterosalpingogram. The additional value of hysteroscopy is that at the same time that the diagnosis is made, appropriate treatment can be carried out, such as removal of polyps, small fibroids, adhesions, or a uterine septum.

CONGENITAL ANOMALIES

Many of the serious maldevelopments of the uterus manifest themselves at the onset of menses. These are conditions where there is an obstruction to the outflow of menstrual blood from a horn of the uterus that does not connect with the vagina. The resultant hematometra and hematosalpinx, unless discovered early, can cause destruction of sensitive epithelial linings or can end in surgery, both with permanent damage to reproductive potential.

More commonly, however, the uterine abnormalities are nonobstructive and are discovered incident to normal delivery, cesarean section, or a problem in reproduction. The more common maldevelopments are illustrated in Fig. 18-1. The majority of women with these abnormalities have a normal reproductive history; if there is a problem, it is usually that of repeated abortion. The incidence of abortion associated with uterine abnormalities has been reported to be between 25% and 53%.[3]

The deformities most likely to cause problems are the septate and bicornuate uteri. It is perhaps paradoxical that the most minor degree of reduplication, i.e., the septate uterus, is accompanied by more difficulties than the more complete reduplications. Because more than 50% of women with uterine anomalies have no difficulties, it is important to rule out all other causes of infertility or repeated abortion before undertaking surgical correction. One cannot make a valid case for the surgical treatment of uterine abnormalities when there is a primary failure of conception, but sporadic cases have been reported with apparent success.

Treatment

The surgical treatment of congenital anomalies of the uterus has been reviewed and described in detail by Jones and Baramki,[3] and by Kistner and Patton.[4] At present there are three main transabdominal surgical approaches; they are described by Strassman,[5] Jones,[6] and Tompkins.[7]

The Strassman technique is to enter each cavity of the bicornuate uterus from the medial aspect and restructure the walls to make a single cavity. This is the best approach for a true bicornuate uterus.

However, the Tomkins procedure is considered by most to be the procedure of choice for the septate uterus. The septate uterus is incised in the midline down through the septum. The septum is opened into each cavity throughout its length, and the two halves are reunited. The objective in both the Strassman and Tompkins procedures is to divide the septum and not remove any uterine tissue. The results, in terms of live births following habitual abortion, are excellent for both procedures.[8,9]

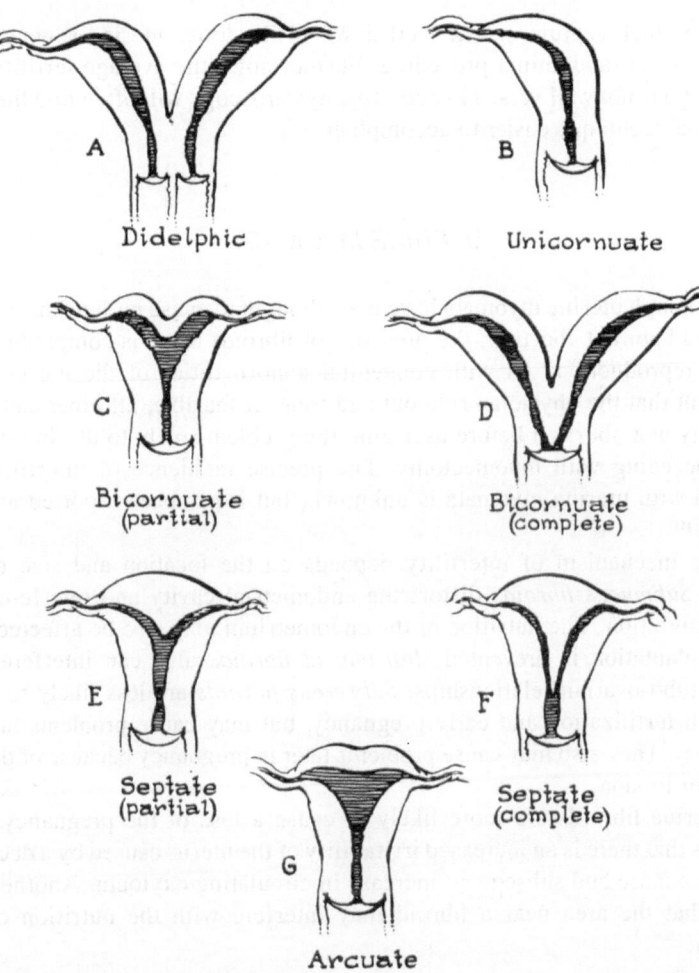

Figure 18-1. Common congenital anomalies of the uterus (from Jones HW: *Progress in Infertility,* 2nd ed. Boston, Little, Brown, 1975).

In the last 7 or 8 years there have been an increasing number of reports on utilization of the hysteroscopic approach for dividing uterine septa, but only in the last few years have large enough series been reported to indicate that this is a feasible therapy for such septa. Uterocautery with a cystoscopic resectoscope or an operating scissors (Daley) can be used. Little bleeding is reported by either method. Success rates are comparable to the Tomkins procedure.

However, not all septa are amenable to this approach, only about two-thirds. A thick septum or one well down in the lower uterine segment still requires a transabdominal procedure. Furthermore, the average fertility specialist who is not well versed in operative hysteroscopy will often find the open abdominal technique easier to accomplish.

UTERINE MYOMATA

Although uterine myomata have been thought to cause both primary infertility and habitual abortion, the presence of fibroids often is compatible with normal reproduction. As with congenital abnormalities of the uterus, it is important that the physician rule out and treat, if feasible, all other causes of infertility and abortion before ascribing the problem solely to uterine tumors and proceeding with myomectomy. The precise incidence of infertility associated with uterine myomata is unknown, but it has been reported as high as 40%.[10]

The mechanism of infertility depends on the location and size of the fibroid. *Submucus fibroids* distort the endometrial cavity and interfere with sperm migration. The nutrition of the endometrium may also be affected, and thus implantation is prevented. *Intramural fibroids* also can interfere with normal tubo-ovarian relationships. *Subserous fibroids* are less likely to interfere with fertilization and early pregnancy, but may cause problems later in pregnancy. They also may cause problems later in pregnancy because of degeneration or torsion.

Uterine fibroids are more likely to cause a loss of the pregnancy. One theory is that there is an increased irritability of the uterus caused by a decrease in oxcytoxinase and subsequent increase in circulating oxytocin. Another theory is that the area near a fibroid may interfere with the nutrition of the placenta.

Diagnosis of Fibroids and Evaluation for Therapy

History, pelvic examination, hysterosalpingogram, hysteroscopy, laparoscopy, and ultrasonography are all aids in the diagnosis and evaluation of uterine fibroids. However, most patients with fibroids seeking help for infertility are asymptomatic. An irregularly enlarged uterus may be the first inkling of a problem, or the fibroids may first show up on a hysterosalpingogram performed to assess tubal patency (Fig. 18-2) or at routine diagnostic laparoscopy. The presence of significant distortion of, or of filling defects into, the uterine cavity in the presence of repeated abortion or even infertility with other cause, dictates surgical removal of the tumors. On the other hand, small filling

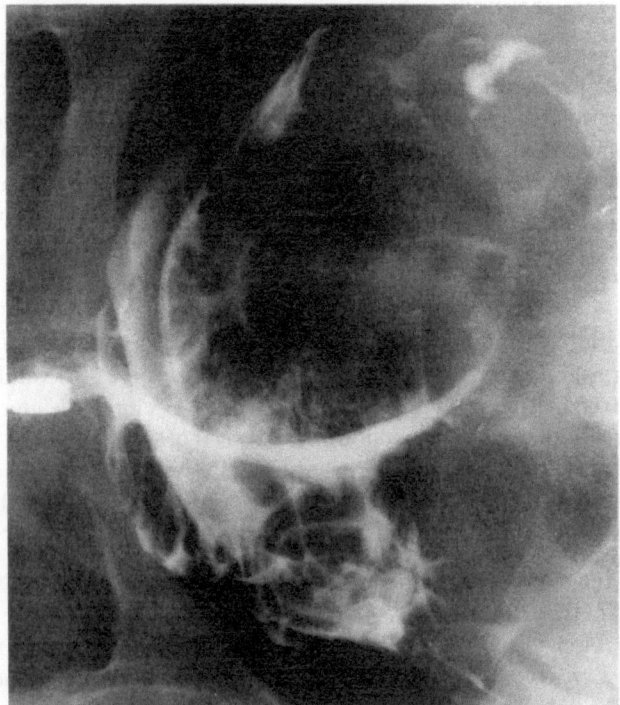

Figure 18-2. Large submucosal fibroid compressing and distorting endometrial cavity. Patient conceived 6 months after myomectomy and delivered a full-term infant by cesarean section.

defects can be further evaluated at hysteroscopy, and appropriate therapy can be carried out at that time. A small polyp or small pedunculated fibroid can be easily removed at hysteroscopy, but even a small sessile fibroid can be quite difficult to remove and requires an experienced hysteroscopist to remove it without damage to the uterus. It is sometimes more prudent to observe such a small fibroid and follow it by a later hysterosalpingogram.

Intramural and subserous fibroids, which are less likely to cause problems, can be followed by serial ultrasound. Significant growth can be the indication for treatment. Such fibroids should be removed primarily only if larger than 5 cm, or if situated in an area where there may be tubal obstruction or distortion of tubal ovarian relationships. Once again, all other causes of infertility should be ruled out and treated. The fibroid tumor greater than 5 cm in diameter should be removed because of the danger of rapid growth and degeneration during pregnancy that could result in pregnancy loss. The smaller fibroids can be followed with accuracy by means of ultrasound. Surgery is not necessarily indicated.

Indications for Treatment

A complete infertility workup should be carried out prior to the recommendation of operative removal of the fibroid. Unless the fibroids are obviously interfering with fertility, or size alone indicates early removal, or if the fibroids are asymptomatic, other factors should be corrected first, and a trial at conception allowed. Even then, surgery should not be carried out solely for an asymptomatic fibroid that is positioned so that it does not contribute to the infertility.

Treatment

The operative principles of myomectomy were described by Bonney more than 25 years ago,[11] and many of his recommendations are still valid.

Hemostasis, utilizing a tourniquet or clamp that occludes the uterine arteries at the level of the cervix, is vital for the removal of large myomata. Bulldog clamps on the infundibulopelvic ligaments are also helpful, but are not always necessary. I have found four principles important in reducing the chances of adhesion formation that would then compromise future fertility:

1. The incision should be planned to remove a number of fibroids through one incision.
2. For removal of a posterior fibroid, particularly one that is relatively large, the incision should be transverse and high in the fundus (Fig. 18-3). Adhesions of bowel or of the adnexa to the scar of a posterior vertical incision can compromise fertility. This would not be a problem with an anterior incision that can be vertical or transverse as the position of the fibroid dictates.
3. To remove a large intramural fibroid that is close to the endometrium, the tumor itself can be bivalved after being 75% dissected free (Fig. 18-4). The bivalving is carried down to the very bottom of the tumor; the lower border of each half is grasped with an Allis clamp and carefully dissected off the submucosa of the endometrium.
4. The myometrium should be approximated with one or two layers of absorbable sutures to obliterate dead space. However, the serosa should be closed with fine suture material, either nonreactive absorbable or nonabsorbable. Microsurgical techniques should be used throughout in handling the peritoneal surfaces.

Results

Ingersoll, in 1970, reported a 50% conception rate in his series of myomectomies associated with infertility.[12] Ten percent of the patients required subsequent hysterectomy. Later reports have shown similar results. Babaknia,

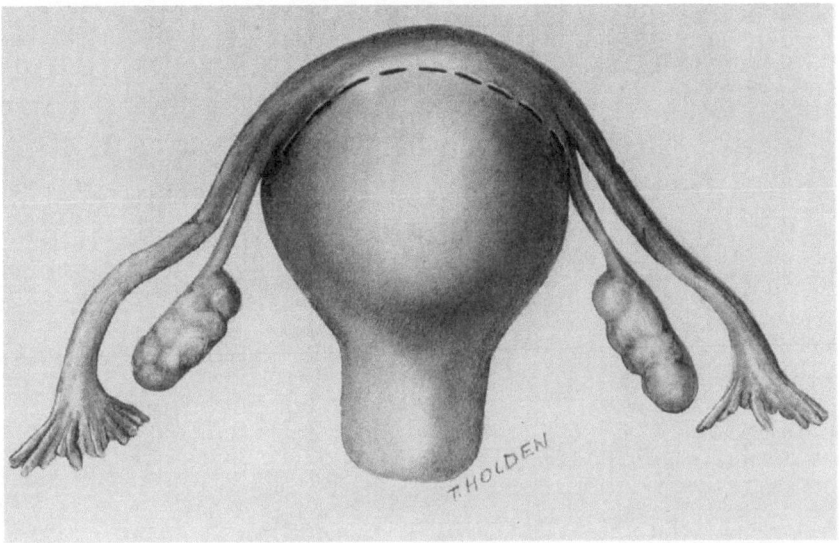

Figure 18-3. Cervical incision near top of uterus for removal of large posterior wall fibroids.

in 1978, reported a 54% conception rate with a 42% term delivery rate.[13] In 1981, Buttram and Reiter reported a 40% to 50% pregnancy rate. In 1984, Garcia and Tureck reported a 53% pregnancy rate for submucus fibroids[15] and in 1986, Rosenfeld reported a 67% pregnancy rate in otherwise unexplained infertility.[16]

Recently, attempts have been made to shrink fibroid tumors with analogues of gonadotropin-releasing hormones.[17] Shrinkage does occur but prompt regrowth also occurs after the medication is discontinued. At the present time, the therapy seems to have its greatest benefit in shrinking tumors before surgery and thus making the procedure less hazardous.

UTERINE SYNECHIAE (ASHERMAN'S SYNDROME)

A rare cause of secondary infertility, but one that appears to be increasing, is partial or complete obliteration of the endometrial cavity by adhesions between the opposing walls; it is known by the eponym, Asherman's syndrome.[18] Since the majority of cases occur when there is an infection during dilation and curettage (D&C) in the postabortal and postpartum period, the majority of patients have, in the past, proven their reproductive capacity. In a smaller percentage of women, the curettage is not associated with pregnancy. When the abortion occurs in the first pregnancy, then the complaint is infertility.

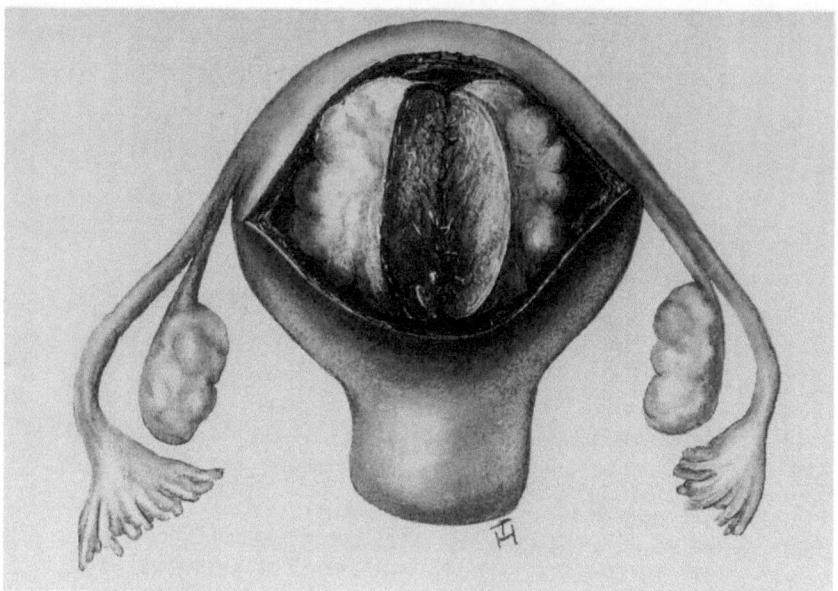

Figure 18-4. Incision through fibroid to expedite removal of a tumor close to the endometrium.

The increasing numbers of therapeutic abortions, as well as the availability of better diagnostic techniques, have caused an apparent, if not real, increase in the incidence of Asherman's syndrome. The presenting complaint in most cases, is secondary amenorrhea or severe oligomenorrhea. Infertility is often only an incidental finding. There are some instances where only minor degrees of endometrial adhesions exist. These adhesions may not cause oligomenorrhea, but can result in infertility or repeated abortion.

In amenorrhea, the diagnosis of Asherman's syndrome is strongly supported by an endocrine workup that demonstrates normal pituitary–gonadal function, along with failure to have withdrawal bleeding after the cyclic administration of estrogen and progestogen. The diagnosis is confirmed by hysteroscopy (Fig. 18-5).[19] In lesser degrees of menstrual disturbance, the diagnosis is often unsuspected and is only discovered by the clinician at routine hysterosalpingography. Hysteroscopy confirms the presence of known adhesions and will often uncover unsuspected adhesions.[20]

Treatment

The extent of the disease influences the approach and the results of treatment, but all treatments are directed toward reestablishing and maintaining the

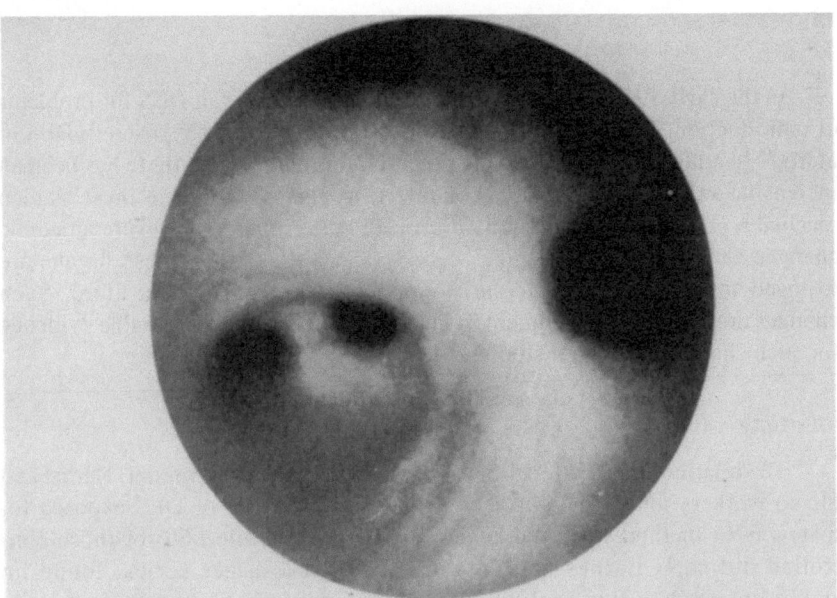

Figure 18-5. A view of intrauterine adhesions via the hysteroscope (from Neuwirth RS: *Hysteroscopy*. Philadelphia, WB Saunders, 1975).

endometrial cavity, and toward stimulation of the regeneration of the endometrial lining. In very severe cases, it may be necessary to carry out hysterotomy along with cervical D&C to identify safely the uterine cavity.[21] In less severe cases, D&C from below should suffice.

Hysteroscopy provides a more thorough approach to the dividing of adhesions than that provided by a uterine curette. The adhesions can be seen directly and divided with a scissors. Usually no coagulation is required. More recently, a report of a series utilizing hysteroscopy described a 93% pregnancy rate with mild adhesions, 78.3% with moderate, and 57.4% with severe. The term pregnancy rates for mild and severe adhesions were 81.3% and 31.9%, respectively.[22]

Some methods must be used to keep the endometrial walls apart while healing. Wallach recommends a Foley catheter,[1] and others recommend an intrauterine device for this purpose.[23] Estrogen treatment, with or without progestin, is given for one or two cycles to promote healing of the endometrium.[24] A recommended dosage is 2.5 mg of conjugated estrogen twice daily for 26 days with 10 mg of medroxyprogesterone acetate during the last 6 days. Klein and Garcia in a 1973 review have reported on a carefully treated group of women with Asherman's syndrome with a 56% pregnancy rate.[19]

DIETHYLSTILBESTROL

In the early 1950s a large number of women were given DES for problems of reproduction. It is estimated that 2 million females were exposed to DES in utero.[25] In addition to an increasing potential for malignancy, there has been an increasing awareness of an impact on infertility that was noted as these women reached reproductive age in the 1970s and 1980s. Apparently, severe anatomic changes can occur in the vagina, cervix, and uterus when these organs are exposed to estrogens, particularly nonsteroidal estrogens, in utero. Such changes are difficult to document in humans but there is considerable evidence for such changes in animal studies.[26]

Infertility

The relationship of infertility to DES exposure is controversial. Herbst and his co-workers found a slight decrease in the infertility of DES-exposed females; 67% of those exposed achieved pregnancy while 86% of those controlled did so.[27] Barnes and co-workers, with a larger series, found no significant increase in infertility following DES exposure.[28] At the present state of knowledge, if the physical findings or hysterosalpingogram demonstrates changes characteristic of DES exposure, and infertility persists without other causes, it is reasonable to assign the cause to DES exposure. It is of interest that in a small series treated with in vitro fertilization, the pregnancy outcome for DES exposed-females was comparable to the nonexposed larger control group.

Pregnancy Loss

On the other hand, there is clear evidence that DES exposure leads to an increased incidence of early spontaneous abortion. Overall, there appears to be a doubling of the abortion rate in DES-exposed women.[29] The increased pregnancy loss seems to be related to the classic T-shaped uterus that may be found in association with DES exposure (Fig. 18-6). It must be emphasized that not all patients exposed to DES have a T-shaped uterus and that the degree of deformity can range from very slight to extreme. The degree of deformity from mild to severe appears to correlate with the chances of pregnancy loss.

There also appears to be increased evidence of cervical competence associated with DES exposure. Cerclage has been recommended for these patients.[30]

OTHER LESIONS

Bacterial invasion rarely causes permanent damage to the uterus but it

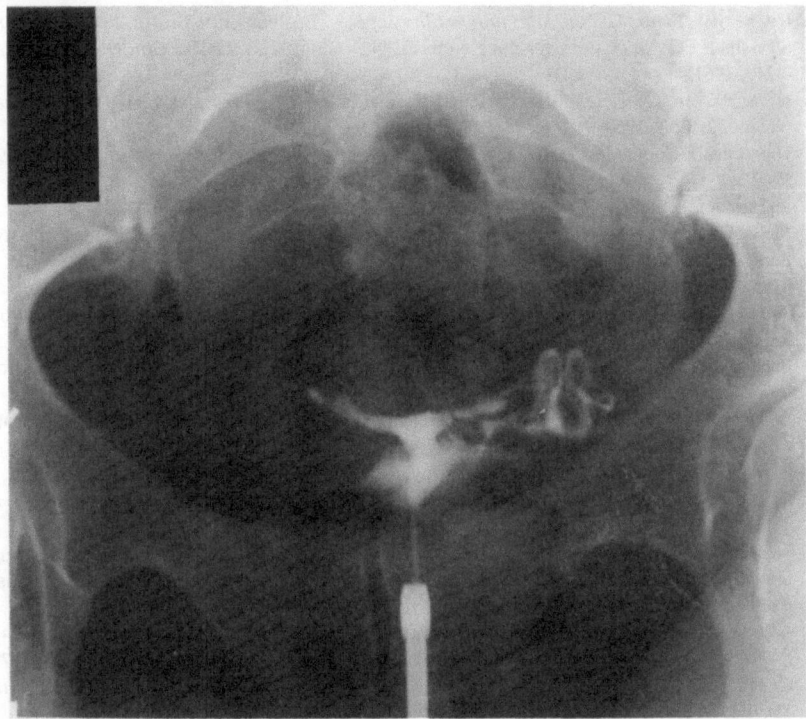

Figure 18-6. T-shaped or staghorn uterus associated with repeated abortion. The patient had four spontaneous first-trimester abortions and one tubular pregnancy. On her fifth pregnancy a cerclage was performed. She went to term.

can occur incident to surgical invasion by D & C, conization, and, more recently and significantly, by the intrauterine device.

Tuberculous endometritis is less common in the United States. Since the use of antibiotics, the reported incidence is 0.2% here and between 5% and 8% in foreign areas. The suspected diagnosis is usually made by the pathologist incident to routine endometrial biopsy; bacteriologic methods are than required to confirm the diagnosis.

REFERENCES

1. Wallach E: The uterine factor in infertility. *Fertil Seril* 23:138, 1972
2. Patton GW Jr: The uterus in infertility evaluation. In Behram SJ, Kistner RW, Patton GW Jr(eds): *Progress in Infertility*, 3rd ed., Boston, Little, Brown, 1988, p 197
3. Jones HW, Baramki TA: Congenital anomalies. In Behrman SJ and Kistner RW (eds): *Progress in Infertility*, 1st ed. Boston, Little, Brown, 1968

4. Kistner RW, Patton GW Jr: *Atlas of Infertility Surgery.* Boston, Little Brown, 1975, pp 65–93
5. Strassman EO: Operations for double uterus and endometrial atresia. *Clin Obstet Gynecol* 4:210, 1961
6. Jones HW Jr: Operations for congenital anomalies of the uterus and vagina. *Clin Obstet Gynecol* 2:1053, 1959
7. Tompkins P: Comments on the bicornuate uterus and twinning. *Surg Clin North Am* 42:1049, 1962
8. Strassmann E: Fertility and unification of double uterus. *Fertil Steril* 17:165, 1966
9. McShane PM, Reilly RS, Schiff I: Pregnancy outcomes following Tompkins metroplasty. *Fertil Steril* 40:190, 1983
10. Rubin IC: Uterine fibromyomas and sterility. *Clin Obstet Gynecol* 1:501, 1958
11. Bonney V: Abdominal myomectomy. In: *Gynecologic Surgery.* London, Cassell, p. 328, 1963
12. Ingersoll FM: Fertility following myomectomy. *Fertil Steril* 14:596, 1963
13. Babaknia A, Rock JA, Jones HW: Pregnancy success following abdominal myomectomy for infertility. *Fertil Steril* 30:644, 1978
14. Buttram VC, Reiter RC: Uterine leiomyomata: Etiology, symptomology and management. *Fertil Steril* 36:433, 1981
15. Garcia CR, Tureck RW: Submucosal leiomyomata and infertility. *Fertil Steril* 42:16, 1984
16. Rosenfeld DL: Abdominal myomectomy for otherwise unexplained infertility. *Fertil Steril* 46:328, 1986
17. West CP, Lumsden WA, Lawson S, Williamson J, Baird DT: Shrinkage of uterine fibroid during therapy with goselerin (Zoladex): A leutinizing hormone-releasing hormone agonist administered as a monthly subcutaneous depot. *Fertil Steril* 48:45, 1987
18. Asherman JG: Amenorrhea traumatica (atretica). *J Obstet Gynecol Br Commonw* 55:23, 1948
19. Klein S, Garcia CR: Asherman's syndrome: A critique and review. *Fertil Steril* 24:905, 1973
20. Cohen MR, Dmowshi WP: Modern hysteroscopy: Diagnostic therapeutic potential. *Fertil Steril* 24:905, 1973
21. Bergman P: Traumatic intrauterine lesions. *Acta Obstet Gynecol Scand* 40 (Suppl 4):1, 1961
22. Valle RF, Sciarra JS: Intrauterine adhesions: Hysteroscopic diagnosis classification, treatment and reproductive outcome. *Am J Obstet Gynecol* 158:1459, 1988
23. Louros NC, Danezis JM, Pontifix G: Use of intrauterine devices in the treatment of intrauterine adhesions. *Fertil Steril* 19:509, 1968
24. Wood J, Pena G: Treatment of traumatic uterine synechiae. *Int J Fertil* 9:405, 1964
25. Glebatis DM, Janerich DT: A statewide approach to diethylstilbestrol—the New York Program. *N Engl J Med* 304:47, 1981
26. DeCherney AH, Naftolin F: Diethylstilbestrol effect in fertility. In Behrman SJ, Kistner RW, Patton GW Jr (eds): *Progress in Infertility*, 3rd ed. Boston, Little, Brown, 1988, p 227
27. Herbst AL, Hubby MM, Blough RR, Azizi FA: A comparison of pregnancy experience in DES-exposed and DES-unexposed daughters. *J Reprod Med* 24:62, 1980
28. Barnes A, Colton T, Gunderson J, et al: Fertility and outcome of pregnancy in women exposed in utero to diethylstilbestrol. *N Engl J Med* 303:281, 1980
29. Muasher ST, Garcia JE, Jones HW Jr: Experience with diethylstilbestrol-exposed infertile women in a program of in-vitro fertilization. *Fertil Steril* 42:20, 1984
30. Goldstein DP: Incompetent cervix in offspring exposed to diethylstilbestrol in utero. *Obstet Gynecol* 52:738, 1978

CHAPTER 19

Amenorrhea and Anovulation

When the temperature chart and biopsy show a lack of ovulation, more intensive investigation must be carried out to identify the cause, so that appropriate therapy might be instituted.

ETIOLOGY

Anovulation may result in either amenorrhea or anovulatory cycles. These two variables have a common etiologic background: amenorrhea often is a more advanced stage of anovulation. In amenorrhea, not only is follicle rupture inhibited, but ovarian secretion of estrogen is diminished to where insufficient stimulation of the endometrium never results in bleeding associated with episodic endometrial breakdown. With anovulatory cycles, on the other hand, although follicle rupture and corpus luteum function are inhibited, there still is sufficient ovarian stimulation and estrogen secretion to result in irregular proliferation and breakdown of the endometrium. This results in either grossly irregular uterine bleeding or periodic bleeding in cycles of short duration.

Both amenorrhea and anovulatory bleeding should be considered symptoms of an underlying endocrine imbalance. A normal hypothalamic–pituitary–ovarian–uterine axis must be intact and functioning to result in rhythmic ovarian stimulation, ovulation, and menstruation. Amenorrhea, itself, may result from a number of factors interfering with this process. These include genetic causes, nutritional deficiencies, emotional disturbances, systemic disease, and disturbances of the ovary, pituitary, thyroid, or adrenal glands. Deficiencies, or inhibiting influences arising in any of these area, can block the necessary flow of nervous stimuli or hormones and bring about amenorrhea. The specific disease entities and the basic anatomic areas wherein they might exert their influence are outlined in Fig. 19-1. These areas are not always known and might not always be understood clearly; for example, the mechanism by which obesity brings about amenorrhea remains explained. Nor is it clear whether masculinizing tumors of the ovary or the adrenals, as well as functional adrenal overactivity, produce amenorrhea by inhibition of the hypothalamus and pituitary gland function by a direct effect upon the ovary, or by a combination of all of these. Nevertheless, an attempt to classify amenorrhea helps clinicians understand the problem better as they begin their diagnostic approach.

Anovulatory cycles indicate the presence of functioning endometrium, so the search for causes of anovulation lies in the hypothalamus, pituitary, or ovary, with the same possible factors, genetic, nutritional, emotional, as described for amenorrhea. Anovulatory cycles usually represent a lesser degree of interference with these normal pathways than does amenorrhea.

DIAGNOSIS IN AMENORRHEA

Besides indicating a logical approach to therapy, an accurate diagnosis of the cause of amenorrhea is imperative to rule out the presence of a serious

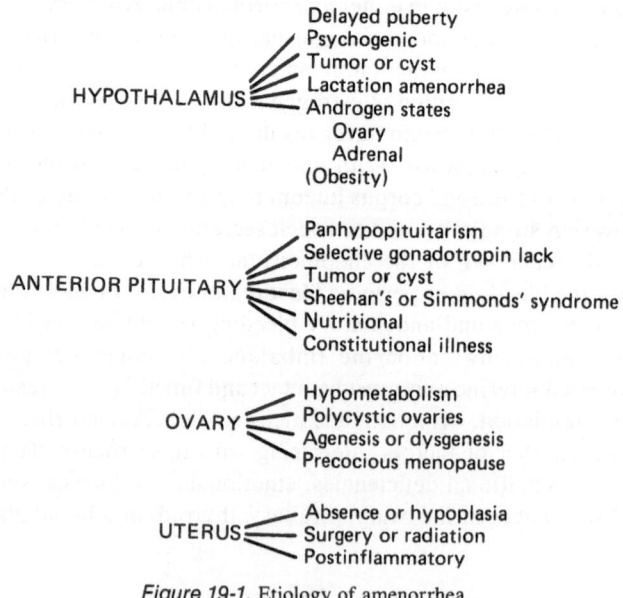

Figure 19-1. Etiology of amenorrhea.

underlying disturbance, of which ovulatory failure may be only a symptom. Primary amenorrhea calls for a genetic survey because approximately 40% of such cases have a chromosomal defect.

Figure 19-2 demonstrates an approach to diagnosis in secondary amenorrhea and in those cases of primary amenorrhea without a genetic cause. Uterine and ovarian causes of amenorrhea are ruled out when withdrawal flow after progesterone indicates the presence of a functioning endometrium and ovaries capable of secreting estrogen. In most instances, withdrawal flow after progestin rules out a large pituitary tumor. Since there are instances where there is functioning tissue associated with a small pituitary tumor, and gonadotropin and estrogen secretion continues, an x ray of the pituitary fossa should be made in all cases of amenorrhea.

If there is ovarian production of estrogen, follicle-stimulating hormone (FSH) production must be in the normal range and there is no need to measure it. On the other hand, if luteinizing hormone (LH) is elevated, even without hirsutism, this will point toward polycystic ovarian disease. Signs and symptoms of increased androgenicity also suggest polycystic ovarian disease or adrenal hyperactivity, and these should be investigated with adrenal function studies. Although thyroid gland disorders rarely cause amenorrhea, thyroid studies also should be carried out if there are suggestive symptoms.

If there has been withdrawal bleeding after progesterone, if the sella x ray is negative, if there is a normal LH level, if there are no signs and symptoms of increased androgenicity, if adrenal function studies are normal, and if there is no disturbance of thyroid function, the diagnosis of *moderate hypothalamic* amenorrhea, with only a nonfunctioning cyclic center, can be made. Such patients are ideal candidates for clomiphene citrate therapy.

If there is a lack of withdrawal flow after progesterone administration, a cycle of estrogen-progestin is administered after which a result of no flow indicates a *uterine* cause of the amenorrhea. If there is withdrawal flow after estrogen-progestin, an FSH determination is carried out; if the results are high, the diagnosis of *ovarian failure* is made.

Despite many contrary reports, a normal or low FSH level does not discriminate between primary pituitary hypofunction and severe hypothalamic amenorrhea. In the latter condition, the pituitary gland may appear nonfunctional because it has failed to be stimulated by the hypothalamic-releasing hormones over a long period of time. Sometimes, but not always, an LH-releasing hormone stimulation test, particularly if combined with a thyrotropin-releasing hormone test, can make that differentiation.[1,2]

The diagnosis of *pituitary amenorrhea* can be made when pituitary x rays are positive. A coned-down view of the sella turcica should be the first approach and one should be able to visualize a tumor or cyst 10 mm in diameter or greater. If a microadenoma or cyst is not seen, but there is erosion or calcification of the

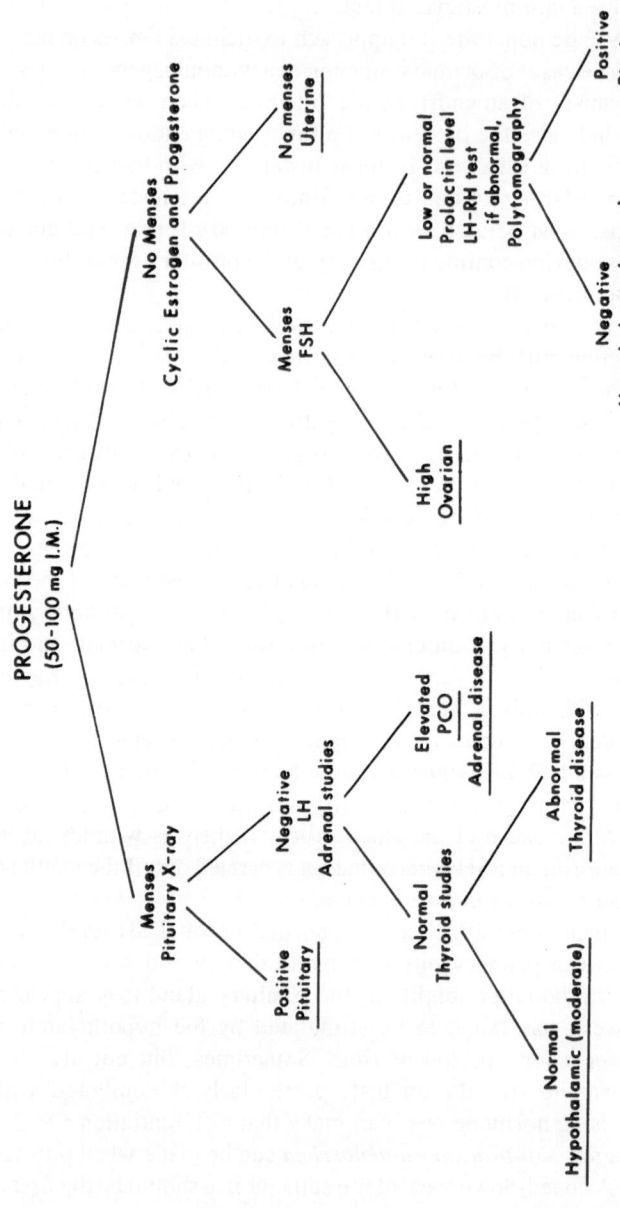

Figure 19-2. A flow sheet for diagnosis in amenorrhea and anovulation.

sella, or a prolactin level greater than 50 ng/ml, a computerized tomographic (CT) scan should be utilized. At this point, if the patient does not withdraw from progesterone, if she has an FSH that is low or normal, a prolactin level that is normal and pituitary x rays that are negative, the diagnosis of *severe hypothalamic amenorrhea* can be made.

Hyperprolactinemia can be found with or without galactorrhea,[3] so a prolactin level should be a part of the workup of every case of amenorrhea or anovulation. Such elevated prolactin levels can be caused by a macroadenoma or a microadenoma of the pituitary gland, or by idiopathic hyperfunction of the pituitary gland.[4] Prolactin levels are often elevated by stress or meals so that the best time to measure prolactin levels is during late morning before lunch.[5]

There appears to be little need to perform CT scans with a prolactin level of less than 50 µg/ml, and these patients can be treated and then followed with coned-down x rays. However, patients with prolactin levels over 50 µg/ml should have CT scans to rule out a microadenoma. These patients are no longer purely infertility patients but need additional tests to delineate the problem and additional treatment to control the microadenoma.[6]

DIAGNOSIS IN ANOVULATION

In anovulation, as in amenorrhea, emotional and nutritional factors are extremely common etiologic factors. The diagnosis of anovulatory bleeding is suggested by the history of a grossly irregular bleeding pattern, although cycles of 21 days or less also may be characteristic of anovulation. A basal body temperature chart is the most practical tool for confirming the diagnosis of anovulation; also diagnostic are the findings of proliferative endometrium and low serum progesterone. It is important, however, to be certain that these two latter tests are carried out just before menstrual flow.

Anovulatory cycles represent a less serious level of disturbance, and usually one need study only thyroid, ovarian, or adrenal function to rule out contributing factors that may be amenable so specific therapy. If some uterine bleeding occurs, normal levels of gonadotropin excretion can be expected.

REFERENCES

1. Taymor ML: The use of LH-RH in gynecology. Wynn RM, ed. *Obstet Gynecol Annual*, New York, Appleton Century Crofts.
2. Lufkin EG, O'Fallon WM, et al: Combine testing of anterior pituitary gland with insulin thyrotropin releasing hormone and luteinizing hormone releasing hormone. *Am J Med* 75:383, 1983
3. Bohnet HG, Dahlen HG, Wuttke W, Schneider HPG: Hyperprolactinemia anovulatory syndrome. *J Clin Endocrinol Metab* 42:132, 1975

4. Archer DF, Sprong JW, Nankin HR, Josimovich JB: Pituitary gonadotropin response in women with idiopathic hyperprolactinemia. *Fertil Steril* 27:1158, 1976
5. Yen SCC: Prolactin in human reproduction. In Yen SCC, Jaffee RB (eds): *Reproductive Endocrinology*, 2nd ed. 1986, p 246
6. Jaffee RB: Pathologic alterations in prolactin production. In Yen SCC, Jaffee RB (eds): *Reproductive Endocrinology*, 2nd ed. Philadelphia, WB Saunders, 1986, p 560

CHAPTER 20

Special Tests in the Male

The finding of a poor postcoital test, accompanied by normally estrogenized mucus and essentially normal semen parameters calls for additional testing of the male.

MUCUS PENETRATION AND IMMUNOLOGIC TESTING

The ability of the sperm to penetrate and survive in normally estrogenized mucus may be caused by cervical mucus antibodies, antibodies carried by the sperm itself, or by unknown factors inherent in the sperm or mucus. Immunologic testing has been dealt with in chapter 19. To further test the ability of the sperm to penetrate cervical mucus, a double cervical mucus penetration test can be performed. The female partner's mucus and a control mucus of bovine cervical mucus is used.[1] The technique is described in Chapter 10. If sperm cannot penetrate the human mucus but does penetrate the bovine mucus, the problem is in the mucus of the female partner. If the sperm penetrates neither mucus, the problem lies within the sperm. If the sperm penetrates both mucus samples, we have an unexplained poor postcoital test.

SPERM PENETRATION ASSAY

In 1976, Yanagimachi described a test in which the ability of human sperm to penetrate hamster eggs from which the zona pellucida that had been removed

163

was quantified.[2] The sperm penetration assay (SPA) has been described by Makler.[3] This test was at first believed to be a valid one for evaluation of the fertilizing ability of sperm. It is indeed a relative indicator of fertility. In a prospective study, a 68% pregnancy rate occurred in those patients with an abnormal test result of 27% or less. Only 1 of 14 men with a zero SPA conceived.[4] A review of the world literature reveals variable results. An abnormal test (less than 20% penetration) was a high predictor of infertility, but not absolute. The pregnancy rates for those with poor tests varied from 0% to 10%.[5] In an in vitro fertilization series, four pregnancies occurred in men with zero penetration.[6]

The test, then, is only a general indicator of a poor fertility index, and it is not absolute.

Before proceeding to therapy in the male with severe oligospermia or complete azoospermia, there are also a number of other diagnostic tests that should be carried out.

TESTICULAR BIOPSY

The extensive use of testicular biopsy in the past has provided us with an understanding of the varying types and degrees of testicular deficiency, or impaired spermatogenesis, associated with degrees of semen deficiency.[7] While this work has been necessary and vital, until some new information is available, there appears to be little place for the routine use of testicular biopsy in all problems of male infertility. It can only be hoped that further advances, such as the utilization of electromicroscopy, will increase the value of this very informative tool.[8]

For the present, however, complete azoospermia associated with normal sized-testes provides the most potentially treatable indication for testicular biopsy. In this situation, the demonstration of normal spermatogenesis will suggest the possible usefulness of an epididymovasostomy. Suspicion of hypophyseal hypogonadism is another indication for testicular biopsy. Physical examination will reveal diminished secondary sex characteristics; deficient gonadotropin excretion is also suggestive. The findings of immature testes on testicular biopsy will confirm the diagnosis and lead to specific replacement therapy with gonadotropins.

However, the vast majority of cases of azoospermia, associated with small or atrophic testes, or oligospermia with either small or normal testes, are associated neither with a block of the efferent ductal system nor with a remedial spermatogenesis defect. It is hoped that this will change. All that can presently be achieved with testicular biopsy in these cases is a pathologic classification of the disorder. Often one cannot give a satisfactory explanation of the etiology other than to note the presence of hypospermatogenesis or maturation arrest. Prognosis is also not aided in most cases. Therefore, when oligospermia, or azoospermia with atrophic testes is present, there is little to be gained by testicular biopsy unless the patient desires a complete evaluation of the picture. It is with extreme rarity that oligospermic men are found to have obstructive lesions.[9]

Technique

The technique, including recommendations for fixation and staining, has been thoroughly described by Rowley and Heller.[10] Because occasionally different pathology exists on either side, the procedure should be bilateral. Testicular biopsy can be performed under general or local anesthesia.

The testis is grasped and held firmly between the second and third fingers of the left hand. A ½- to ⅓-inch incision divides the skin, dartos layers, and tunica vaginalis (Fig. 20-1). The tunica albuginea is then incised and, by exerting pressure on the testicle, tubular tissue is extruded from the tunica. This is excised (Fig. 20-2). Unless there is considerable bleeding, it is best not to place sutures around bleeding vessels in the tunica albuginea or testicular tissue, as considerable postoperative pain results. A clamp that crushes the blood vessels for 5 minutes usually suffices. The tunica vaginalis and scrotal layers are closed, and the procedure is repeated on the other side.

The testicular tissue is best placed in a fixative that does not cause

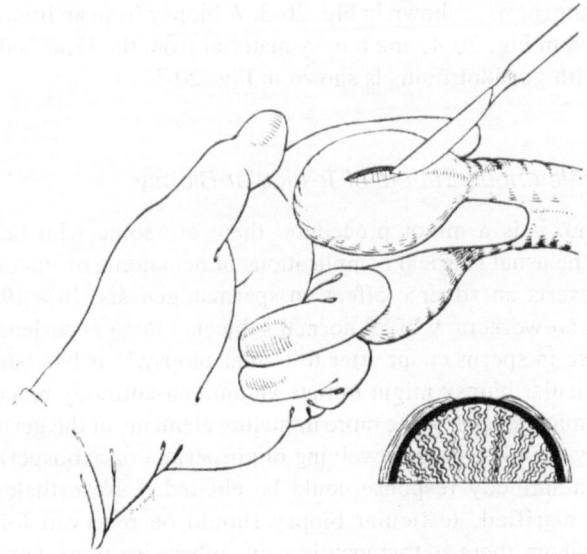

Figure 20-1. Testicular biopsy: Initial incision.

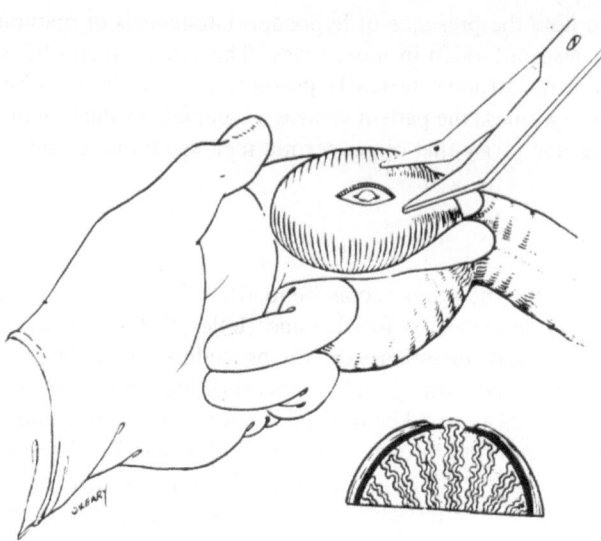

Figure 20-2. Removal of testicular tissue.

shrinkage of tissue such as Bouin's or Zenker's solution. Histologic details of testicular biopsies in various condition have been extensively described.[9] Normal spermatogenesis is shown in Fig. 20-3. A biopsy from an immature testis is demonstrated in Fig. 20-4, and biopsy material from the same individual after treatment with gonadotropins is shown in Fig. 20-5.

Possible Deleterious Effects of Testicular Biopsy

Although it is a minor procedure, there are some who believe that in addition to the usual surgical complications of hematoma or infection, testicular biopsy exerts an adverse effect on spermatogenesis. In a 1965 study by Gordon and co-workers, 9 of 20 normal subjects (45%) experienced a significant decrease in sperm count after testicular biopsy.[11] It has been suggested that the testicular biopsy might initiate an antigen-antibody reaction directed against spermatogenesis or the more immature elements of the germinal epithelium. However, in one study involving oligospermia or azoospermic men, no such antigen-antibody response could be elicited.[12] Nevertheless, until the situation is clarified, testicular biopsy should be reserved for only those patients in whom there is therapeutic gain, otherwise more harm than good might result.

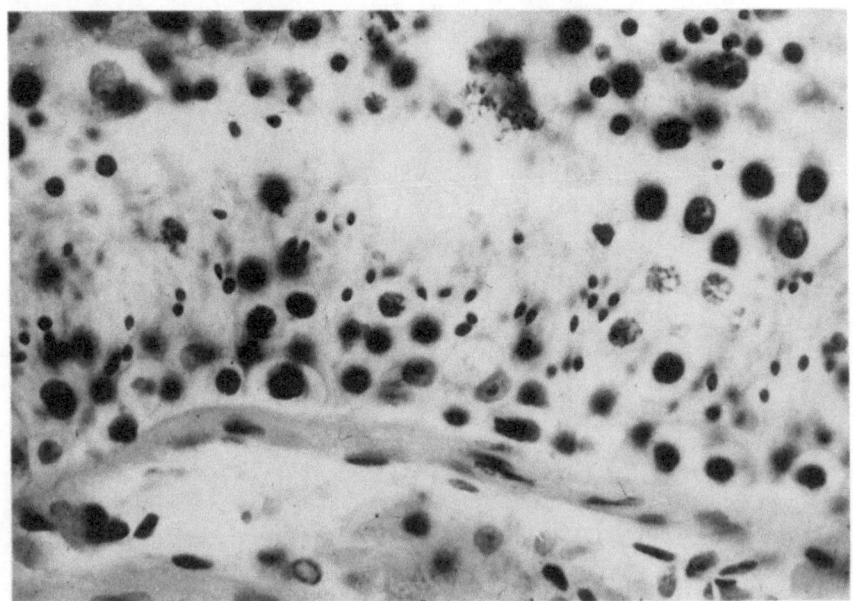

Figure 20-3. Testicular biopsy: Normal spermatogenesis.

HORMONAL STUDIES

The same low yield of useful information obtained from routine testicular biopsy holds for *routine* hormonal studies in the evaluation of the male factor.

Gonadotropins

The majority of patients with oligospermia and even azoospermia will have normal follicle-stimulation hormone (FSH) and luteinizing hormone (LH) levels in the serum or urine. The usual situation involves a deficiency of semen, but the subject is usually androgenic and the testes are of normal size. In such cases there is little to be gained from gonadotropin studies. There are situations, however, where gonadotropin levels are meaningful.

In the male who is obviously hypogonadal (and these are rare), or in whom there are clinical and laboratory evidences of deficient Leydig cell production of testosterone, measurements of serum FSH and LH can differentiate between primary testicular disease and hypothalamic-pituitary failure. If serum FSH and LH are elevated, the problem is in the testes. If low or normal, the problem is in the pituitary or hypothalamus. A luteinizing hormone-releasing hormone test may help to differentiate between pituitary and hypothalamic disease.[13]

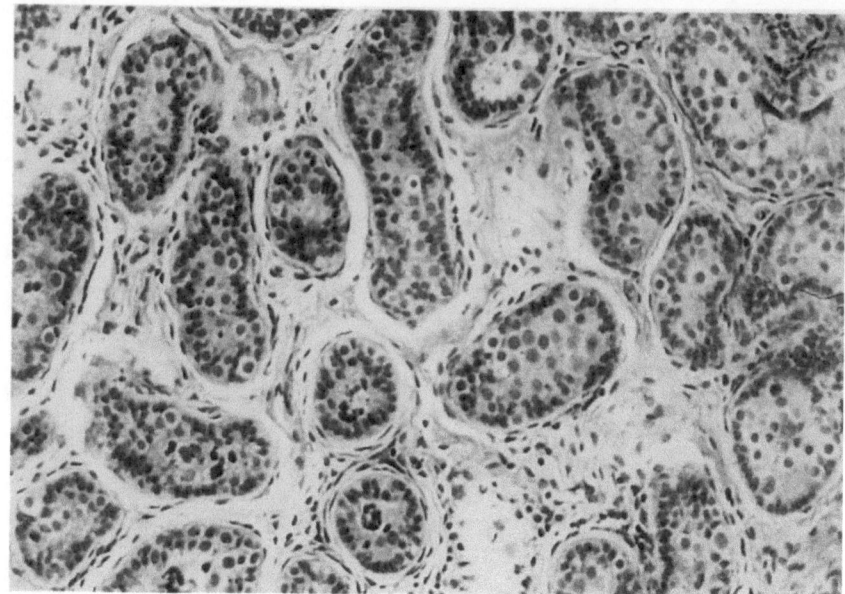

Figure 20-4. Testicular biopsy: Immature testis associated with hypopituitary function. Failure of maturation.

As indicated, most patients with oligospermia have normal testosterone and LH levels. However, isolated damage to the seminiferous tubules causes an isolated increase in FSH levels.[14–16] Usually, this is associated with small testes and is an irremedial lesion.

The Adrenal Cortex

MacLeod has suggested that some cases of male infertility are associated with abnormal adrenal function.[17] Of six patients with immature cells studied, four were found to have abnormal levels of 17-ketosteroids or 17-ketogenic steroids. A male form of congenital or acquired adrenal hyperplasia has been postulated.[9] The diagnosis of adrenal genital syndrome is difficult in the male because there are no symptoms of masculinization so readily noted in the female. The patient is well developed with normal hair distribution and normal secondary sex characteristics. However, the testes may be somewhat small or soft. Elevation of 17-ketosteroids excretion or of dehydroepiandrosterone-sulfate levels in blood is the key to the diagnosis. However, there have been few reports with well-controlled laboratory studies before and after therapy. It is my feeling that this is a fairly rare condition, and that the routine use of cortisone should be avoided.

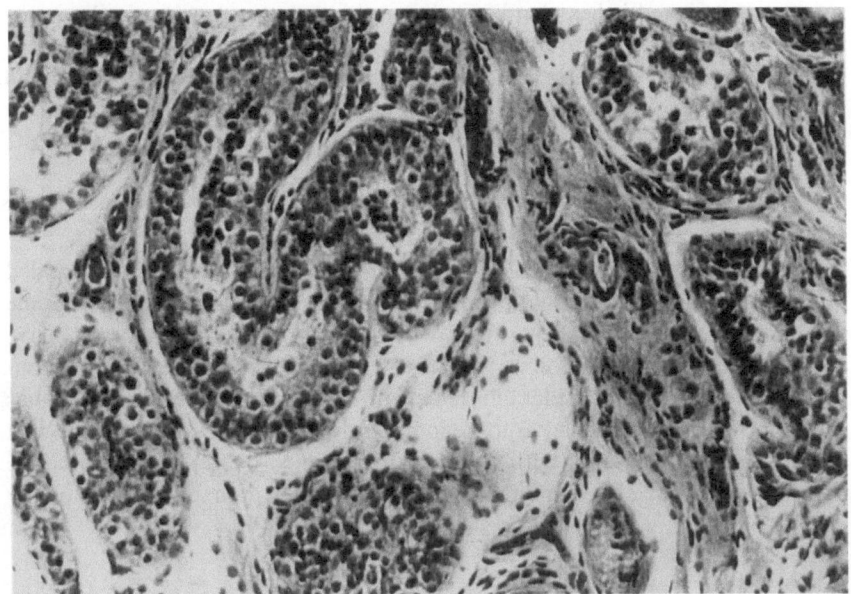

Figure 20-5. Testicular biopsy: Same patient as in Figure 20-4 after treatment with gonadotropin. Maturation has resumed.

SEX CHROMATIN DETERMINATION

In males with azoospermia, sex chromatin determination can be a screening method before testicular biopsy. Sohval has pointed out that paternity has not been reported in a chromosome-positive male. In such cases, testicular biopsy can be avoided.[18] However, a chromatin-negative pattern does not rule out Klinefelter's syndrome, 25% of which will be chromosome negative.[9]

SEMINAL FRUCTOSE LEVELS

Fructose is specifically secreted by the seminal vesicles. In men with congenital bilateral aplasia of the epididymides and vasa deferentia, (and presumably seminal vesicles), there is absence of fructose in the semen.[19,20] Fructose is present when the azoospermia is due to obstruction in the epididymis or vas deferens, or there is failure of spermatogenesis. Therefore, a routine test for fructose is indicated in all males found to have complete azoospermia.

Some reports indicate that fructose production varies inversely with the sperm count,[20] and it has also been shown that fructose levels correlate positively with androgen levels.[21,22] However, other studies could find no significant differences in fructose concentration between normal oligospermic and azoospermic seminal plasma exclusive of congenital absence.[23]

THERMOGRAPHY AND VENOGRAPHY

The increased importance of varicocele in male infertility has expanded interest in methods that might aid in the diagnosis.[24] Selective retrograde venography of the internal spermatic vein has been described as a conclusive approach to the diagnosis of varicocele.[25] However, venography is time consuming and requires considerable technical skill. Scrotal thermography has been offered as an alternative to venography with the added advantage that it can select out patients with a subclinical (nonpalpable) varicocele. The presence of a varicocele in these individuals can then be confirmed by venography.[26]

REFERENCES

 1. Gaddum-Rosse P, Blandau R, Lee W: Sperm penetration into cervical mucus in vitro: II. Human spermatozoa in bovine mucus. *Fertil Steril* 33:644, 1980
 2. Yanagimachi RJ, Yanagimachi H, Rogers BJ: The use of zone-free animal ova is a test for the assessment of fertilizing capacity of human spermatozoa. *Biol Reprod* 15:471, 1976
 3. Makler A: Modern methods in semen analysis evaluation. In Behrman SJ, Kistner RW, Patton GW Jr (eds): *Progress in Infertility*, 3rd ed. Boston, Little, Brown, 1988, p 633
 4. Shy KK, Stenchever M, Maller CH: Sperm penetration assay and subsequent pregnancy: A prospective study of 74 infertile man. *Obstet Gynecol* 71:685, 1988
 5. Mao C, Grimes DA: The sperm penetration assay: Can it discriminate between fertile and infertile men? *Am J Obstet Gynecol* 159:279, 1988
 6. Kuzan FB, Muller CH, Zarutskie RW, Dixon CC, Soules MR: Human sperm penetration assay as an indicator of sperm function in human in-vitro fertilization. *Fertil Steril* 48:282, 1987
 7. Howard RR, Shiffren RC, Simmons FA, Albright F: Testicular deficiency: A clinical and pathologic study. *J Clin Endocrinol Metab* 10:121, 1950
 8. Pederson H, Rebbe H, Hammen R: Human sperm fine structure in a case of severe asthenospermia-necrospermia. *Fertil Steril* 22:56, 1971
 9. Amelar R: Infertility in men. Philadelphia, FA Davis, 1966, p 90
10. Rowley M, Heller C: The testicular biopsy: Surgical procedure, fixation and staining techniques. *Fertil Steril* 17:177, 1966
11. Gordon D, Barr A, Herrigel J, Paulsen C: Testicular biopsy in man: I. Effect upon sperm concentration. *Fertil Steril* 16:522, 1965
12. Ansbacher R, Gangai M: Testicular biopsy: Sperm antibodies. *Fertil Steril* 26:12, 1975
13. Roth JC, Kelch RP, Kaplan SL, Grumbach MM: FSH and LH response to luteinizing hormone-releasing factor in prepubertal and pubertal children, adult males and patients with hypogonadotropin and hypogonadotropic gonadism. *J Clin Endocrinol Metab* 35:926, 1972

14. Van Thiel DH, Sherins RJ, Meyers GH Jr, DeVita VT Jr: Evidence for a specific seminiferous tubular factor affecting follicle stimulating hormone levels in oligospermia. *J Clin Invest* 51:1009, 1972

15. DeKrester DM, Burger HG, Hudson B: The relationship between germinal cells and serum FSH levels in males with infertility. *J Clin Endocrinol Metab* 38:787, 1974

16. Hunter WM, Edmond P, Watson GS, McLean N: Plasma LH and FSH levels in subfertile men. *J Clin Endocrinol Metab* 39:740, 1974

17. MacLeod J: A possible factor in the etiology of human male infertility: Preliminary report. *Fertil Steril* 13:29, 1962

18. Sohval AR: Sex chromatin chromosomes and male infertility. *Fertil Steril* 14:180, 1963

19. Amelar RD, Hotchkiss RS: Congenital aplasia of the epididymides and vasa deferentia: Effects on semen. *Fertil Steril* 14:44, 1962

20. Phadke AM, Samant NR, Shubbada DD: Significance of seminal fructose studies in male infertility. *Fertil Steril* 24:894, 1973

21. Landau RL, Loughead R: Seminal factors as index of androgenic activity in man. *J Clin Endocrinol Metab* 11:1411, 1951

22. Mauss J, Borsch G, Torok L: Differential diagnosis of low or absent seminal fructose in man. *Fertil Steril* 24:411, 1974

23. Gregoire AT, Moran MJ: The enzyme activity, protein and fructose content of normal, oligospermic, postvasectomy, and infertile azoospermic men. 24:208, 1973

24. Dubin L, Amelar RD: Surgery of male infertility. In Behrman SJ, Kistner RW, Patton GW Jr (eds): *Progress in Infertility*, 3rd ed. Boston, Little, Brown, 1988, p 689

25. Comhaire F, Kunnen M: Selective retrograde venography of the internal spermatic vein: A conclusive approach to the diagnosis of varicocele. *Andrologia* 8:11, 1976

26. Comhaire F, Monteyne R, Kunnen M: The value of scrotal thermography as compared with selective retrograde venography of the internal spermatic vein for the diagnosis of "subclinical" varicocele. *Fertil Steril* 27:6, 1976

PART VI

Therapy

CHAPTER 21

Treatment of the Male

There is a great deal of pessimism concerning the potential for significant therapy in the male. The reason, I believe, is that therapy in the past has often been limited to the male with marked oligospermia (i.e., sperm count less than 20 million/ml). At these low levels the condition is usually irreversible. Influenced by MacLeod and Gold's report,[1] therapists considered the subfertile male, with 20 to 40 million/ml, as "normal" or "fertile," and treatment was often withheld from this group. If, however, one accepts the concept of the couple as a unit, and that a sperm count of 20 to 40 million/ml cc represents subfertility, treatment of this subfertile male could be meaningful as far as the couple is concerned. Ironically, this is the group of males for whom the most can be done, and yet who often go without treatment.

The salutary effect of various regimens and medications on spermatogenesis can be overemphasized and undoubtedly have been in many reports published over the past 35 years. Even after a careful reading of a report, one is usually uncertain as to the efficacy of the recommended medication or program. This is often due to the failure to use controls, although this may be difficult when it comes to therapy. Other pitfalls are present; first, the natural variation in sperm count that may vary spontaneously by 20 to 30 million. When reporting results in terms of improved semen quality, most authors do not take this variation into sufficient consideration. Another factor is the spontaneous pregnancy rate, even with sperm counts of less than 20 million/ml. Table 21-1 is a composite of three studies of fertile populations of men. Within these fertile populations, 5% to 21% had sperm counts of less than 20 million/ml, and

Table 21-1. Frequency Distributions of Sperm Counts Found in 2000 Allegedly Fertile Men Requesting Vasectomy Compared with Previous Reports

Sperm count (millions/ml)	MacLeod and Gold[1] (%)	Nelson and Bunge[2] (%)	Rehan et al.[3] (%)
<10.1	2	4.7	2
10.1–20.0	3	15.5	5
20.1–40.0	12	30.8	16
40.1–60.0	12	21.0	18
60.1–80.0	14	14.3	21
80.1–100.0	13	6.7	13
>100.0	44	7.0	24
Number of subjects	1000	386	1300
Source of patients	Prenatal clinic	Vasectomy clinic	Vasectomy clinic

between 12% and 31% had counts ranging between 20 and 40 million/ml. Too often the issue is clouded when therapists include males in both groups of sperm counts and do not statistically compare the results with the known fertility rates in these groups. This does not mean that the regimens proposed are not without merit, but the therapist should use them in the light of the present state of infertility knowledge and its limitations.

HORMONE THERAPY

In the past, approaches to hormone therapy have mainly been attempts to administer exogenous hormones to stimulate spermatogenesis. Since, in the majority of cases, subfertility and oligospermia are not associated with any hormonal deficiency, or at least a demonstrable one, it is not surprising that the results have not been too promising. However, there are times when hormone therapy is indicated, or can at least be utilized as a last resort.

Androgens

In 1950, studies by Heller and co-workers showed that, if spermatogenesis was depressed by testosterone administration, there was a rebound of spermatogenesis to levels "significantly" higher than those before treatment.[4] When high doses of testosterone propionate or long-acting testosterone are administered over a 10-week period, if a rebound occurs it will usually appear within 3 to 6 months.

In Rowley and Heller's follow-up report, 110 of 163 courses of therapy resulted in a rise in sperm concentration.[5] In 41% of the couples, conception followed therapy. These are promising figures, but the expected variation in sperm count, the natural fertility in oligospermic males, and the failure to break down the results by various levels of count make the work difficult to interpret. A few other investigators also cautiously reported success,[6] but the fact that this treatment has failed to become firmly established after 35 years speaks for its questionable nature. One drawback is that in a small number of individuals—2% in one series—there is a permanent decrease in spermatogenesis.[6] One should therefore be cautious about utilizing this therapy in men with subfertile specimens (20 to 40 million) where there is a significant spontaneous conception rate until all other approaches have been exhausted.

The use of low-dose androgens has also been recommended. Since exogenous testosterone will reduce the production of testosterone by the testicles through hypothalamic pituitary inhibition, this form of therapy does not appear to have any scientific rationale. Rowley and Heller pointed out that it required, on the average, 11.2 g of exogenous testosterone daily to result in direct stimulation of the testes.[7] Nevertheless, reports on its use persist, and a recent report states that it may help sperm motility when other parameters are not effective.[8]

Clomiphene Citrate

The reports considering the effectiveness of clomiphene citrate in improving sperm quantity and quality are also conflicting. As in most studies, the number of cases is small and the definitions of oligospermia are variable. Medical treatment in the male has the additional problem of requiring long courses of treatment to note improvement in spermatogenesis, and this is not always followed. In Mellinger and Thompson's preliminary report, improvements in counts in 10 of 13 oligospermic males were noted, but conception did not occur.[9] The study of Wieland and co-workers revealed variable results in 11 men who were treated with cisclomiphene.[10] Schellen and Beck treated 101 patients with clomiphene for 40, 60, or 90 days.[11] Ozoospermic patients gave no response, although some with oligospermia showed improvement. There were 19 pregnancies.

Paulson and Wacksman believe that the best candidates for clomiphene therapy are those men with oligospermia and normal follicle-stimulating hormone levels but who show some evidence of spermatic hypoplasia on testicular biopsy.[12] The suggested regimen is 25 mg daily, with 5-day rest periods and with therapy maintained for up to 9 months. Heller and his co-workers have summarized their conclusions concerning clomiphene: while low doses (25 to 50 mg daily) stimulate sperm production in normal men, higher doses have a higher toxic effect on spermatogenesis.[13] Recent studies utilizing placebos as a control failed to show any improvement with clomiphene on semen parameters, the sperm penetration test, or the occurrence of pregnancy.[14-16]

Human Chorionic Gonadotropin

The ability of human chorionic gonadotropin (HCG) to bring about improved spermatogenesis in individuals with hypogonadotropic hypogonadism is well accepted.[17] The same ability for improved spermatogenesis in relation to oligospermia in eugonadotropic males is controversial. Table 21-2 summarizes some of the reports over the past 30 years. A critical evaluation of these papers reveals that some of the patients had initial sperm counts of more than 30 million, and a few of more than 40 million, making one wish that the authors had been more selective. In this group, the improvement in pregnancies that occurs in oligospermia (see Table 21-2), make it difficult to establish the reliability of these reports.

Despite a cursory view suggesting improvement, Rowley and Heller conclude that HCG does not stimulate spermatogenesis in normal men.[21] It should also be noted in these studies that there is often an initial depression of spermatogenesis followed in 2 to 4 months by a rebound or "overproduction." There is general agreement that when the initial sperm count is less than 10 million, there is universal failure. It would appear that the HCG can be given as a last resort, provided that expectations for significant improvement are not high.

Human Menopausal Gonadotropin

The results of human menopausal gonadotropin (HMG), are similar to those for HCG. For those few patients in whom there is oligospermia, or azoospermia, due to pituitary failure (hypopituitary hypogonadism), HMG provides a significant replacement therapy. Even then, for good results, it is best combined with chorionic gonadotropin.[22]

Various reports on the use of HMG in oligospermia accompanied by normal pituitary function are summarized in Table 21-3, but the small number of cases in each report and the difficulty in differentiating between increasing sperm count due to therapy or only that seen as the normal variation makes

Table 21-2. Results with Human Chorionic Gonadotropin
in the Treatment of Male Infertility

Study	Year	Number of cases	Dose (IU)	Sperm count (million)	No. of cases improved	Pregnancies
Dorner et al.[18]	1960	10	32,000	2–35	8	Not reported
Glass and Holland[19]	1963	17	180,000	—	12	7
Futterweight and Sobrero[20]	1968	27	195,000	<35	15	10

Table 21-3. Effect of Human Menopausal Gonadotropin
in the Treatment of Male Infertility

Study	Number of cases	Initial sperm count (million)	Number of cases improved	Pregnancies
Lytton and Mroueh[23]	16	rare to 21	3	2
Polishuk et al.[24]	23	0 to 21	4	1
Danezis and Batrinos[25]	11	1 to 22	5	2
Mroueh et al.[26]	8	rare to 33	1	Not reported
Schwartzstein[27]	12	rare to 20	5	Not reported

them difficult to interpret. The report by Danezis and Batrinos was the most optimistic, with 5 of 11 cases showing improvement in sperm count, and improved motility noted in 7.[25]

In view of the expense and prolonged therapy involved, more conservative approaches should be attempted before resorting to gonadotropin therapy for oligospermia associated with normal pituitary gonadotropin levels.

Gonadotropin-Releasing Hormone

A few reports are now available concerning the clinical use of gonadotropin-releasing hormone (GnRH) in normal gonadotropin oligospermic males.[28,29] Initially, injections were given two or three times daily over a lengthy period of time. In one study, three of six subjects, and in another study two of four subjects with oligospermia, showed an increase in sperm count. Despite these somewhat optimistic preliminary reports, the multiplicity of injections, as well as other pitfalls of evaluation, still make this a questionable approach; this is further complicated by a recent report of antibody formation to releasing hormones after prolonged administration required in the male. More recently, a study utilizing a pulsatile infusion pump demonstrated that this approach was more effective than multiple injections.[30]

Other Hormones

Stewart postulated that cortisone may be of value in the treatment of selected cases of male infertility, particularly in patients with congenital or acquired adrenal-genital syndrome.[31] It is recommended, therefore, that when there is a good sperm count with low motility, dehydroepiandrosterone-sulfate be measured. To find actual adrenal hyperplasia in the male is quite rare, so this kind of treatment is not often indicated. Indeed, there are reports of suppression of spermatogenesis by corticosteroid administration.[32]

Thyroidal Therapy

Therapy is effective in true hypothyroidism, but this, too, is rare. The use of triiodothyronine, 25 to 50 μg daily, seems to be of some empirical value when there is lowered motility in association with a normal sperm count.[33]

TREATMENT OF ENVIRONMENTAL FACTORS

The most promising approach to therapy for the male factor is to modify the male's environmental status. In many instances the subfertile male (with a sperm count of 20 to 40 million) plays a significant etiologic role in the couple's infertility. Treating the subfertile male helps the couple because primarily the subfertile male, and not the infertile one, will respond to modification of environmental factors.

The adverse effects of heat on spermatogenesis has been appreciated for some time.[34] Therefore, avoidance of skin-tight underwear, prolonged sitting, hot baths, whirlpool baths, or saunas have been shown to result in improvement of seminal characteristics.[35] Specialized cooling supports have also resulted in significant improvement.[36]

Excellent studies have now demonstrated the harmful effects of tobacco and alcohol on spermatogenesis, and these should be avoided. The role of caffeine is being investigated. Recent in vitro studies have shown that caffeine stimulated ejaculated human spermatozoa,[37,38] but this has not been carried over to in vitro studies.[39] At present, there is no evidence to indicate that vitamins significantly enhance semen quality.

SURGICAL TREATMENT

Varicocele Ligation

The efficacy of varicocele ligation remains controversial (see Chapter 5). Since the optimistic reports from Great Britain in the 1950s,[40,41] enthusiasm over the effectiveness of this procedure has continued. In the United States, Charny initially reported a 64% improvement in semen quality; he restricted his therapy to include only men with sperm counts of less than 20 million.[42] In 36 patients, 14 pregnancies resulted—a significant success rate. In 1970, Dubin and Amelar reported an 81% improvement in sperm quality and a 48% pregnancy rate in 111 cases.[43] In their study, the size of the varicocele appeared to have no influence on the outcome of the therapy. Other reports have not only demonstrated that this is one of the most promising treatments for the male (with significant improvement in semen quality even in patients with counts less than 10 million/ml),[44-46] but have recommended ligating the left spermatic vein when oligospermia exists even without clinical evidence of varicocele.[47,48] In contrast to these optimistic reports, one more recent study failed to demonstrate a significant improvement from internal spermatic reinligation and called for a large-scale prospective study.[49]

The technique is to ligate the internal spermatic vein just above the internal inguinal ring through an incision just above, and parallel to, Poupart's ligament.[50] If there are multiple branches, these are ligated as well. Care must be taken to avoid damage to the spermatic artery. Hydrocele is an occasional complication, but this should not affect fertility.

Epididymovasostomy

When there is complete azoospermia and a biopsy shows normal spermatogenesis, obstruction is diagnosed, and an operation to reestablish continuity can be considered. The technique has been thoroughly described by Amelar.[51] For the operation to be successful, there has to be normal sperm production, the obstruction must be in a relatively small segment of the vas distal to the epididymis, and the vas must be otherwise normal. Only problems of azoospermia fall into this category. Once these criteria have been satisfied, the operation itself is technically successful in only 20% of patients,[52] and thus, yield in pregnancies is not great. Balanced against this is the relative innocuousness of the procedure. The recent introduction of microsurgery, less reactive suture material, and constant irrigation may improve results.[53]

Vasovasostomy

Along with the increased use of vasectomy for contraception has also come an increase in the number of men requesting reanastomosis. Where in the past this was an operation of a limited success, modern techniques using microsurgery, a nylon stent, and fine sutures produce some improvement in results.[54,55]

RETROGRADE EJACULATION

Retrograde ejaculation is associated with disruption of the physiologic closure of the proximal end of the posterior urethra concomitant with emission. By employing the sequence of emptying the bladder, ejaculation, and immediate catheterization to remove the ejaculate followed by insemination of the female partner, conception becomes a distinct possibility. Recently, the addition of specialized buffers and the use of intrauterine insemination have increased the effectiveness of treatment of this relatively rare condition.[56]

ASSISTED REPRODUCTIVE TECHNOLOGY

The techniques and medications described above are utilized, for the most part, in an attempt to improve the quantity and quality of sperm delivered by the male. Unfortunately, the results of such treatments are not always effective, and we must turn to techniques of concentration and improved delivery that will further increase the chances of conception. The new techniques of assisted reproductive technology (intrauterine insemination, gamete intrafallopian transfer, and in vitro fertilization) are now widely used[57,58] and will be described in the following chapters. These approaches are more exotic. It is hoped that the young therapists of today will not foresake the less exciting therapeutic approaches as described in this chapter, and that add their small part to the improvement of sperm quality.

REFERENCES

1. MacLeod J, Gold RA: The male factor in fertility and infertility. *J Urol* 66:436, 1951
2. Nelson CMK, Bunge RG: Semen analysis: Evidence for changing parameters of male fertility potential. *Fertil Steril* 25:503, 1974
3. Rehan NE, Sobrero AH, Fertig JW: The semen of fertile men: Statistical analysis of 1300 men. *Fertil Steril* 26:492, 1975
4. Heller G, Nelson WO, Hill IB, et al: Improvement in spermatogenesis following depression of the human tests with testosterone. *Fertil Steril* 1:415, 1950
5. Rowley MJ, Heller CG: The testosterone rebound phenomenon in the treatment of male infertility. *Fertil Steril* 23:498, 1972
6. Lamensdorf H, Compere D, Begley G: Testosterone rebound therapy in the treatment of male infertility. *Fertil Steril* 26:469, 1975
7. Rowley MJ, Heller CG: Inhibition and stimulation of human spermatogenesis. In Behrman SJ, Kistner RW (eds): *Progress in Infertility*, 2nd ed. Boston, Little Brown, 1975, p 719
8. Brown S: The effect of orally administered androgens on sperm motility. *Fertil Steril* 26:305, 1975
9. Mellinger R, Thompson R: The effect of clomiphene citrate in male infertility. *Fertil Steril* 17:94, 1966
10. Wieland R, Ansari A, Klein D, et al: Idiopathic oligospermia: Control observations and response to cisclomiphene. *Fertil Steril* 23:471, 1972
11. Schellen T, Beck J: Use of clomiphene treatment for male sterility. *Fertil Steril* 25:407, 1974
12. Paulson DF, Wacksman J: Clomiphene citrate in the management of male infertility. *J Urol* 115:73, 1976
13. Heller CG, Rowley MJ, Heller GV: Clomiphene citrate: A correlation of its effect on sperm concentration and morphology; Total gonadotropins, ICSH, estrogen and testosterone excretion and testicular morphology in normal men. *J Clin Endocronol Metab* 29:638, 1969
14. Charny CW: Clomiphene therapy in male infertility: A negative report. *Fertil Steril* 32:551, 1979
15. Newton R, Solinfeld JS, Schiff I: Clomiphene treatment of infertile men: Failure of response with idiopathic oligospermia. *Fertil Steril* 34:399, 1980
16. Sokol RZ, Steiner BS, Bustillo M, Peterson G, Swerdloff RS: A controlled comparison of the efficacy of clomiphene citrate on male infertility. *Fertil Steril* 49:865, 1988

17. Turner H, Zanartu J, Nelson W: Effect of chorionic gonadotropin therapy on fertility in males with scrotal tests. *Fertil Steril* 15:24, 1964

18. Dorner TG, Moch G, Zabel H: The "over production effect" of these tests after cessation of human chorionic gonadotropin administration in men with oligoasthenospermia. *Fertil Steril* 11:457, 1960

19. Glass S, Holland H: Treatment of oligospermia with large doses of human chorionic gonadotropin: A preliminary report. *Fertil Steril* 14:500, 1963

20. Futterweit W, Sobrero AJ: Treatment of normogonadotropic oligospermia with large doses of chorionic gonadotropin. *Fertil Steril* 19:971, 1968

21. Rowley MJ, Heller CG: Inhibition and stimulation of human spermatogenesis. In Behrman SJ, Kistner RW (eds): *Progress in Infertility*, 2nd ed. Boston, Little, Brown, 1975, p 719

22. MacLeod J, Pazianos A, Ray B: The restoration of human spermatogenesis and of the reproductive tract with urinary gonadotropins following hypophysectomy. *Fertil Steril* 17:7, 1966

23. Lytton B, Mroueh A: Treatment of oligospermia with urinary human menopausal gonadotropin: A preliminary report. *Fertil Steril* 17:696, 1966

24. Polishuk W, Palti Z, Laufer A: Treatment of defective spermatogenesis with human gonadotropins. *Fertil Steril* 18:127, 1967

25. Danezis J, Batrinos M: The effect of human postmenopausal gonadotropins on infertile men with severe oligospermia. *Fertil Steril* 18:788, 1967

26. Mroueh A, Lytton B, Kase N: Effects of human chorionic gonadotropin and human menopausal gonadotropin (Pergonal) in males with oligospermia. *J Clin Endocrinol Metab* 27:53, 1967

27. Schwartzstein L: Human menopausal gonadotropins in treatment of patients with oligospermia. *Fertil Steril* 25:813, 1974

28. Zarate A, Valdes-Vallina F, Gonzalez A, et al: Therapeutic effect of synthetic luteinizing hormone-releasing hormone (LH-RH) in male infertility due to idiopathic azoospermia and oligospermia. *Fertil Steril* 24:485, 1973

29. Schwartzstein L, Aparicio NJ, Turner D, et al: Use of synthetic luteinizing hormone-releasing hormone in treatment of oligospermic men: A preliminary report. *Fertil Steril* 26:331, 1975

30. Shargle AA: Treatment of idiopathic hypogonadism in men with luteinizing hormone-releasing hormone: A comparison of treatment with daily injections and with a pulsatile infusion pump. *Fertil Steril* 47:492, 1987

31. Stewart BH: Infertility in the male: Method of Bruce H. Stewart. In Conn HF (ed): *Current Therapy*. Philadelphia, WB Saunders, 1971, p 442

32. Mancini R, Lavieri J, Muller F, et al: Effect of prednisone upon normal and pathologic human spermatogenesis. *Fertil Steril* 17:500, 1966

33. Taymor ML, Selenkow HA: Clinical experience with L-triiodothyronine in male infertility. *Fertil Steril* 9:560, 1958

34. MacLeod S, Hotchkiss RS: The effect of hyperpyrexia upon spermatozoa counts in man. *Endocrinology* 28:760, 1941

35. Lynch R, Lewis-Jones DI, Machlin DG, Desmond AD: Improved seminal characteristics in infertile men after a conservative treatment regimen based on the avoidance of testicular hypothermic. *Fertil Steril* 46:476, 1986

36. Zorgniotti AW, Cohen MS, Sealfon AI: Chronic scrotal hypothermia: Results in 90 infertile couples. *J Urol* 135:944, 1980

37. Haesungeharern A, Chulavatnatol M: Stimulation of human spermatozoal motility by caffeine. *Fertil Steril* 24:662, 1973

38. Schoenfeld C, Amelar RD, Dubin C: Stimulation of ejaculated human spermatozoa by caffeine. *Fertil Steril* 24:662, 1973

39. Dougherty KA, Cockett ATK, Urry RI: Caffeine theophylline and human sperm motility. *Fertil Steril* 27:541, 1976

40. Davidson HA: Testicular temperature and varicocele. *Practitioner* 173:703, 1955
41. Hanely HG: The surgery of male subfertility. *Ann R Coll Surg Engl* 17:159, 1955
42. Charny C: Effect of varicocele on fertility: Results of varicocelectomy. *Fertil Steril* 13:47, 1962
43. Dubin L, Amelar R: Varicocele size and results of varicocelectomy in selected subfertile men with varicocele. *Fertil Steril* 21:606, 1970
44. Dubin L, Amelar R: Varicocelectomy as therapy in male infertility: A study of 504 cases. *Fertil Steril* 26:217, 1975
45. Mehan D: Results of ligation of internal spermatic vein in the treatment of infertility in azoospermic patients. *Fertil Steril* 27:110, 1976
46. Brown JS: Varicocelectomy in the subfertile male: A ten-year experience with 295 cases. *Fertil Steril* 27:1046, 1976
47. Palti Z, Kedar S, Polishuk W: Ligature of left spermatic vein in the treatment of oligospermia. *Fertil Steril* 19:631, 1968
48. Fogh-Anderson P, Nielson NC, Rebbe H, et al: The effects on fertility of litigation of external spermatic vein in men without clinical signs of varicocele. *Acta Obstet Gynecol Scand* 54:29, 1975
49. Vermeulen A, Vanlewegle M: Improved fertility after varicocele correction: Fact or fiction. *Fertil Steril* 42:249, 1984
50. Winer JH: The surgery of male infertility. In Behrman SJ, Kistner RW (eds): *Progress in Infertility*, 2nd ed. Boston, Little, Brown, 1975, p 729
51. Amelar R: *Infertility in Men*, Philadelphia, FA Davis, 1966, p 124
52. Kar J, Phadke A: Vaso-epididymal anastomasis. *Fertil Steril* 26:743, 1975
53. Pardanani DS, Kothari MS, Pradhan SA, Mahendrakar MN: Surgical restoration of vas continuity after vasectomy: Further clinical evaluation of a new operation technique. *Fertil Steril* 25:319, 1974
54. Amelar RD, Dublin L: Male infertility, current diagnosis and treatment. *Urology* 1:1, 1973
55. Amelar RD: Medical management of male infertility. In Crockett ATK, Urry RL (eds): *Male Infertility*. New York, Grune and Stratton, 1976, p 249
56. Zavos PM, Wilson EA: Retrograde ejaculation: Etiology and treatment via the use of a new non-invasive method. *Fertil Steril* 42:627, 1984
57. Arny M, Quaglianello J: Semen quality before and after processing by a swim-up method: Relationship to outcome of intrauterine insemination. *Fertil Steril* 48:643, 1987
58. Matson PL, Blackledge DG, Richardson PA, Turner SR, Yovich JM, Yovich JL: The role of gamete intrafallopian transfer (GIFT) on the treatment of oligospermic infertility. *Fertil Steril* 46:608, 1987

CHAPTER 22

Treatment of the Cervical Factor

The treatment of the cervical factor is essentially the treatment of the poor postcoital test. However, the standards for a good or poor postcoital test are not well defined, and the significance of the test itself is questioned by many. Nevertheless, some observations appear to have some basis in pathophysiology.

ASSESSMENT OF THE POSTCOITAL TEST PRIOR TO THERAPY

From Table 9-1 in Chapter 9, it appears that the presence of less than five active sperm per high-powered field is accompanied by a relative decrease in fertility, and this level can be taken as the indication of a poor postcoital test. A "poor postcoital test" first calls for a careful review of semen analysis. *Deficient semen quality is probably one of the most common causes for a poor postcoital test, and probably the most overlooked.* It is not only the count, but the motility and longevity of the sperm that are the important factors to observe.

Second, before assigning the cause of the poor postcoital test to a hostile cervix, the physician must be certain that the test was carried out during the *preovulatory period.* This can be ascertained only by waiting for the date of the onset of the next menstrual flow, and then analyzing the basal body temperature chart.

Thus, if the semen quality is good, if the test was carried out during the preovulatory period, and if an immune study and mycoplasma culture are negative, one might then assign the cause to a "hostile cervix" and initiate appropriate therapy.

CERVICAL STENOSIS

Stenosis of the cervix is usually caused by overzealous cauterization of the endocervical canal; less commonly it is of congenital origin. In the iatrogenic type, the problem is due more to the destruction of endocervical glands resulting in inadequate mucus, rather than to a narrowing of the passageway itself. Indeed, if menstruation can occur, it is difficult to conclude logically that the passage of the tiny sperm can be aided by widening the passage, yet dilatation of the stenosed cervix appears to be helpful. Dilatation should first be done under anesthesia, incident to laparoscopy or D & C, and then, once dilated, the enlargement should be maintained by two or three monthly preovulatory dilatations under paracervical block at office visits.

Low doses of estrogen may be added to the dry cervix in the hope that not all glands have been destroyed and that those remaining will respond with an increased secretion of mucus. When these attempts fail, intrauterine insemination is the treatment for this condition[1,2] (see Chapter 23).

INADEQUATE CERVICAL MUCUS

The type of problem most amenable to therapy is where there is inadequate production of preovulatory mucus by the endocervical glands caused neither by overcauterization nor by chronic infection. Although the cause itself is unknown, there is often a good response to small doses of estrogen. Conjugated estrogens, 0.3 mg, or ethinyl estradiol, 0.02 mg daily, are given daily from the 8th to the 18th day of a 28-day cycle; however, these preparations occasionally cause a delay in ovulation. If ovulation is postponed, the physician can delay starting the medication until the 10th day of the cycle, or prescribe the medication every other day. Once estrogen therapy has been initiated, it should be maintained for a minimum of 6 months.

Although there are no scientific reports available, the use of cough medicines* that are designed to loosen bronchial secretions often do cause an increase in cervical secretions at midcycle.

*Robitussin®, A.H. Robbins Company, Richmond, Virginia.

CERVICITIS

The role of cervicitis in infertility and its treatment is extremely controversial. First, it is often overdiagnosed. The cellular thick mucus found associated with a poor postcoital test is more likely due to poor timing in relation to ovulation or to inadequate secretion of the mucus by the endocervical glands, rather than to true chronic inflammation.

To rush in with the cautery is counterproductive since cauterizing the inner cervix destroys the endocervical glands and more often does more harm than good. Therapists, aware of this damage, recommend gentle cryosurgery of the exocervix,[3,4] but it is difficult to see how cryosurgery can help to improve either mucus or endocervical origin or sperm survival and migration. Furthermore, most "erosions" treated by cryosurgery are in actuality low-lying endocervical glands, which so many gynecologists erroneously interpret as chronic inflammatory process.

In years past, fertility specialists recommended the use of local or systemic antibiotics for patients with a chronic inflammatory process. Many years ago, Buxton and his co-workers cast considerable doubt on the effectiveness of antibiotics in improving pregnancy rates,[5] and in their excellent review of the cervical factor in infertility, Davajan and Nakamura do not even mention the use of antibiotic therapy.[4]

When the physician finally makes a firm diagnosis of chronic infection, by first ruling out other causes of poor cervical mucus, the best approach appears to be the use of careful high endocervical or intrauterine homologous insemination.[6]

OTHER MODALITIES

Coital position in infertility is usually overemphasized, although it may, rarely, be an etiologic factor in faulty insemination. What may be more significant is the position of the uterus itself. *Third-degree retroversion* of the uterus causes the external os to point to the anterior vaginal wall and, with the female in the recumbent position, the os may lie outside the seminal pool. When the male partner has a low-volume ejaculate, this deficiency is enhanced further. Homologous insemination is the treatment of choice.

Too often there is *no explanation* for persistent poor post coital tests despite normal semen analysis, good timing, adequate mucus, and negative immune tests. At this point one is tempted to fall back on unproven methods, such as the use of precoital alkaline douche, which is part of the folklore of infertility treatment. It is impossible to say whether such a douche will be of any value, but since there is little harm it can be used. Similarly, it is difficult to prove that *homologous artificial insemination* is of value in this situation, but it, too, can be employed before resorting to more complicated techniques of intra-uterine insemination[7] (see Chapter 23) or gamete intrafallopian tube transfer (see Chapter 31).

REFERENCES

1. Barwin BN: Intrauterine insemination of husband semen. *J Reprod Fertility* 36:101, 1974
2. Hall ME, Magyar DM, Varquea JM, Hayes MF, Moghissi KS: Experiences with intrauterine insemination for cervical factor and oligospermia. *Am J Obstet Gynecol* 151:1333, 1986
3. Roland M: Comments on cervical factor in infertility. *J Reprod Med* 3:3, 1969
4. Darvajan V, Nakamura RM: The cervical factor. In Behrman SJ, Kistner RW (eds): *Progress in Infertility*, 2nd ed. Boston, Little, Brown, 1975, pp 17–46
5. Buxton L, Southam A, Herrmann W, Girvin G, Nadel H: Bacteriology of the cervix in human sterility. *Fertil Steril* 5:493, 1954
6. Cohen M: The cervix factor: Its significance in reproductive processes. *J Reprod Med* 3:133, 1969
7. Check JH, Adelson BS: Improvement of cervical factor by high dose estrogen and human menopausal gonadotropin therapy with ultrasound monitoring. *Obstet Gynecol* 63:179, 1984

CHAPTER 23

Homologous Artificial Insemination (AIH and IUI)

A discussion of artificial insemination using the husband's semen logically follows the chapters on the treatment of the male factor and the cervical factor. Husband insemination is one method of treating oligospermia, faulty sperm delivery, the "hostile cervix" that does not respond to hormonal or antibiotic therapy, and an unexplained poor postcoital test.

Artificial insemination has been known to man for centuries. Since the late 18th century, the literature has contained sporadic reports of human insemination therapy utilizing the husband's sperm. Our present knowledge of the history of artificial insemination can be credited to Rohleder, who in 1934 wrote *Test Tube Babies*[1] and to Schellen, who in 1957 reviewed artificial insemination, particularly in relation to animal insemination.[2] Both authors agree that John Hunter was the first to perform husband artificial insemination (AIH) sometime between 1776 and 1779. Aside from the American, Marion Sims, who reported successful AIH in 1886, France was the scene of the major activity in the 19th century. Cervical insemination has been used extensively in the United States for the past 50 years, and a number of excellent reviews have been published.[3,4]

GENERAL CONSIDERATIONS

Except in those few cases where AIH is clearly indicated (such as failure of normal semen to be deposited at the cervical os because of hypospadias, impotency, vaginismus, or a third-degree retroverted uterus), its value must be weighted against its adverse effects. It has been questioned by some as to whether AIH for oligospermia or for the hostile cervix is a significant contribution to a problem of infertility.[5] Yet, pregnancies do occur, and it is difficult for the therapist to deny a particular couple an approach that has been successful for others. Against this, the physician must weigh the psychological drawbacks of AIH. It places tremendous pressure on the husband to produce a specimen at a particular time, on a given date. The wife must maintain her basal body temperature chart, clear her own schedule, make excuses to avoid embarrassment, and keep her appointments once or twice a month. Added to these pressures may be the mounting month-to-month failures, all of which exert adverse emotional effects on both the couple's sex life and their marriage as a whole. Very few couples can maintain the equanimity needed for 6 months, the minimum time period that should be considered for an AIH trial. Couples undergoing AIH often need the benefits of infertility counseling before and during therapy.

INTRACERVICAL INSEMINATION (AIH)

Faulty delivery of sperm due to hypospadias, retrograde ejaculation, impotence, vaginitis, and, occasionally, third-degree retroversion uterus are the absolute indications for cervical insemination and provide the best success rates.[5] The two other main indications for its use are in oligospermia and cervical hostility, and many question that AIH makes a significant contribution to the treatment of these factors of infertility.[6] The problem has been in the variation standards of oligospermia and lack of controls.

The Split Ejaculate

In the treatment of oligospermia, however, the use of the split ejaculate, at least theoretically, gives intracervical insemination some advantages over coitus. It is a natural method of sperm concentration. Having delivered the semen by split ejaculate, insemination must then be utilized to place sperm in proximity to the female reproductive tract. A concentrate reaches the endocervical canal.

Harvey was the first to point out that when a man ejaculates, approximately 80% of the sperm, and usually the more active ones, come out in the first half of the ejaculate, and the second half contains relatively few sperm.[7] Subsequently, many reports have confirmed this finding.[8,9] This process is reversed in about 5% of cases, so both partitions must still be examined before using one or the other. One study showed that postcoital tests were improved when the better portion of a split ejaculate was utilized for cervical insemination.[10] Therefore, there is not much to be gained in performing cervical insemination for oligospermia or a poor postcoital test without utilizing split ejaculate.

Technique

The purpose of AIH is to deposit semen into the intracervical canal. No more than 0.5 ml of semen should be placed into the cervix. Greater amounts than 0.5 ml may make their way into the endometrial cavity and cause severe cramps as well as an occasional episode of endometritis. One of the functions of the cervix is to act as a filter. If the physician uses a hollow cannula with an acorn tip (Fig. 23-1), the acorn can be held against the external os for 2 to 3 minutes after instilling the 0.5 ml. This ensures thorough mixing of the semen with the endocervical secretions in situ. The remainder of the semen is sprayed against the external os, and then the external os is positioned so as to rest in the pool of semen that collects in the lower blade of the Graves speculum. The patient remains in this position with the speculum in place for 10 to 15 minutes. At the end of that time the speculum is removed, and the patient remains in the resting position for another 10 to 15 minutes before leaving the treatment room.

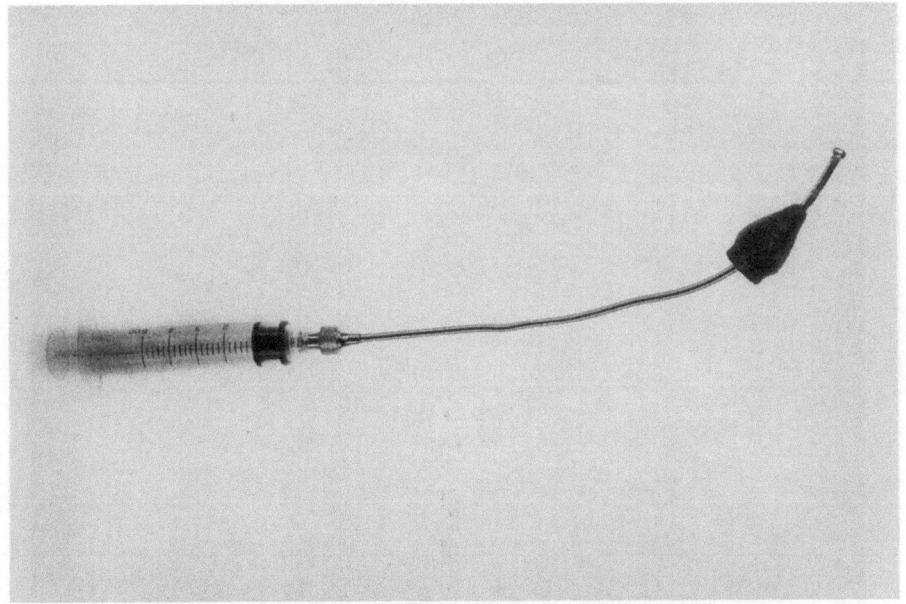

Figure 23-1. Cannula with acorn tip for use in cervical insemination.

The use of a cervical cap is an alternate approach. The cervical cap is placed on the cervix, the cap is filled by means of the stem that protrudes from the vaginal opening. This does not allow for direct intracervical insemination, and there is little evidence that the sperm in the cap are capable of causing fertilization after more than a few hours' residence in the cap.

Many physicians have stopped using the cap because the patients often have difficulty removing it, necessitating an emergency medical visit 6 to 8 hours later. An alternative is to insert a Fertilopack® as the speculum is removed (Fig. 23-2). The patient is instructed to remove this herself 3 or 4 hours later. There are no studies to indicate superiority of either method.

Ovulation timing

The careful assessment of ovulation timing is a prerequisite for artificial insemination, whether by donor or husband semen. Because often we are dealing with semen of less than optimal quality, this timing is probably more important in AIH. When dealing with oligospermia, because it takes 36 to 72 hours for semen quality to return to an optimum state after ejaculation, the physician is often limited to only one insemination a month. The sperm also probably does not survive as long as the high-quality semen used in donor insemination.

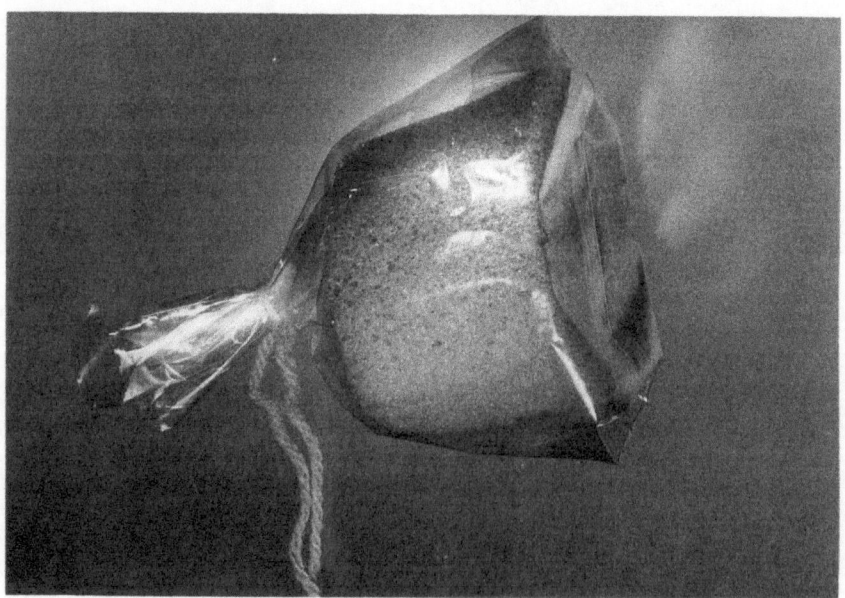

Figure 23-2. Fertilopak to maintain semen in contact with external os.

The patient must be on a basal body temperature chart, not to predict ovulation in a particular cycle, but to know that one has not gone beyond ovulation and to select the appropriate time for therapy in a subsequent cycle. Weir and Downs, in their description of the fertile period based on 200 conception cycles with a single exposure, described a fertile period extending from 4 days before temperature rise to 1 day after.[11] Ideally, one should use two treatments, the first, 2 days before the low point of the basal body temperature chart, and the second, on the day of the low point. When only one treatment is available, one should try to coincide the treatment with the low point of the basal temperature chart. If the cycle length varies by no more than 2 or 3 days, and two treatments a month are possible, one should attain proper timing in approximately four of six planned cycles. If there is more variance in cycle length, and thus, variability of the time of ovulation, the physician must resort to additional methods of predicting the onset of ovulation for purposes of insemination (see chapter 16).

Cervical Mucus

Changes in cervical mucus provide the simplest approach to predetermining ovulation. These changes are dependent on the preovulatory increase in estrogen production, which stimulates the endocervical glands to produce a rich watery mucus, high in glycogen mucin and salts. Thus, an assessment of spinnbarkeit, increased ability to stretch the mucus,[12] sodium chloride concentration,[13] glucose concentration,[14,15] and viscosity[16] are all methods that have been recommended. These are all quite helpful when there is not too much variation in cycle length. The end points are quite definite when cycles vary from only 25 to 35 days in length. In markedly irregular cycles, i.e., more than 35 days in length, there may be several peaks of estrogen secretion from the ovary, each not enough to trigger the preovulatory rise of luteinizing hormone (LH), but each still sufficient to cause preovulatory changes in cervical mucus. This is a failing common to all methods of ovulation production based on estrogen-related phenomena.

LH Assay

In 1946, Farris described a test for the predetermination of ovulation based on the occurrence of hypermia in rat ovaries that had been injected with an extract of midcycle urine.[17] Presumably, this represented a response to the preovulatory surge of LH. For the next few years, Farris described this as a successful method of predicting the day of ovulation. Although some therapists have utilized this test with some success,[18] others have been unable to duplicate his results,[19] and so this method to determine ovulation has been neither widely accepted nor continued.

The use of home LH assays, based on monoclonal antibodies has been reviewed in chapter 17, and it is the most practical aid at the present time as well as for advice concerning coitus.

The use of clomiphene citrate, menopausal gonadotropins, and human chorionic gonadotropins should be reserved for intrauterine insemination (IUI) where ovulation timing is more critical because of the loss of the reservoir function of cervical mucus.

Indications for AIH and Results

Among infertility specialists, the use of AIH remains controversial because in so many instances the results of therapy are so variable and in some instances seem discouraging (Table 23-1). A review of the literature published in 1979 gave an 18% mean pregnancy rate for oligospermia, while the mean spontaneous pregnancy rate in six other studies was 14%.[4] One reason for differences may be the variation of indications and the techniques utilized for AIH. Another important reason is that the various indications for therapy are not individually analyzed. Results related to faulty delivery of essentially normal sperm are, as would be expected, generally good; there is little controversy concerning its use in this area. But using AIH because of a cervical factor (hostile cervix), or because of oligospermia, is more open to question.

We reviewed our experience with AIH over an 8-year period, 1967 to 1975, and, along with the findings of others, have summarized them herewith.[5]

Faulty Delivery. Faulty delivery due to hypospadias, impotence, retrograde ejaculation, vaginismus, retroverted uterus, or small volume constitute ideal indications for AIH; unfortunately, these are not the common conditions. From a total of 57 patients treated with AIH over an 8-year period, only three cases fell into this category. Two conceived (Table 23-2). Larger studies also have reported pregnancy rates varying from 62.5% to 85% when AIH was carried out because of impotence.[22,23]

Table 23-1. AIH Results from the Literature

Author	Year	Total number of patients	Number pregnant	Percent	Technique
Mastroianni et al.[20]	1957	113	7	6	Vaginal cannula
Amelar and Hotchkiss[21]	1965	39	22	56	Split ejaculate
Perez-Pelaez and Cohen[22]	1965	38	10	26	Split ejaculate
Speichinger and Maddox[23]	1976	24	1	4	Cervical cap
Dixon et al.[24]	1976	158	15	10	Cap or split
Steiman and Taymor[5]	1977	57	17	29	Split ejaculate

Oligospermia and Subfertility. In oligospermia, the use of a split ejaculate lends some rationale to AIH.[7-9,25,26] Sperm density is usually higher in the first partition, although in 6% of cases, density was higher in the second. When one obtains a concentrate of sperm in a small volume, insemination is necessary. The fertility of the couple is often greatly improved when sperm concentration is doubled and there is no interference with motility. In our series, 5 of 22 couples with oligospermia (sperm count less than 20 million) conceived (see Table 23-2). This is not a startling result, and it is difficult to know what would be the spontaneous pregnancy rate at this level of sperm count. The data do suggest that it may be helpful in one out of four couples. Most reports include sperm counts of less than 40 million, and the incidence of pregnancies with split ejaculate AIH varied between 26.3% and 56%.[21,22]

Poor Postcoital Test. The use of AIH in couples with persistently poor postcoital tests is also controversial. If there is a dry or stenotic cervix, it is appropriate to bypass the lower cervix and perform high cervical insemination. When there is no stenosis and the mucus is normal, when there is a normal sperm count and no immune factor, it is difficult to establish a rationale for the procedure. To identify the patient who might benefit, the physician should carry out an insemination and, 6 to 8 hours later, a postcoital test. If there has been an improvement in the postcoital test, the physician might proceed. A split ejaculate is not required.

In couples with persistently poor postcoital tests, despite fertile semen specimens, 8 of 25 (32%) conceived (see Table 23-2). The results from the literature vary from 6.2%[19] to 70%.[26] It is exceedingly difficult to evaluate the results of cervical insemination treatment because of the difference in technique. Indications vary and length of treatment is an important determinant of success. Split ejaculation may or may not be used. In a review of the literature Corson noted an overall 17.5% rate with AIH treatment, along with a spontaneous pregnancy rate of 12.2%.[3] This does not seem to be a great difference, but it must be taken into consideration that the treated patients conceived within a few months while the spontaneous pregnancy rate occurred over a 2-year follow-up. The ability to accelerate the process, at least, is meaningful to the

Table 23-2. Indications for AIH and Resultant Pregnancies[a]

Indications	No. of cases	No. of pregnancies
Faulty delivery	3	2
Oligospermia (sperm count less than 20 million)	22	5
Subfertile semen	7	2
Poor postcoital test	25	8
Total	57	17 (29.8%)

[a]From Steinman and Taymor.[5]

couple. It would appear then that with proper indications and technique AIH has a role in infertility therapy.

INTRAUTERINE INSEMINATION

IUI has been utilized sporadically through the years, but has been avoided by most physicians because of the fact that whole semen in the uterus can cause severe cramping as well as an infection. Barwin reported a 67% conception rate for oligospermia utilizing IUI, but the cervical canal was also injected with semen in these patients. Three patients had to be hospitalized for severe cramps.[27]

The recent development of advanced techniques for handling sperm utilized in in vitro fertilization programs has eliminated the problem of cramps and infection and has reawakened interest in the use of IUI.[28]

Indications

The purpose of IUI is either to bypass an endocervical canal that is not functioning or, as in cases of oligospermia, to bring about an increased concentration of motile sperm closer to the fallopian tubes.

The indications for IUI are listed in Table 23-3. By cervical factor, one means a poor postcoital test arising from various causes in the face of normal semen, good timing, and lack of antibodies. These causes could be cervical stenosis, lack of preovulatory cervical mucus secretion, or an unexplained poor postcoital test.

There is no consensus as to what constitutes oligospermia, and the variation in the patient selection in the literature adds to the difficulty in assessing the efficacy of this form of treatment.[29] Most reports involve sperm counts under 40 million, but some use 20 million or even 10 million as the top level to be included. Patients with poor sperm motility, asthenospermia, with or without oligospermia, are usually treated as well.

Table 23-3. Indications for Intrauterine Insemination

Cervical factor
Oligospermia or oligoasthenia
Immune factor
Unexplained infertility

Table 23-4. Flow Sheet for IUI

Divide semen into two Falcon tubes (unless <1 ml)
Add equal amounts of media
Mix thoroughly (particularly if there is much mucus)
Centrifuge 5 minutes at 300 G. Increase to 10 minutes if pellets are poor
Draw off supernatant (use sterile pipette)
Add 1 ml media to each, mix, combine pellets
Centrifuge 5 minutes
Remove supernatant
Add 0.75 ml media for insemination
Rinse Tef-Cat with media
Pick up semen directly with rinsed Tef-Cat
Examine postwash motility

Immune factors include both male and female. Until recently, testing has been uncertain, so in older studies the case selection may be uncertain as well.

The definition of unexplained infertility also varies, but usually assisted reproductive technology such as IUI has been reserved for couples who remain infertile for at least 3 years after a complete negative infertility workup.

Technique of IUI

The basic steps of technique are to "wash" the sperm by centrifuging the mixture of semen and sterile nutritive media once or twice, decanting the supernatant, and suspending the sperm in a small amount of media. There are variations in the type of media used, and in the number of washings. Some centers use the swim-up method for collecting only the active sperm; others do not. For normal sperm that is to be utilized in cervical cases or unexplained infertility, no special handling other than centrifuging is required. Specialized techniques, such as Percoll® gradients, are often utilized to concentrate oligospermic specimens. It is important to use sterile technique and to avoid too strong a force with centrifugation.

A typical flow is shown in Table 23-4. The media used in this system is a Hams F-10 media containing Hepes solution to protect against a change in pH (Irvine Scientific). The final pellet is mixed with approximately 0.5 ml of media for insemination. Many types of catheters have been designed and are available commercially. A flexible polyethylene catheter (Tef-Cat™)* suffices for the majority of cases. For patients with sharp angulation or with marked cervical stenosis, a hollow plastic tube with a hollow steel insert may be needed (Shephard)*. A tenaculum applied gently to the cervix to straighten out the uterine angle often aids in a difficult insertion. The patient lies on her back for 10 or 15 minutes and is then ready to leave the office or clinic. No cap or pack is necessary.

*Cook Ob/Gyn, Spenser, Indiana.

Timing of Insemination

Cervical insemination has one advantage over IUI in that if the cervical mucus is adequate, the reservoir function of cervical mucus is present. Sperm can survive for a day or two in the mucus, and they can make their way from time to time up into the uterus and tubes. Accuracy of timing is not as vital. In IUI, however, this reservoir function is not utilized, and some form of ovulation detection or augmentation is required.

The simplest approach at the present time is to use the home LH kits. The first color change occurs usually 28 hours before ovulation. Therefore, the optimum time for insemination is the next morning. Since there is a 25% error in this form of ovulation prediction, it probably would be more prudent to also treat on the day of the first color change as well as daily over the next 2 days.

Ovulation timing with clomiphene citrate (CC) or human menopausal gonadotropins (HMG) combined with human chorionic gonadotropin (HCG) along with ultrasound monitoring is a more certain way to have accurate insemination timing.

CC is given in a dose of 100 mg daily, from the 5th to the 9th day of the cycle. Starting on day 12, ultrasound examination of the ovary is performed every other day until the lead follicle reaches 20 mm. At this point HCG is given, 5000 IU, usually in the evening. Insemination can then be carried out 32 to 35 hours after the administration of HCG, two mornings later. To be more certain, the insemination can be carried out the day after the HCG administration as well.

The use of HMG/HCG seems to be more effective. However, this approach requires daily injections, closer monitoring to prevent multiple pregnancies and ovarian hyperstimulation, and is more expensive. Table 23-5 demonstrates one study in which there was a marked increase in fecundity in patients given HMG/HCG (14% per cycle) over cc treatment and the natural cycle (2% per

Table 23-5. Treatment and MPO with IUI during Spontaneous Cycles, CC Cycles, CC or HMG/HCG Cycles, and HMG/HCG Cycles[a]

Ovulation	Patients	Cycles	Pregnancy	MPO
Spontaneous	76	186	4	0.022[b]
Ovulation management	44	105	9	0.085[b]
Clomiphene citrate (CC)	9	13	1	0.077
CC or HMG/HCG	34	64	4	0.063
HMG/HCG	14	28	4	0.143

[a]From Kemmann et al.[40] MPO = monthly probability of frequency occurrence.
[b]$P<0.02$.

cycle).[41] This increase is undoubtedly due to both improved timing and the availability of more than one mature oocyte. Another possible beneficial effect of HMG may be its stimulating effect on cervical mucus. The patients should be advised to have coitus on the morning after the HCG injection and then the IUI the following morning, essentially 35 hours after the HCG. Coitus the day before may cover an early ovulation due to a spontaneous surge of LH.

Results

As in AIH, the results of IUI are often difficult to evaluate because of the variation in case selection, the variation in methodology, and the failure to use controls. Therefore, there is still a degree of controversy as to the efficacy of this time-consuming and expensive form of treatment.[26]

Tables 23-6 to 23-9 demonstrate the results from some of the many reports that have been published since 1985 on the four main indications for IUI: cervical factor, oligospermia, immune infertility, and unexplained infertility.

The best results are obtained in the treatment of cervical factor and unexplained unfertility, with overall success rates of 31% and 32%, respectively (Tables 23-6 and 23-9). It usually takes a minimum of three cycles to reach these rates.

The results of oligospermia are the most difficult to evaluate because some centers use sperm counts of less than 40 million as an indication, while others use less than 20 million or even less than 10 million as the indicator for treatment. Still others use even higher counts than 40 million. Others will treat patients if the motility is less than 40% (oligoasthenia). It is not surprising, then, that the results vary from 0% to 43% (overall 21%) (Table 23-7). More rigidly selected and controlled studies will be required to assess the true worth of IUI in oligospermia.

Table 23-6. IUI Results in Cervical Factor

Author	Year	Number of cases	Pregnancies	Percent	Ovulation augmentation
Toffler et al.[30]	1985	10	2	2	No
Wiltbank et al.[31]	1985	20	5	25	No
Confino et al.[32]	1986	18	12	67	No
Hall et al.[33]	1986	19	3	16	No
Quagliarello and Arny[34]	1986	30	6	20	No
Byrd et al.[35]	1987	29	10	34	No
Total		125	38	31	

Table 23-7. IUI Results in Male Factor

Author	Year	Number of cases	Pregnancy	Percent	Ovulation augmentation
Toffler et al.[30]	1985	10	2	20	No
Wiltbank et al.[31]	1985	17	0	0	No
Hoing et al.[36]	1986	53	9	14	Yes
Cruz et al.[37]	1986	7	1	14	Yes
Byrd et al.[35]	1987	21	9	43	No
Cummings[38]	1988	20	5	20	No
Pardo et al.[39]	1988	99	21	21	No
Total		227	47	21	

The results of IUI for immune factors are also marginal, but pregnancies do occur (Table 23-8). It appears to be more successful if the antibodies are in the female tissues, whereas there is less success when antibodies are attached to the sperm.

Ovulation augmentation is now frequently used in the treatment of unexplained infertility.[40–42] The reports suggest a real advantage when this approach is utilized, probably because of the better timing of the insemination and the availability of multiple mature oocytes. It is possible that ovarian augmentation in connection with the other indications might improve the results for these indications as well.

In summary, despite the controversy and uncertainty, IUI appears to yield a significant number of pregnancies in certain conditions, and it should be a treatment step in many patients before proceeding to in vitro fertilization, gamete intrafallopian tube transfer, or AID.

Table 23-8. IUI Results in Immune Factors

Author	Year	Number of cases	Pregnancy	Percent	Ovulation augmentation
Toffler et al.[30]	1985	6	1	16	No
Wiltbank et al.[31]	1985	8	2	25	No
Confino et al.[32]	1986	18	5	28	No
Byrd et al.[35]	1987	15	1	6.7	No
Total		47	9	19	

Table 23-9. IUI Results in Unexplained Infertility

Author	Year	Number of cases	Pregnancy	Percent	Ovulation augmentation
Byrd et al.[35]	1987	14	6	38	No
Dodson et al.[40]	1987	46	12	26	Yes
Kemmann et al.[41]	1987	14	4	25	Yes
Serhal et al.[42]	1988	22	9	41	Yes
Total		96	31	32	

REFERENCES

1. Roehleder H: *Test Tube Babies*. New York, Vantage, 1934
2. Schellen AMCM: *Artificial Insemination in the Human*. New York, Elsevier, 1957
3. Corson SL, Batzer FF: Homologous artificial insemination. *J Reprod Med* 26:231, 1981
4. Nachtigall RD, Faura N, Glass RH: Artificial insemination of husband's sperm. *Fertil Steril* 32:141, 1979
5. Steinman RP, Taymor ML: Artificial insemination homologous and its role in the management of infertility. *Fertil Steril* 28:146, 1947
6. Glass RH, Ericcson RJ: Spontaneous cure of male infertility. *Fertil Steril* 31:305, 1979
7. Harvey C, Jackson MJ: A method of concentrating spermatozoa in human semen. *J Clin Path* 8:341, 1955
8. Amelar RD, Hotchkiss RS: The split ejaculate: Its use in the management of male infertility. *Fertil Steril* 16:46, 1965
9. Eliasson R, Lindholmer C: Distribution of spermatozoa in different fractions of split ejaculates. *Fertil Steril* 23:252, 1972
10. Adoni A, Palti Z: Better post-coital tests for oligospermic patients using split ejaculate artificial insemination. *Fertil Steril* 31:587, 1979
11. Weir W, Downs T: The optimal time for conception. *Fertil Steril* 19:64, 1968
12. Marcus LS, Marcus CC: Cervical mucus and its relation to infertility. *Obstet Gynecol Survey* 18:749, 1963
13. McSweeney DJ, Sbarra AJ: A new cervical mucus test for hormonal appraisal. *Am J Obstet Gynecol* 88:705, 1964
14. Doyle JB, Ewers FJ, Sapit D: A new fertility testing tape. *JAMA* 172:1744, 1960
15. Siegler AM: The cervical glucose as an indicator of ovulation. *Am J Obstet Gynecol* 79:1169, 1960
16. Kosasky HJ: A tackimeter for the determination of tackiness of cervical mucus. *Fertil Steril* 28:354, 1977
17. Farris EJ: A test for determining the time of ovulation in conception in women. *Am J Obstet Gynecol* 52:14, 1946
18. Murphy D, Torrano E: Day of conception in relation to length of menstrual cycle: A study of 65 conceptions resulting from isolated coitus. *Fertil Steril* 15:385, 1964
19. Levin L, Buxton CL, Engle ET: On the validity of the hyperemia method for determining ovulation time in women. *Am J Obstet Gynecol* 58:795, 1945
20. Mastroianni L, Laberge JL, Rock J: Appraisal of the efficacy of artificial insemination with husband's sperm and evaluation of insemination techniques. *Fertil Steril* 8:620, 1957
21. Amelar RD, Hotchkiss RS: The split ejaculate. Its use in the management of male infertility. *Fertil Steril* 16:46, 1965

22. Perez-Pelaez M, Cohen MR: The split ejaculate in homologous insemination. *Int J Fertil* 10:25, 1965
23. Speichinger JP, Mattox JH: Homologous artificial insemination and oligospermia. *Fertil Steril* 27:135, 1976
24. Dixon RE, Buttram VC, Schum CW: Artificial insemination using homologous semen: A review of 158 cases. *Fertil Steril* 27:647, 1976
25. Lindholmer CH: Survival of human spermatozoa in different fractions of split ejaculate. *Fertil Steril* 24:521, 1973
26. Farris EJ, Murphy DP: The characteristics of the two parts of the partitioned ejaculate and the advantages of its use for intrauterine insemination. *Fertil Steril* 11:465, 1960
27. Barwin BW: Intrauterine insemination of husband's semen. *J Reprod Fertil* 39:101, 1974
28. Marro RP, Varguas JM, Saito H, Gibbons WE, Berger T, Mishell DRV: Clinical applications of techniques used in human in-vitro research. *Am J Obstet Gynecol* 146:477, 1983
29. Allen NC, Herbert CM, Maxson WS, Rogers BJ, Diamond MP, Wentz AC: Intrauterine insemination: A critical review. *Fertil Steril* 44:569, 1985
30. Toffler RC, Nagel TC, Tagetz GE, Phansly SA, Okagaki T, Warrin CA: Intrauterine insemination: The University of Minnesota experience. *Fertil Steril* 43:743, 1985
31. Wiltbank MC, Kosasa S, Rogers B: Treatment of infertile patients by intrauterine insemination of washed spermatozoa. *Andrologia* 17:22, 1985
32. Confino E, Friberg J, Dudbiewicz AB, Gleicher N: Intrauterine insemination with washed human spermatozoa. *Fertil Steril* 46:155, 1986
33. Hall ME, Magyar DM, Vasquea JM, Hayes MF, Moghissi KS: Experience with intrauterine insemination for cervical factor and oligospermia. *Am J Obstet Gynecol* 151:1333, 1986
34. Quagliarello J, Arny M: Intracervical versus intrauterine insemination: Correlation of outcome with antecedent post-coital testing. *Fertil Steril* 46:870, 1986
35. Byrd W, Ackerman GS, Carr BR, Edman CD, Gazick DS, McConnell JD: Treatment of refractory infertility by transcervical intrauterine insemination with washed sperm. *Fertil Steril* 48:921, 1987
36. Hoing L, Devroey P, Van Steirtoghen AC: Treatment of infertility because of oligosasthenoteratospermia by transcervical intrauterine insemination of motile spermatozoa. *Fertil Steril* 45:388, 1986
37. Cruz RI, Kemmann E, Brandeis VT, Becker KA, Beck M, Beardsley L, Sheldon R: A prospective study of intrauterine insemination of processed sperm for males with oligoasthenospermia in super ovulated women. *Fertil Steril* 46:673, 1986
38. Cummings DC: Pregnancy rates following intrauterine insemination with washed or unwashed sperm. 49:745, 1988
39. Pardo M, Barr PN, Bancella N, Cordeu B, Buxaderas J, Pomerol JM, Sabater J: Spermatozoa selection on discontinuous Percoll grolants for use in artificial insemination. *Fertil Steril* 49:505, 1988
40. Dodson WC, Whitesides DB, Hughes CL, Easley HA, Haney AF: Superovulation with intrauterine insemination in the treatment of infertility: A possible alternative to gamete intrafallopian transfer and in-vitro fertilization. *Fertil Steril* 48:444, 1987
41. Kemmann E, Bohrer R, Sheldon G, Fiascorro G, Beardsley L: Active ovulation management increases the monthly probability of pregnancy occurrence in ovulatory women who receive intrauterine inseminating. *Fertil Steril* 48:916, 1987
42. Serhal PF, Katz M, Little V, Woronowski H: Unexplained infertility—the value of Pergonal superovulation combined with intrauterine insemination. *Fertil Steril* 49:602, 1988

CHAPTER 24

Therapeutic Donor Insemination (Artificial Insemination Donor)

Artificial insemination has been known to man for centuries. Since the late 19th century it has been utilized extensively for breeding of farm animals. In humans, the experience until this century was primarily with husband insemination. When, in the early part of this century, the first reports of the use of a donor appeared, they were greeted by a storm of indignation. Only in the last 50 years has therapeutic donor insemination (TDI) been sufficiently widespread that it is now accepted as more than just a controversial medical curiosity. In the Western world, the number of children available for adoption has decreased because of changing attitudes toward abortion and toward single parenthood. This has led many couples to view TDI as the only source for the relief of their childlessness.

This procedure—charged as it is with emotional, cultural, and religious overtones—places a tremendous responsibility on the physician.[1] He or she has, first of all, the responsibility to the patient, and must respect and attempt to satisfy the woman's great desire to bear a child, as well as the mutual desire of the couple. Equally important is the responsibility to the child, to ensure that the child will grow up in a climate of affection and emotional stability. Finally, the physician is responsible to the therapy itself; his or her standards and ethics should be such that therapeutic donor insemination will continue to be a respected form of scientific therapy.

Since the decision to have donor insemination involves such emotionally laden areas as sexuality, marriage, and the husband's self-image, the physician is justified in being concerned about the possibility of psychological sequelae.

PSYCHOLOGICAL CONSIDERATIONS

Most women have a strong drive toward the significantly emotional events of pregnancy and motherhood.[2,3] One Freudian observer, noting that 40% of women conceiving by TDI believed that their child resembled their father, uncle, or brother, interpreted this as indicating latent fears of incestuous behavior.

On the positive side, for the female, this is her opportunity to physically experience pregnancy, labor, and motherhood, and lay to rest any lingering doubts concerning her femininity.[4]

For the husband, of course, the situation is more difficult. He can take comfort in the thought that, by agreeing to donor insemination, he is giving his wife the supreme sign of his love and concern. One would thus expect that on such a firm basis, a good marital relationship can continue.

There are few studies on the long-term outcome of TDI, chiefly because the treatment works better with secrecy. In 1959, however, Haman reported on a follow-up of 216 insemination babies and cited fewer parental problems than with adoption.[5] In 1966, Behrman and Gosling reported only two cases of emotional disturbance in 393 successful pregnancies,[6] although a report 10 years later indicated a higher degree of emotional consequences.[7] Eighty percent of the husbands interviewed had guilt feelings about what they perceived as their ability to fulfill the expectations of their families and society. Most of the wives also felt guilty because they did not share their husband's failure in the reproductive process. During pregnancy, most couples reported a decrease in the frequency of coitus. Nevertheless, here, as in other studies, there were few long-term problems.

These studies demonstrate that, with the proper selection of only strongly motivated couples who mutually arrive at the decision for TDI in full accord, there should be few serious psychological dangers.

LEGAL ASPECTS

TDI is an acceptable form of therapy in most Western countries. Until recently, few states have had any laws pertaining to this form of treatment. However, in 1987 Andrews published an extensive summary of new legislation that has taken place over the past few years.[8] Half of the states require written consent from the husband, and a majority indicated that the husband is the legal father. Other state laws legislate that the donor is not the legal father, and that the physician is required to file information with the state about acquired immune deficiency syndrome (AIDS) as well as provide processes for confidentiality. It can be hoped that more and more states will pass these laws, which for the most part are necessary for the physician, patient, and donor. Pending this, a physician must take steps to protect himself. The best protection is the proper selection of patients, and limiting the procedure to situations where both the husband and wife not only fully agree but are anxious to have the therapy. Some form of consent or agreement from both husband and wife should be obtained, even though there is some question about the legal implications of such documents. It is best for the women to be delivered by an obstetrician who is unaware of the method of insemination, so that he can sign the birth certificate without committing perjury.

SECRECY FOR ARTIFICIAL INSEMINATION DONORS

For many years most physicians have felt that secrecy is an important part of TDI for emotional health for both the child and for the couple. Except in azoospermia, there is always a possibility that the husband is the father and the couple should be encouraged to recognize this possibility. In recent years there has been a somewhat changing attitude concerning secrecy, particularly among geneticists and a number of social workers. Also because of the recognition of more transmissible diseases, there has been a move toward long-term record keeping. There is no evidence of increased incidence of congenital abnormalities,[9] and to risk emotional problems on such rare conditions that are usually untreatable seems like an overreaction. As far as record keeping is concerned, one would hope that such records would be kept in a manner to respect the secrecy of the child, parents, and donor. In my experience, secrecy has helped in the stability of the family unit as attested to by frequent requests for a second or third child.

INDICATIONS

The most common indication for TDI is severe oligospermia or azoospermia. It is estimated that 15% of marriages are sterile, and in 20% of these there is a serious male factor. This theoretically places the number of potential patients for donor insemination in the millions. As far as oligospermia is concerned, it is impossible to set any arbitrary level of semen quality. With moderate oligospermia, after a series of trials with homologous insemination, donor therapy is often requested, and this is reasonable. Rh compatibility has been a recognized indication, more so in the past than now. Hereditary congenital anomalies in the husband constitute one group of indications. Another group would be males with circulating antibodies. Indications from a series of 107 cases are shown in Table 24-1.

SELECTION OF DONORS

Until recently, most physicians utilized selected groups of young professionals. Aside from taking a history of chronic familial diseases and matching the husband as far as hair and eye coloring was concerned, little attention was paid to screening for a wide variety of sexually transmitted diseases.

One still does match physical characteristics to the husband, but the problem of acquired immunodeficiency syndrome (AIDS) has awakened the profession to the potential infections with a host of pathogens.[10] In a recent review, Greenblatt and her co-workers listed the potential infections, the likelihood of each having an effect upon the pregnancy fetus, along with their recommendations for screening.[11] In 1986, the American Fertility Society (AFS) published extensive guidelines for screening donors for TDI.[12] The history taking involves screening in order to eliminate groups that are at high risk for AIDS, and those with a long history of genital infections. They recommend initial screening tests for cytomegalovirus, *Neisseria, Chlamydia*, and hepatitis B. When fresh semen is to be used they recommend an initial serum screening for AIDS antibodies. If negative, repeated tests are to be performed every 6 months for active donors. If frozen semen is to be utilized, they recommend an initial screening test for AIDS. If negative, specimens can be collected and frozen. The donor is tested again in 60 days, and the specimens released only if the results at this time are negative. In 1988, however, because of the increasing awareness of the risk of AIDS, the AFS recommended that only frozen sperm be utilized in TDI, and that the quarantine period be increased to 180 days.[13]

Table 24-1. TDI Applied in Various Indications[a]

Indication	Number of cases
Azoospermia	56
Severe oligospermia	42
Ejaculatory incompetence	1
Retrograde ejaculation	1
Impotence	2
X-ray exposure	2
Rh or ABO incompatibility	3
Total	107

[a]From Chong and Taymor.[23]

There is no doubt about the fact that the potential for transmitting the AIDS virus by donor insemination has made a tremendous impact on this mode of therapy.[12] Before the risk was known, a number of women had been infected with the use of semen from apparently men infected with AIDS. With recognition of the problem, it is now a rare although still serious hazard of therapeutic donor insemination.

For physicians who use fresh semen, donors who are at risk for AIDS should still be excluded: homosexuals, drug users, men with numerous sexual partners. Indeed, married men with proven fertility are the best donors. An initial test for the human immunodeficiency virus (HIV) is carried out for any donation, and then the test should be repeated at 6-month intervals. Even this does not exclude the danger of infections since seroconversion may take up to 12 weeks.[11] Although it has been stated that a negative HIV test in an individual with no risk factor can virtually exclude HIV infection,[14] one may have to resort to the use of frozen sperm to achieve even more confidence of safety.

FRESH VERSUS FROZEN SPERM

In the early 1960s, with advances in methodology came a surging interest in the use of frozen semen and sperm banks, although the practice had been with us since the 18th century.[15] Over the next 20 years, frozen sperm was used with varying frequency. It certainly has been proved to be effective and safe with acceptable anomaly and abortion rates.[16] The advantages of frozen sperm are the increased safety as far as AIDS is concerned, and the availability for those practitioners who do not have access to fresh sperm. The disadvantages are the lower success rates (see results) and inability of the physician to personally select the donor.

TECHNIQUE

The technique of insemination for donor semen is essentially the same as that for husband's semen (see chapter 23). Intracervical instillation of no more than 0.5 ml is carried out, and the remainder is left in the vagina. A Fertilopak may be used if desired. There is no need for split ejaculate, intrauterine insemination, or cervical caps. After removal of the speculum, the patient lies on the table for an additional 15 to 20 minutes.

Some authors recommend mixing the husband's semen to that of the donor so that the couple will not know which spermatozoa actually fertilized the ovum. Encouraging coitus on the evening of the treatment would seem not to dilute the sperm and yet provide some psychological and possible physiologic benefits. However, Quinlavin and Sullivan described immobilizing and agglutinating effects of husband's semen on donor sperm and not only recommended avoidance of mixing, but even abstinence for a few days.[17]

TIMING

Ideally, insemination should be carried out 2 days before the low point of the basal body temperature chart and on the day of the low point.[18] This should cover a 4-day period and should suffice in most regular cycles (26 to 30 days). When the cycles are more irregular, there is nothing to prevent the use of more frequent insemination. With a greater degree of irregularity of ovulation, the methods of determining and forcing ovulation described in chapter 17 can be utilized. With continued failure intrauterine insemination along with ovulation enhancement may ultimately be needed. In one study the use of the home luteinizing hormone kits did not improve the results.[19]

RESULTS

Table 24-2 lists six of the larger series reported from 1959 to 1982 in which the overall results are fairly uniform, ranging from 67% to 76% success provided that preliminary infertility screening had been carried out. In contrast, in a report where no screening was done, the success rate was only 45%. The majority of conceptions occur within the first three cycles and 86% to 95% by the sixth cycle. If the physician is persistent, conceptions do occur later, and patience ultimately may be rewarded. A number of patients who would conceive fail to do so if they do not go at least six cycles. However, before proceeding beyond six cycles, a laparoscopy is indicated.

As experience has developed with the use of frozen sperm, sufficient data have become available to compare the results of frozen sperm with fresh. At the

Table 24-2. Overall Results of TDI

Study	Year	Total	Conceptions (%)
Behrman[20]	1959	168	75
Haman[5]	1959	399	76
Murphy and Torrano[21]	1966	112	68
Warren[22]	1974	490	69
Chong and Taymor[23]	1975	107	72
Dixon and Buttram[24]	1975	171	44
Aiman[25]	1982	78	67

present time, the majority of studies do find that frozen sperm is less effective,[26,27] although one report suggested that the thawed specimen contained a minimum of 40 million sperm with grade 3 motility—frozen sperm was as good as fresh.[28] No doubt, with time, the methodology will improve sufficiently to bring the efficacy of frozen sperm on a par with fresh.

REFERENCES

1. Rubin B: Psychological aspects of human artificial insemination. *Arch Gen Psychiatry* 13:121, 1965
2. Beck W: A critical look at the legal, ethical and technical aspects of artificial insemination. *Fertil Steril* 27:1, 1976
3. Benedeck T: The organization of reproductive drive. *Int J Psychoanal* 41:1, 1960
4. Deutsch H: Psychology of pregnancy, labor and puerperiun. In Greenhill JP (ed): *Obstetrics*, 11th ed. Philadelphia, WB Saunders, 1955
5. Haman JO: Therapeutic donor insemination. *Calif Med* 90:130, 1959
6. Behrman SJ, Gosling J: *Fundamentals of Gynecology*, 2nd ed. New York, Oxford University Press, 1966, p 35
7. Avidan D: Artificial insemination donor: Clinical and psychological aspects. *Fertil Steril* 27:528, 1976
8. Andrews LB: Ethical and legal aspects of in-vitro fertilization and artificial insemination by donor. *Urol Clin North Am* 14:633, 1987
9. Verp M, Cohen MR, Simpson L: Necessity of genetic screening in AID. *Obstet Gynecol* 62:474, 1983
10. Peterson EP: Artificial insemination by donor: A new look. *Fertil Steril* 46:4, 1986
11. Greenblatt RM, Handsfield HH, Sawyers MH, Holmes KK: Screening therapeutic insemination donors for transmitted diseases: Overview and recommendations. *Fertil Steril* 46:351, 1986
12. American Fertility Society: New guidelines for the use of semen donor insemination. *Fertil Steril* 46 (Suppl 2), 1986
13. American Fertility Society: Revised new guidelines for the use of semen-donor insemination. *Fertil Steril* 49:211, 1988
14. Ho DI, Sarngadhram MG, Resnick L, Dimarzo-Veronesa F, Rota T, Hirsch M: Primary human T-lymphotrophic virus type III infection. *Ann Intern Med* 103:880, 1985
15. Sherman J: Research on frozen human semen: Past, present and future. *Fertil Steril* 15:485, 1964
16. Sherman JK: Synopsis of the use of frozen human semen since 1964: State of the art human semen banking. *Fertil Steril* 24:397, 1973
17. Quinlavin WL, Sullivan H: The immunologic effects of husband's semen on donor spermatozoa during mixed insemination. *Fertil Steril* 28:448, 1977
18. Murphy D, Torrano E: The day of conception: A study of 48 women having 2 or more conceptions by donor insemination. *Fertil Steril* 14:410, 1963
19. Kossoy LR, Hill GA, Herbert CM, Brodes BL, Dalgish CS, Dupont WD, Wantz AC: Therapeutic donor insemination: The aspects of insemination timing with the aid of a urinary luteinizing hormone immunoassay. *Fertil Steril* 49:1626, 1988
20. Behrman SJ: Artificial insemination. *Fertil Steril* 10:248, 1959
21. Murphy D, Torrano E: Donor insemination: A study of 112 women. *Fertil Steril* 17:273, 1966
22. Warren MP: Artificial insemination: Review after 32 years of experience. *NY State J Med* 74:2538, 1974

23. Chong AP, Taymor ML: Sixteen years' experience with therapeutic donor insemination. *Fertil Steril* 26:791, 1975
24. Dixon R, Buttram VC: Artificial insemination using donor semen: A review of 171 cases. *Fertil Steril* 27:2, 1975
25. Aiman J: Factors affecting the success of donor insemination. *Fertil Steril* 37:94, 1982
26. Smith KD, Rochriguez-Rigau LJ, Steinberger E: The influence of ovulatory dysfunction and timing of insemination on the success of artificial donor (AID) with fresh or cryopreserved sperm. *Fertil Steril* 36:496, 1981
27. Richter M, Haning RV, Shapiro SS: Artificial donor insemination: Fresh versus frozen semen: The patient as her own control. *Fertil Steril* 41:277, 1984
28. Bordson BL, Ricci E, Dickey RP, Dunaway H, Taylor SN, Curole DN: Comparison of fecundability with fresh and frozen semen in therapeutic donor insemination. *Fertil Steril* 46:466, 1986

CHAPTER 25

Treatment of Luteal Phase Defect

In the chapter on the workup of the ovulatory factor, the difficulty in the diagnosis of the disturbed luteal phase was emphasized. Not only do multiple physiologic disorders probably cause the upset, but often the upset apparently comes and goes, occurring during one cycle but not another. These create difficulties in diagnosis, make rational therapy problematic, and, in particular, its evaluation almost impossible. Nevertheless, the luteal phase deficiency factor in infertility has been recognized for many years, and a number of treatment programs have been recommended.[1,2]

GENERAL THERAPY

Before resorting to direct treatment of the deficient corpus luteum, or the endometrium, the physician should make every effort to cure any underlying general disorder if it is the cause of this relative ovulatory defect.

Polycystic ovarian disease, or milder forms of adrenal androgenic hyperplasia, is usually accompanied by anovulation or amenorrhea, because of the inhibiting action of excess androgens at the hypothalamic or pituitary level. Occasionally the inhibitory effect is incomplete; ovulation occurs, but there is sufficient inhibition to affect the quality of corpus luteum function. Thyroid deficiency, nutritional deficiency, and emotional tension are other causes of luteal phase deficiency that are amenable to treatment. Hyperprolactinemia is another cause of luteal phase deficiency, and it responds well to Parlodel®* 2.5 to 5.0 mg daily.[3]

If no *specific* causes are found, as in most cases, the two present treatments of choice are clomiphene citrate and progesterone. It is impossible to say which of these two methods is superior. No parallel series have been reported; probably the previously mentioned inconsistencies in diagnosis make such a study impossible.

CLOMIPHENE CITRATE

Clomiphene citrate stimulates ovulation by allowing the release of gonadotropins, follicle-stimulating hormone (FSH), and luteinizing hormone (LH). The logical reason for using clomiphene in the treatment of luteal phase deficiency is based on those studies demonstrating a deficiency of FSH in the follicular phase of the cycle in cycles with short luteal phases[4] (see Fig. 11-7). It has been postulated that the low levels of FSH in the first part of the cycle result in an inadequate follicle that ovulates but becomes a poor corpus luteum with deficient progesterone production. Treatment with clomiphene increases FSH, which improves folliculogenesis. This results in a more normal corpus luteum with more suitable progesterone production.[5] However, the majority of cycles in which treatment has been carried out are not significantly shortened. The diagnosis is usually made by a combination of poor basal body temperature chart, lowered progesterone levels, or an endometrium that is out of phase. On the contrary, cycles such as these are often found to have a relatively low LH surge at midcycle following normal FSH stimulation. Still others show a lowered tonic release of LH during the luteal phase.[6]

The definitive work of Downs and Gibson demonstrated that clomiphene was only effective when the endometrial biopsy was 5 days or more out of phase,[7] the situation more frequently found with short luteal phase (Fig. 25-1). Milder degrees of luteal phase deficiency did not respond as well to clomiphene therapy.

Thus, in selecting clomiphene therapy, the therapist should be aware of the variability of the pathophysiology, the length of the luteal phase, as well as the mechanism of action of the different medications involved and, with this in mind, should select clomiphene as the optimal therapy only in the short luteal phase. Poor results—and a pessimistic attitude toward all clomiphene citrate therapy—are more likely if clomiphene is used for *all* types of luteal phase defects. There are few studies available that have really evaluated its efficacy.[7] One study in which eight patients with short luteal phase were treated with clomiphene, seven pregnancies occurred.[8] In another where no attention was

*Parlodel®, Sandoz, East Hanover, New Jersey.

paid to the luteal phase, the success rate with clomiphene was only 21%.[9] Furthermore, as in all therapy with clomiphene, the therapist must be alert to its adverse effects on the cervical mucus,[10] and if this occurs, treat the condition with small doses of estrogen or even intrauterine insemination.

PROGESTERONE

In luteal phase deficiency, there is a degree of progestational endometrial effect, but the endometrium is not sufficiently stimulated. Here, the condition is obviously associated with a progesterone deficiency.

Jones was one of the earliest to prescribe progesterone for luteal phase deficiency.[2] In an excellent review of the subject, she outlined the pathophysiology in treatment of this condition.[6] She believes strongly that progesterone, itself, should be administered, since synthetic progestins have been shown to suppress corpus luteum function.[11] Therefore, she recommends the use of progesterone vaginal or rectal suppositories, 25 mg, twice daily, starting 2 or 3 days after the basal body temperature rise.

My preference is to start with one suppository daily beginning 2 or 3 days

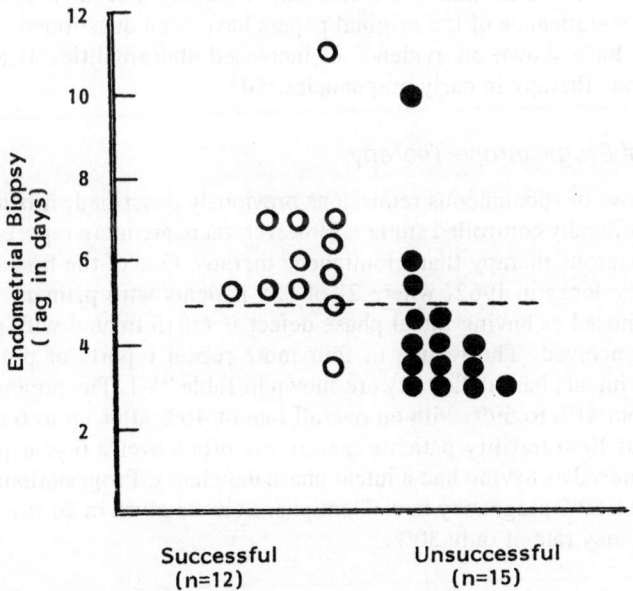

Figure 25-1. Relationship of success of clomiphene citrate therapy to endometrial lag >5 days versus <5 days. Twenty patients underwent 27 courses of therapy (*P*<.001) (from Downs and Gibson,[7] reproduced with permission).

Table 25-1. Progesterone Suppositories
in the Treatment of Luteal Phase Deficiency

Study	Year	Number of patients	Pregnancies	Percent
Garcia et al.[17]	1977	14	6	43
Soules et al.[18]	1977	17	7	41
Wentz et al.[19]	1984	54	23	43
Rosenberg et al.[20]	1980	13	9	69
Total		98	45	46

after the rise in basal body temperature. An endometrial biopsy is performed 2 or 3 months later to see if additional progesterone is needed.

Once pregnancy has been established and diagnosed, it is advantageous to continue exogenous steroids for 3 or 4 months. Studies in the early 1970s raised the possibility of increased incidence of congenital heart problems in the offspring of mothers given progestational steroids in early pregnancy.[12] The Food and Drug Administration recommended discontinuing the use of *routine* progesterone treatment in early pregnancy.[13] Luteal phase deficiency, however, is a condition in which there is a definite indication for progesterone therapy. In the early 1970s and early 1980s the couple was made aware of the supposed risks, and the pros and cons had to be carefully weighed. Recently, however, the statistical significance of the original papers have been questioned. A number of studies have shown no evidence of increased abnormalities as a result of progesterone therapy in early pregnancies.[14,15]

Results of Progesterone Therapy

Because of spontaneous remissions previously described, it is difficult to have scientifically controlled studies. However, there are more reports concerning progesterone therapy than clomiphene therapy. One of the first series was reported by Jones in 1962, where 21 of 555 patients with primary infertility were diagnosed as having luteal phase defect.[16] Of 15 treated with progesterone, 12 conceived. The results of four more recent reports of progesterone therapy in luteal phase deficiency are shown in Table 25-1. The pregnancy rates ranged from 41% to 69% with an overall rate of 46% after up to 6 months of therapy. Of 1000 fertility patients seen in my office over a 6-year period, 62 were diagnosed as having had a luteal phase deficiency. Progestational therapy resulted in a 60% pregnancy rate. Clomiphene citrate given in 20 cases resulted in a pregnancy rate of only 30%.

GONADOTROPIN THERAPY

When both clomiphene and progesterone treatment fail, one can then consider the use of gonadotropins. Human chorionic gonadotropin can be used in a dose of 2000 to 4000 IU every other day, starting 2 or 3 days after the basal body temperature rise. This form of treatment is expensive and inconvenient because it requires injections every other day. This treatment can delay menses. Since there is no way to diagnose pregnancy because the chorionic gonadotropin will interfere with the pregnancy test, one must arbitrarily stop the treatment to see whether menses will occur; thus the advantages of sustained stimulation of the corpus luteum are lost. No significant studies of its efficacy are available. Postmenopausal gonadotropin (Pergonal) may play a role in the treatment of the short luteal phase, but here too, the treatment is expensive and inconvenient. Postmenopausal gonadotropin has the added problem of hyperstimulation with ovarian enlargement and multiple pregnancies. Thus far, only preliminary reports have been published. One study described the use of pituitary FSH for luteal phase deficiency—5 of 15 women conceived.[21] The patients were not given progesterone beforehand, so theoretically a better percentage could have been obtained with the much simpler medication. In addition, pituitary FSH is no longer available for even investigative use.

REFERENCES

1. Rock J, Bartlett M: Biopsy studies of human endometrium criteria of dating and information about amenorrhea, menorrhea, and tissue of ovulation. *JAMA* 108:2022, 1937
2. Jones GES: Some newer aspects of management of infertility. *JAMA* 146:212, 1951
3. De Pozo E, Wyss H, Tolis G, Acaniz J, Campana A, Naftolin F: Prolactin and deficient luteal function. *Obstet Gynecol* 53:282, 1979
4. Ross GT, Cargille CM, Lipsett MB, et al: Pituitary and gonadal hormones in women during spontaneous and induced ovulatory cycles. *Rec Prog Horm Res* 26:1, 1970
5. DiZerega GS, Hodgen GD: Luteal phase dysfunction infertility: A sequel to aberrant folliculogenesis. *Fertil Steril* 35:489, 1981
6. Jones GES: Luteal phase defects. In Behrman SJ, Kistner RW, (eds): *Progress in Infertility*, 2nd ed. Boston, Little Brown, 1975, p 299
7. Downs KA, Gibson M: Clomiphene citrate therapy for luteal phase defect. *Fertil Steril* 39:34, 1983
8. Quagllianello J, Weiss G: Clomiphene citrate in the management of infertility associated with shortened luteal phase. *Fertil Steril* 31:373, 1979
9. Huang K: The primary treatment of luteal phase inadequacy: Progesterone versus clomiphene citrate. *Obstet Gynecol* 155:824, 1986
10. Graff G: Suppression of cervical mucus during clomiphene therapy. *Fertil Steril* 22:209, 1971
11. Johansson EDB: Depression of progesterone levels in women treated with synthetic gestagens after ovulation. *Acta Endocrinol* 68:779, 1971
12. Levy EP, Cohen A, Fraser FC: Hormone treatment during pregnancy and congenital heart defects. *Lancet* 1:611, 1973
13. Warnings on use of sex hormones in pregnancy. *FDA Drug Bulletin* 5:4, Jan–March, 1975
14. Check JH, Ranber A, Teichman M: The risk of fetal anomalies as a result of progesterone therapy during pregnancy. *Fertil Steril* 45:575, 1987
15. Katz Z, Lancet M, Skornik J, Chemke J, Magilner BM, Klinberg M: Teratogenecity of progestogens given during the first trimester of pregnancy. *Obstet Gynecol* 65:755, 1985

16. Jones GS: Luteal phase defects. In Gold JJ (ed): *Gynecologic Endocrinology*. Hagerstown, MD, Harper and Row, 1975, p 301
17. Garcia J, Jones GS, Wentz AC: The use of clomiphene citrate. *Fertil Steril* 28:707, 1977
18. Soules MR, Wiebe RH, Askel S, Hammond CB: The diagnosis and therapy of luteal phase deficiency. *Fertil Steril* 28:1033, 1977
19. Wentz AC, Herbert CM, Maxson WS, Garver CH: Outcome of progesterone treatment of luteal phase inadequacy. *Fertil Steril* 41:856, 1984
20. Rosenberg SM, Luciano AA, Riddick DH: The luteal phase defect: The relative frequency of, and encouraging response to treatment of vaginal progesterone. *Fertil Steril* 34:17, 1980
21. Huang KE, Muechler EK, Bonfiglio TA: Follicular phase treatment of luteal phase defect with follicle stimulating hormone in infertile women. *Obstet Gynecol* 64:32, 1984

CHAPTER 26

Induction of Ovulation

The patient who desires to ovulate in order to conceive should first be given specific therapy for the underlying etiologic factor, i.e., psychotherapy for emotional causes, improved nutrition and thyroid supplements, corticosteroids for adrenal hyperplasia, or surgical removal of androgen-producing tumors.

However, in a large number of women who fall, usually by exclusion, into the category of hypothalamic or pituitary hypofunction, a specific diagnosis cannot be made. It is possible that some women requiring ovulation induction may represent the low end of a normal spectrum of hypothalamic pituitary function. Probably other women have mild emotional disturbances causing anovulation, but do not seem to require psychotherapy. In some patients, a specific cause of hypothalamic inhibition can be found, as in galactoamenorrhea syndromes, post-pill amenorrhea, and profound emotional disturbances. In still others, according to laboratory tests, the cause of the amenorrhea appears to be a functional disturbance of the pituitary gland. All of these cases, added together, make up the large percentage of women with problems of amenorrhea requiring ovulation induction.

Before 1960 little effective therapy was available for this group of patients. Pituitary irradiation,[1] small doses of estrogen,[2] or cyclic estrogen and progesterone[3] had been administered with little or no success. Furthermore, in one recent study, Evans and Townsend demonstrated that, in true anovulation there is no place for cyclic therapy.[4] More than 30 years ago, however, two approaches were developed that significantly improved our ability to induce ovulation: clomiphene citrate and gonadotropin derived from pituitary glands or the urine of postmenopausal women. In the last decade, two more agents have been added to the list: bromocriptine for anovulation or amenorrhea associated with high prolactin levels and gonadotropin-releasing hormone (GnRH).

CLOMIPHENE CITRATE

Clomiphene citrate is neither a gonadotropin nor a steroid. Although structurally related to diethylstilbestrol, it does not possess significant estrogenic or progestational activity in the human. The chemical structure is shown in Fig. 26-1. The initial experimental work was carried out with a related product, ethamoxytriphetol (MER-25). Because this compound demonstrated pituitary gonadotropin-inhibiting effects in rats, it was tried in humans to suppress estrogen production. Contrary to expectations, pituitary gonadotropin stimulation was observed. Utilizing MER-25, Tyler and co-workers in 1960[5] and Kistner and Smith in 1960[6] reported successful induction of ovulation and pregnancy in patients with suspected Stein-Leventhal syndrome. In 1961, Greenblatt and co-workers[7] reported the apparent stimulation of ovulation with clomiphene citrate (MRL-41) in 70% of 36 patients treated for secondary amenorrhea. Since that time, the years have confirmed its effectiveness. And since that time clomiphene has become one of the most widely used medications in infertility management.[8]

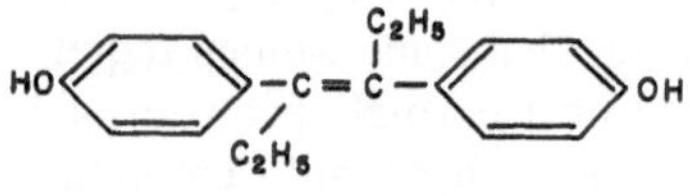

STILBESTROL

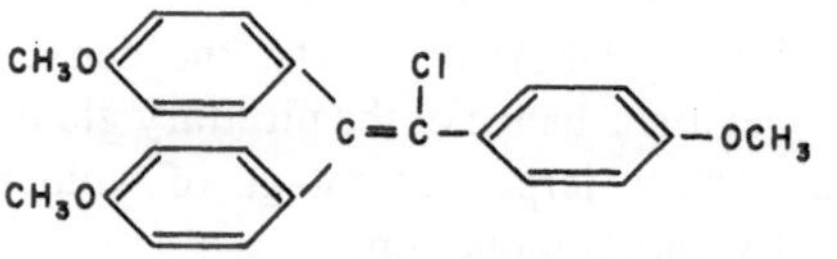

CHLOROTRIANISENE (TACE)

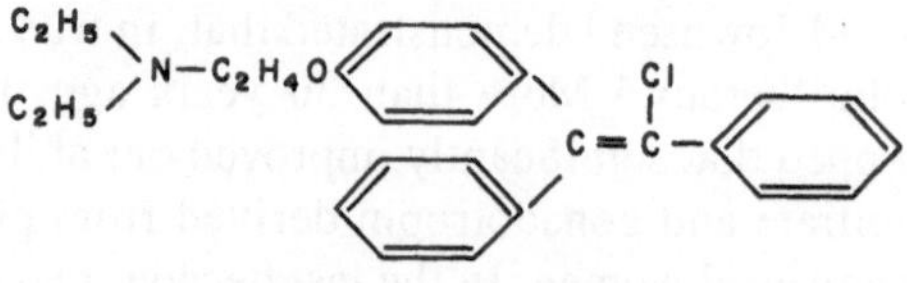

CLOMIPHENE

Figure 26-1. Chemical structure of clomiphene and related compounds.

Mechanisms of Action

Clomiphene citrate, because of its chemical structure, competes with estrogen for binding sites in the hypothalamus and possibly the pituitary[9] (Fig. 26-2). Being a weak estrogen, it has a weaker negative feedback effect on both GnRH and gonadotropins, so that the secretion of these two factors is increased.[10] During the administration of clomiphene, there is a moderate rise in follicle-stimulating hormone (FSH) and luteinizing hormone (LH) secretion and a gradual accelerating increase in estrogen production by the ovary. If hypothalamic–pituitary–ovarian function is potentially functional, the rising level of estrogens triggers an LH release similar to that seen in a normal cycle, and ovulation ensues.

Indications

The major indication for clomiphene treatment is in the infertility patient who is anovulatory, and in whom specific causes of anovulation have been ruled out. The woman most likely to respond to moderate doses of clomiphene is the one with mild hypothalamic amenorrhea. Only the cyclic center is not functioning. However, there has been sufficient discharge of releasing factor from the tonic center to maintain pituitary synthesis of gonadotropins and at least a low-normal level of estrogen. As a result, during clomiphene administration there is a further increase in FSH and LH. Patients with irregular ovulation, mild emotional amenorrhea, most cases of post-pill amenorrhea, and cases of polycystic ovaries fall into this category.

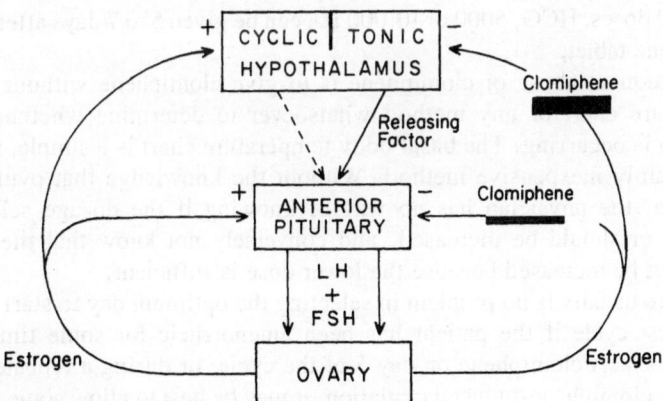

Figure 26-2. Mechanism of action of clomiphene. Clomiphene blocks the inhibitory effect of estrogen on gonadotropin synthesis and release, resulting in an increase of FSH and LH that stimulates follicle growth and initiates the cycle.

Dosage

The spectrum of hypothalamic hypofunction, ranging from mild to severe, is confirmed by knowing that there is a dosage range required to produce an ovulatory response in a large group of patients with amenorrhea. The milder disturbances respond to 50 to 100 mg daily for 5 days. More severe degrees of hypothalamic dysfunction require up to 200 mg daily for 5 days. The patients requiring human chorionic gonadotropin (HCG) to imitate the midcycle surge of LH are those in whom higher doses of clomiphene may cause some FSH and LH release with some follicular development, but there is not enough LH stored in the pituitary for an ovulatory surge.

Unfortunately, laboratory tests cannot always clearly identify the degree of hypothalamic dysfunction, although clinical evidence of circulating estrogen (anovulatory bleeding, fern formation, a positive progesterone test) usually suggests the milder degree of hypofunction.

Therefore, a program of increasing dosage provides an approach whereby maximum results with clomiphene citrate can be achieved with safety.[11] One starts with a low dose of one tablet (50 mg) daily for 5 days. As patients with obvious polycystic ovaries are occasionally very sensitive to clomiphene, with these patients it is best to start them with one tablet daily for only 3 days. If, by basal body temperature chart, an ovulatory response is noted, this dosage is maintained for 6 to 12 months. Even if conception does not occur, there is nothing to be gained by further increasing the dosage. However, if "ovulation" is not apparent by the temperature chart, the dosage should be increased by one pill a day, up to as high as four tablets, 200 mg a day, for 5 days if necessary to achieve an ovulatory response. Some physicians increase the length of therapy from 7 to 10 days as well. If an ovulatory response does not follow with these increased doses, HCG, 5000 or 10,000 IU, can be given 5 to 7 days after the last clomiphene tablet.

A frequent abuse of clomiphene is to give clomiphene without using a temperature chart or any method whatsoever to determine whether or not ovulation is occurring. The basal body temperature chart is a simple, reliable, and certainly inexpensive method. Without the knowledge that ovulation is occurring, the physician has no way of knowing if the dosage selected is adequate or should be increased, and conversely not know that the dosage should not be increased because the lower dose is sufficient.

There usually is no problem in selecting the optimum day to start therapy in the first cycle if the patient has been amenorrheic for some time. Most physicians start clomiphene on day 5 of the cycle, or during a repeated cycle following clomiphene-induced ovulation, it may be best to allow some time for endogenous gonadotropins to stimulate at least a degree of follicular development. Therefore, one could wait as long as 8 days after an episode of uterine bleeding before initiating therapy.

Monitoring

The basal temperature chart provides an ideal method for monitoring the response to clomiphene. Although it is recognized that this is not an absolute determinant of the presence or absence of ovulation, it provides a practical and simple approach. One looks for a thermal response of 12 to 16 days in length. A thermal response of less than 12 days may well represent only luteinization of the theca, and calls for the next step up in dosage. Once the patient is on a dose providing good thermogenic response, it is maintained.

If the treatment is successful and the patient ovulates, the basal body temperature will rise within 3 to 10 days after the last dose of clomiphene. Frequent intercourse during that interval is advisable.

Results

It is difficult to assess the effectiveness of clomiphene because of the variety of menstrual disorders for which it has been prescribed. These have ranged from irregular ovulation, in which conception may occur without therapy, to cases of primary amenorrhea, in which no benefits can be anticipated. Utilizing this stepwise increase in dosage, in the appropriate type of patient, our ovulatory rate was increased from 47% to 71% and the pregnancy rate from 36% to 43% (Table 26-1). The majority of these patients were treated before it was acceptable to use higher doses; therefore, with such use one could expect an even higher ovulatory and pregnancy rate. The results of therapy with clomiphene citrate have been widely reported. There is an average of 70% to 80% ovulatory rate, and a 40% to 50% conception rate.

Failure to Conceive despite Ovulation

The reasons for the discrepancy between ovulatory and conception rates are multiple. Certainly a large percentage represent the natural difference be-

Table 26-1. Cumulative Ovulatory and Pregnancy Rates
with Increasing Daily Doses of Clomiphene Citrate in 152 Patients

Dose	Number ovulating	Cumulative ovulatory rate (%)	Number of pregnancies	Cumulative pregnancy rate (%)
50 mg	41	27	23	15
100 mg	48	47	31	36
150 mg	9	64	3	38
200 mg	2	66	1	38
Clomiphene (150 mg) and HCG (5000 IU)	12	71	7	43

tween ovulation and pregnancy rate in any infertile population. However, there are in practice a number of specific reasons, and these are listed in Table 26-2.

The failure to carry out an adequate infertility workup before starting treatment is one of the major abuses of clomiphene therapy and one of the causes of ovulation without conception.

Secondly, clomiphene, as an antiestrogen, has an adverse effect on cervical mucus, and consequently can inhibit pregnancy by inhibiting sperm migration through the cervical canal. There is a difference of opinion as to the clinical significance of this effect. There are those reports that suggest a significant effect of clomiphene on cervical mucus,[12,13] and those that feel poor mucus occurs in only 15% of the subjects.[14] Whether it is 15% or more, in my experience it can have a detrimental effect on the cervical factor. Therefore, once a patient is ovulating well on a certain dosage of clomiphene, the postcoital test should be repeated. The recommended therapy for poor cervical mucus in the past has been to prescribe small doses of estrogen after midcycle. There are no studies to indicate that this significantly helps the problem, but there are other methods to assist sperm insemination if this does appear indicated: intrauterine insemination, a change to human menopausal gonadotropin (HMG) therapy, or even the gamete intrafallopian tube transfer procedure.

Another apparent cause for ovulation without conception is the somewhat increased production of androgen by clomiphene, and this is particularly true in patients with borderline elevated dehydroepiandrosterone-sulfate levels. Combining prednisone or dexamethasone with clomiphene in these patients significantly increased both the ovulatory rate and pregnancy rate.[15]

Luteal Phase Defect and Clomiphene

Because of its varied effects upon the hypothalamic–pituitary axis, clomiphene citrate therapy may sometimes result in an ovulatory cycle but one in which a luteal phase deficiency exists.[16] Often this may be due to inadequate dosage. If the basal body temperature chart shows an obvious defect, such as a short luteal phase, one may proceed to the next dosage level. If on the other hand, pregnancy does not occur after a number of apparent ovulations by the

Table 26-2. Causes of Conception Failure
Despite Ovulation with Clomiphene Citrate

Inadequate infertility workup
Adverse effect of clomiphene on cervical mucus
Androgen effect of clomiphene
Inadequate dosage or duration of therapy

chart, an endometrial biopsy is indicated. Doses can then be increased or luteal phase progesterone can be added.

Side Effects

The chief side effects of clomiphene therapy are hot flashes and pelvic discomfort, which occur in 10.7% and 7.4% of patients. A small number of patients complain of a myriad of vague symptoms, including visual disturbances, none of which appears to have any serious implications. The incidence of birth defects does not seem to run higher than the general population.[17] Although there is some evidence that clomiphene remains in the tissue for a considerable time after ingestion, a study by Geier and co-workers demonstrated that 51% was excreted in 5 days, and only a trace was found at 6 weeks of pregnancy, well before organogenesis.[18]

Complications

Complications of clomiphene therapy relate to ovarian overstimulation. This can result in enlargement of the ovary and multiple pregnancies.[19,20] Once again, it is difficult to obtain meaningful incidence of these complications because large series include changing patterns of drug administration, and the later series, utilizing smaller dosages, are too small to be of significance. The figures reported by MacGregor and colleagues include the cumulative experience of numerous workers adding up to more than 4000 patients seen through June 1967.[21] Of 1337 live births, 136 (10%) were multiple. Of 6714 patients, 13.9% were reported as having some degree of ovarian enlargement. Ascites were recorded only rarely.

The above incidence of ovarian overstimulation was compiled during a period when the individual sensitivity of patients to the drug was not fully appreciated, and modifications of dosage were not utilized. There is every reason to believe that, with proper attention to these details, such complications can be significantly reduced.

GONADOTROPINS

When the pituitary gland fails to secret sufficient gonadotropins to result in follicular maturation and ovulation, and when clomiphene citrate is not capable of stimulating the pituitary to perform this function, FSH and LH can be administered.

Human FSH and LH have been available for the induction of ovulation since 1958,[22] with gonadotropins initially derived from pituitary glands removed at autopsy. Later, gonadotropin derived from the urine of post-menopausal females was used.[23] Since the supply of pituitary gonadotropin is limited, it is used in only a few centers. In the United States, only gonadotropin of urinary origin (HMG) is commercially available at the present time.

Mechanisms of Action

HMG comes in an ampule containing 75 IU of FSH activity and 75 IU of LH activity. Apparently both FSH and LH are necessary for development of the follicle. FSH directly stimulates follicle growth. LH acts by promoting the secretion of estrogen, which, in turn, has an enhancing effect on follicle development. Gonadotropin is administered until there is evidence of follicular maturation. An ovulatory dose of chorionic gonadotropin is then administered. Since LH is not commercially available, human chorionic gonadotropin (HCG) is utilized to trigger ovulation, and is effective because one of its main biologic activities is that of luteinizing, or stimulation of ovulation.

The Selection of Patients for Gonadotropin Therapy

It is obvious that in pituitary amenorrhea, where there is insufficient pituitary function to respond to the stimulation of gonadotropin-releasing factors (either naturally or even as a result of the action of clomiphene citrate), gonadotropin can be selected as primary therapy after remedial causes of pituitary failure have been either ruled out or treated.

Patients with severe hypothalamic dysfunction will also ultimately require gonadotropin therapy, because only a small percentage will respond to even the larger doses of clomiphene citrate, with or without HCG added. However, these latter measures should be tried first.

Even among subjects with apparently mild hypothalamic dysfunction, there will be a considerable number who will not respond to clomiphene citrate; however, these should be minimal if the patients are gradually brought up to the maximum dosage of clomiphene. But some of those who have not conceived after 6 to 12 months of clomiphene cycling will conceive on gonadotropin therapy. The reason for this is unclear. In the total management of an infertility patient, rather than have the patient experience persistent failure over many months and years, it is sometimes judicious to change to HMG.

Administration and Dosage

HMG is administered, as a daily intramuscular dose, at a level of 150 to 225 IU of FSH activity (2 to 3 ampules). In using HMG for in vitro fertilization or intrauterine insemination, one wants to maintain a large number of follicles and oocytes to increase the chances of conception. Thus, in this situation, medication is started on the second or third day of the cycle to enhance recruitment of multiple follicles. In treating women with anovulation or amenorrhea, one assumes that there are not other causes for infertility, and that ovulation of only one or two oocytes is required. The desired effect can be obtained without a severe risk of complications. Therefore, treatment can be started 5 to 6 days after the induction of an artificial cycle or after the onset of withdrawal bleeding of an anovulatory cycle. Daily injections of Pergonal are administered until the patient appears to be ready to ovulate. This usually takes 6 to 12 days.

HCG is then administered as a single dose, 5000 to 10,000 IU, to imitate the relatively sharp midcycle rise of LH. In subjects in whom the postovulatory phase appears to be shortened, a second dose of HCG can be administered 5 days after the basal body temperature rises. Theoretically, this would appear to be indicated more often in subjects with complete pituitary failure, in whom there is not sufficient endogenous LH secreted to maintain a corpus luteum, once formed. The optimum time for administration of the ovulation dose will be discussed under monitoring. Knowing that ovulation will occur 37 to 38 hours after the administration of HCG, the couple can be given the appropriate advice as to the time of coitus in order to optimize the chances of conception.

Results: Conception and Complications

With proper selection and with progressive and persistent treatment, HMG therapy is extremely effective. Overall pregnancy rates range from 50% to 70%. However, patients with low-estrogen amenorrhea (World Health Organization, Class I) have success rates close to 80%, while patients with normal estrogen amenorrhea (World Health Organization, Class II), polycystic ovaries, and oligo-ovulation do less well, approximately 35%.

The two serious complications are multiple pregnancies and ovarian enlargement, with or without ascites. A classification of ovarian overstimulation in terms of ovarian enlargement is shown in Table 26-3. Multiple pregnancies should be considered as a complication because of the increased risk to both the mother and the fetus. As shown in a review,[24] this is true even of twin pregnancies, and problems are obviously compounded for pregnancies involving three or more fetuses.

Table 26-3. Classification of Ovarian Overstimulation

Mild—ovarian enlargement <7cm
Moderate—ovarian enlargement 7–10 cm
Severe (hyperstimulation syndrome)—ovarian enlargement >10 cm, with or without ascites

Grade 1 ovarian enlargement is not necessarily serious, but more severe grades are painful and can be potentially harmful to the ovary (Fig. 26-3). Ascites is a serious complication that requires hospitalization, careful monitoring of fluid and electrolyte balance, and occasionally emergency surgery for hemorrhage.[25,26] The theoretical causes of massive enlargement and ascites have been reviewed by Engel and his co-workers.[27] They theorize that the ascites may be due to the high estrogen levels.

Causes of Overstimulation–Variability of Response

Overstimulation, in terms of multiple pregnancies and ovarian enlargement, is undoubtedly due to the maturation and ovulation of too many follicles. Too much and too prolonged administration of HMG brings too many follicles to maturity. Multiple ovulation occurs when HMG is administered. The dose of HCG may be a factor, but this has been difficult to establish.

Extreme variability of individual responsiveness to HMG makes it impossible to establish a rigid dose schedule for HMG, as one can do for clomiphene citrate. Some success with test doses, starting low and gradually increasing until an ovulatory response has been achieved, have been reported.[28] However, because there is often marked variability in the same individual from cycle to

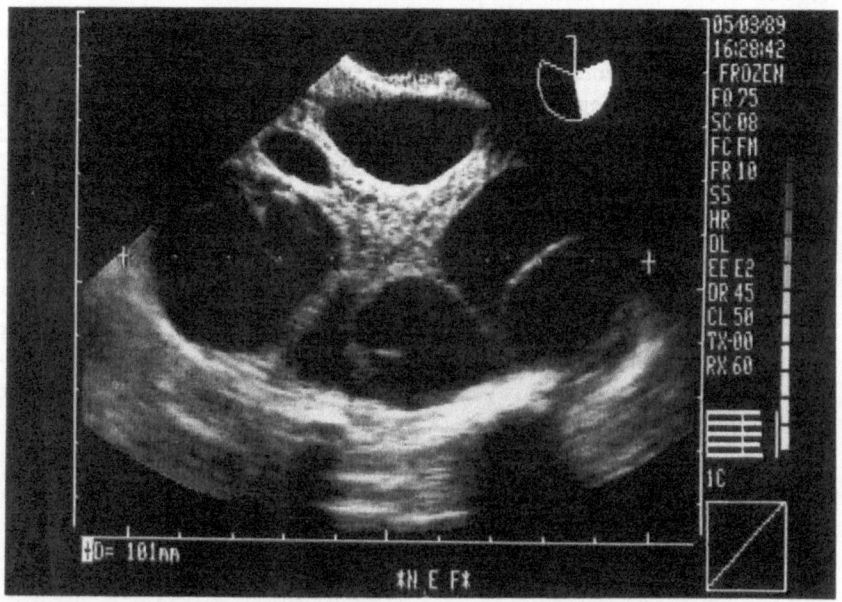

Figure 26-3. Massively enlarged ovary (101 mm) with multiple corpus lutea.

cycle, and the medication is so expensive, this approach remains relatively impractical.

The reason for such variability is that a patient's own gonadotropin often synergizes with the administered gonadotropins. No one ever knows the exact state of FSH, LH, and estrogen levels in a given patient at the start of treatment, nor the state of follicular development, so that the ultimate amount of HMG required cannot be predetermined. That is why subjects with absent gonadotropins seem to have fewer problems with overstimulation, although the total dose required for ovulation is considerably more. This is also why it has been found helpful to bring about an artificial menses one week prior to starting therapy, so that some consistency of follicular maturation will be at hand as each treatment cycle is commenced.

Monitoring the Response

A close relationship between the levels of total estrogen excretion during the 24 hours just prior to the administration of HCG and the occurrence of ovarian enlargement and multiple pregnancies has been demonstrated.[29] Therefore, in the past it was vital to use a therapeutic program in which the HCG was administered as soon as the total estrogen excretion reached physiologic levels, i.e., 100 μg/24 hours. Total estrogen excretion was measured by rapid method, one modified from the technique of Brown and co-workers.[30] However, plasma estrogen are now almost exclusively used.[31] Some individuals place a great deal of weight on the cervical mucus, monitoring a number of changes in the mucus to provide a cervical score.[32] Unfortunately, the changes in the cervical mucus reach a maximum well before optimum follicular maturation is reached, and other methods must be used to supplement the cervical score.

With the development of follicular ultrasound, it was hoped that an accurate method for monitoring follicular maturation would be at hand, one that could be used by all therapists without the need for complicated laboratory assays. However, as experience with ultrasound monitoring grew, it was found that ultrasound alone could not prevent multiple pregnancies[33] nor ovarian hyperstimulation.[34] As a result, the conclusion has developed that ultrasound can play a role in monitoring ovulation induced by gonadotropins, but that it must be used in cooperation with other methods.[35] Cervical mucus can indicate that sufficient gonadotropins are being given early in the cycle. Estradiol levels can indicate that there is an adequate stimulation during the middle course of treatment or that there is too much stimulation. An ultrasound can determine when the follicle(s) are ready to respond to HCG or whether or not there are too many follicles and that HCG should be withheld. The results in terms of high pregnancy rates and low complication rates seem to be considerably greater when all three modalities are utilized.[36] However, even with such monitoring, multiple pregnancies are not completely eliminated,[37,38] and the patient should be so forewarned. A number of reports on the use of selective discontinuation of pregnancy are in the literature, but it would be better if this approach were not required.[39,40]

Two ampules of HMG (150 IU) are administered for 5 days, and monitoring is begun on the 6th day of treatment. If the cervical mucus shows 3 plus ferning, two more ampules are given and plasma estradiol levels and ultrasound examination of the ovaries are planned for the next day. If the cervical mucus shows poor ferning, the dosage of HMG is increased to three ampules daily, and the plasma estradiol and ultrasound are withheld until treatment day 8.

Two or three ampules of HMG are continued daily as indicated until the lead follicle reaches 18 mm, and as long as the estrogen level ranges between 500 and 3000 pg. This allows continuation of HMG until optimum follicle size is reached, at which point 10,000 IU of HCG is administered.

For those patients who are slow to respond and do not have 3 plus ferning on treatment day 6, the dosage is increased to three ampules (225 IU) on day 6 and 7 and the estradiol monitoring and ultrasound is begun on day 8. If the estradiol remains under 500 pg, it may be necessary to increase the dosage to four or five ampules (300 to 375 IU daily). Once again, HCG is administered when the lead follicle is 18 mm and the estradiol levels are between 500 and 3000 pg.

HCG is not administered if three or more follicles reach 17 mm in size or if the estradiol levels go above 3000 pg, particularly when associated with a large number of follicles ranging from 11 to 17.

This plan of therapy has been the one followed by our group for the past 6 years. The results of pregnancy and complications with this approach as compared to our prior endeavors are shown in Table 26-4. With estrogen mon-

Table 26-4. Ovulation Induction Monitored by Daily Fern Test
or by Daily Total Estrogen Excretion

	Fern test		Estrogen excretion	
	Number	Percent	Number	Percent
Patients	35		63	
Cycles	81		153	
Ovulatory	76	94	110	72
Conceptions	20	57	34	54
Multiple	8	40	8	24
Triplet	2		0	
Ovarian enlargement	11	14 of cycles	17	11
Ascites	4		0	

itoring, the pregnancy rate remained high. Although there were still multiple pregnancies, none was greater than twins. Although there were ovarian enlargements in 11% of cycles, there were no cases of ascites. One cannot say that with estrogen monitoring multiple pregnancies and significant ovarian enlargement will be eliminated, but at least the occurrence of these two complications should be minimized. More convincing evidence of the relationship of estrogen monitoring to multiple pregnancies is shown in Table 26-5.

CLOMIPHENE–HMG-HCG

Two of the drawbacks to gonadotropins therapy have been the expense of the medication and the necessity for daily intramuscular injections. One approach that can reduce, although not eliminate, this inconvenience and expense is the sequential use of clomiphene and HMG-HCG in clomiphene failures.

It can be postulated that some patients do not have sufficient stores of FSH in their pituitary gland, and, therefore, follicular development in response to clomiphene citrate is only partial. Furthermore, endogenous estrogen production is insufficient to trigger an LH release that would provoke ovulation. It can be further theorized that some subjects with amenorrhea might respond to clomiphene therapy up to a certain point of follicular development, after which the addition of exogenous gonadotropins might bring the follicle to maturity. If this thesis is correct, less gonadotropins will be required to bring about ovulation than gonadotropin alone.

In a preliminary study, seven patients were first given gonadotropin alone, and then clomiphene-gonadotropin, to induce ovulation.[42] An average of 45% less gonadotropins was required to bring about an ovulatory response in the

Table 26-5. Effect of Estrogen Monitoring on Pregnancy Outcome[a]

	Before estrogen monitoring (1960–1967)	After estrogen monitoring (1969–1973)
No. of patients	290	351
No. of treatment courses	606	759
No. of pregnancies	130	143
No. of single births	63	94
No. of multiple births	31	20
No. of abortions	36	29
Pregnancy rate	45%	41%
Multiple birth rates	33%	17%
Abortion rate	28%	20%

[a]From Gemzell.[41]

cycles in which gonadotropin was preceded by the use of clomiphene. Kistner has reported 23 pregnancies in 40 patients.[43]

Even if this approach is successful in achieving pregnancy with decreased cost and inconvenience to the patient, careful monitoring is still required to prevent ovarian hyperstimulation and to reduce multiple pregnancies.

GONADOTROPIN-RELEASING HORMONE

In 1971 the groups of Schally and Guillemin and their co-workers almost simultaneously reported the isolation and amino acid sequence of luteinizing-releasing factor, now more commonly called GnRH.[44,45] Soon after a synthetic product was available for ovulation induction (Fig. 26-4). The first report was optimistic, but a review of subsequent series demonstrated a mean pregnancy rate of only 15%. This is not surprising when we consider that initially the treatments consisted of two or three injections per day, and now we know from the work of Knobil that GnRH, to be effective, must be administered in pulses almost 90 to 120 minutes apart.[46]

Selection of Patients

Patients with amenorrhea or anovulation with an intact pituitary gland can be subjects for GnRH therapy. HMG therapy combined with HCG remains the agent of choice, but there are certain theoretical advantages to the use of GnRH. Because estrogen feedback mechanisms remain intact, the incidence of hyperstimulation should be greatly reduced with GnRH as compared with

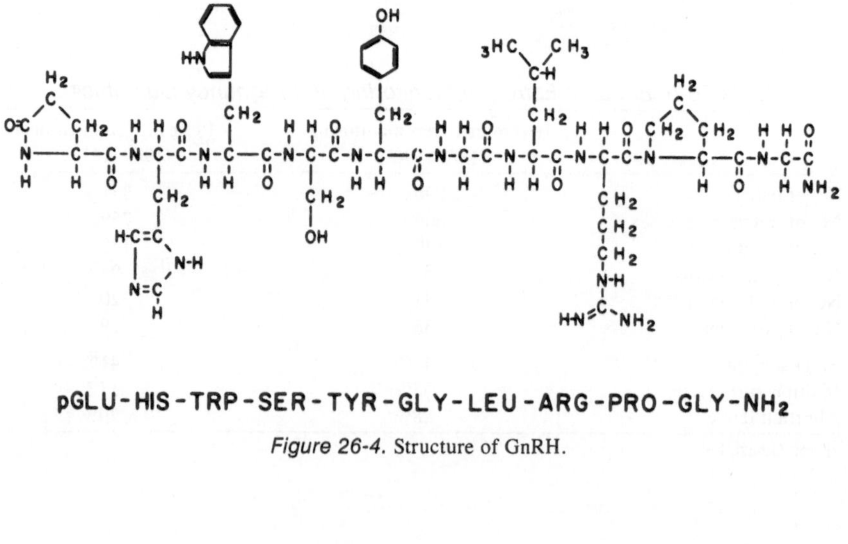

pGLU – HIS – TRP – SER – TYR – GLY – LEU – ARG – PRO – GLY – NH₂

Figure 26-4. Structure of GnRH.

HMG.[47] However, ovarian hyperstimulation does occur occasionally and monitoring is still required.[48]

Technique of Administration

GnRH is administered by means of a computerized pump from which a needle is attached to the patient intravenously or subcutaneously. Each pulse consists of 10 to 20 μg. GnRH is administered at 90- to 120-minute intervals starting on the 2nd or 3rd day at the start of an artificial cycle. The response is monitored by the determination of estradiol levels, and by ultrasound examinations that indicate that ovulation is near. At this point, 10,000 IU of HCG is administered. An alternate approach is to allow ovulation to occur spontaneously, stop the GnRH, and give HCG intermittently after ovulation in order to support the luteal phase.[49]

Results

Individual reports with the subcutaneous rate show ovulatory rates as high as 90% with a pregnancy rate of 59% per cycle.[50,51] The overall results from some surveys in the literature are not as optimistic.[52] In this summary the intravenous route resulted in an overall ovulatory rate of 78% with a 33.5% pregnancy rate per cycle. The subcutaneous route appeared to be not quite as effective, but there were fewer complications.[53] In addition, some claim that the intravenous route appears to be more predictable.[54] In any event, GnRH administration appears to be an alternate to HMG therapy with the special advantage of diminished ovarian hyperstimulation.

BROM-ERGOCRYPTINE

Another addition to our armamentarium for ovulation induction is brom-ergocryptine*. This medication has been used primarily for treatment of the galactorrhea-amenorrhea syndromes.[55] The compound appears to work by inhibiting prolactin release, probably at the pituitary level,[56–58] or by an increase in prolactin-inhibiting factors.[59] Although FSH and LH levels are usually normal, the increased prolactin levels seem to block the episodic release of LH.[60]

There appears to be little doubt concerning its effectiveness in reducing elevated prolactin levels, suppressing galactorrhea, and inducing ovulation and pregnancy. In a study of ten patients, Mroueh and Slier-Khodr reported seven resumptions of ovulation and five pregnancies.[61]

Beyond the galactorrhea-amenorrhea syndrome, Bohnet and co-workers

*Parlodel®, Sandoz Pharmaceuticals, East Hanover, New Jersey.

have shown that of 127 patients with secondary amenorrhea, 13.4% had hyper-prolactinemia, but only half of these had galactorrhea.[62]

Therefore, any patients with elevated prolactin levels and any degree of ovulatory disorder ranging from luteal phase deficiency to amenorrhea should be given bromocriptine, and the results in terms of correcting the ovulatory defect at least should be excellent. An area of controversy has been the administration of bromocriptine to patients with ovulatory defects with normal prolactin levels. Originally, a number of studies reported a return to normal ovulation and pregnancies in a small series of such women.[63-65] However, control studies utilizing placebos have demonstrated that these results were in no way significant.[66] Knowing the relative high degree of remission that occurs with amenorrhea and anovulatory cycles, it would appear to be unjustified to administer bromocriptine to women with normal prolactin levels except in some selective cases of polycystic ovarian syndrome.[67]

POLYCYSTIC OVARIES

Bilateral ovarian wedge resection should be reserved until an adequate trial of medical therapy has been attempted without success, and should be used only in well-documented cases of polycystic ovaries. There have been sufficient advances in diagnostic methods in the past years, i.e., LH assay, androgen assay, and laparoscopy, to virtually eliminate the performance of nonindicated ovarian wedge resection. If possible, surgery should be avoided because of the high incidence of postoperative adhesions that result in infertility.[68] However, with the use of modern techniques of microsurgery along with adjuvants for protection against adhesions, this complication should be minimal.

Once there has been a failure with clomiphene or clomiphene HCG, one may cautiously resort to gonadotropin therapy. Since patients with polycystic ovaries already have high or high-normal LH levels[69] and are relatively deficient in FSH,[70] the "pure" form of FSH* would theoretically be safer. However, even with pure FSH, hyperstimulation occurs and careful monitoring is required.[71]

If repeated ovarian enlargement occurs, it may be better to then proceed to ovarian wedge resection. The surgery itself may be less harmful to the ovary than repeated enlargements. If wedge resection fails, HMG can be given postoperatively with less likelihood of hyperstimulation. Undoubtedly, as our experience has grown with medical treatment, the surgical approach is being used less and less.

*Metrodin®, Serono Laboratories, Norwell, Massachusetts.

REFERENCES

1. Rakoff AE: Hormonal changes following low dosage irradiation of pituitaries and ovaries in anovulatory women. *Fertil Steril* 4:263, 1953
2. Rakoff AE, Plaster EL, Goldfarb AF: Comparison of various therapies for treatment of anovulation. In Rosenberg E, (ed): *Gonadotropin Therapy in Female Infertility.* Amsterdam, Excerpta Medica, 1973, p 128
3. Igarashi M, Matsumoto S, Hosaka H: Further studies on the rebound phenomenon of ovarian function. *Fertil Steril,* 16:257, 1965
4. Evans J, Townsend L: The induction of ovulation. *Am J Obstet Gynecol,* 125:321, 1976
5. Tyler ET, Olsen HJ, Gotlieb MH: Induction of ovulation with an anti-estrogen. *Int J Fertil,* 5:429, 1960
6. Kistner RW, Smith OW: Observations on the use of a non-steroid estrogen antogonist, MER-25. *Surg Forum* 10:725, 1960
7. Greenblatt RB, Barfield WE, Jungck EC, et al: Induction of ovulation with MRL-41: Preliminary report. *JAMA* 178:101, 1961
8. Taymor ML: The use and abuse of clomiphene. *Fertil Steril* 47:206, 1987
9. Kato J, Kiobayashi T, Villee CA: Effect of clomiphene on the uptake of estradiol by the anterior hypothalamus and hypophysis. *Endocrinology* 82:1049, 1968
10. Adashi EG: Clomiphene citrate: Mechanisms and sites of action—a hypothesis revisited. *Fertil Steril* 42:331, 1984
11. Rust LA, Israel R, Mishell DR Jr: An individualized graduated therapeutic regimen for clomiphene citrate. *Am J Obstet Gynecol* 120:785, 1974
12. Graff G: Suppression of cervical mucus during clomiphene therapy. *Fertil Steril,* 22:209, 1971
13. Hammond MG, Halme JK, Talbert LM: Factors affecting the frequency rate in clomiphene citrate induction of ovulation. *Obstet Gynecol* 62:192, 1982
14. Gysler M, March CM, Mishell DR, Bailey EJ: A decade's experience with an individualized treatment regimen including its effect on the post-coital test. *Fertil Steril* 36:161, 1982
15. Lobo RA, Paul W, March CM, et al: Clomiphene and dexamethasone in women unresponsive to clomiphene alone. *Obstet Gynecol* 60:497, 1982
16. Jones, GS, Maffezzoli RD, Strott CA, et al: Pathophysiology of reproductive failure after clomiphene-induced ovulation. *Am J Obstet Gynecol* 99:814, 1967
17. Adashi EG, Rock JA, Sapp KC, Martin EJ, Wentz AC, Jones GS: Gestational outcome of clomiphene related conceptions. *Fertil Steril* 31:620, 1979
18. Geier A, Lumenfeld B, Pariente C: Estrogen reception binding material in blood of patients after clomiphene citrate administration by a radioreceptor assay. *Fertil Steril* 47:778, 1984
19. Scommegna L, Lash SR: Ovarian overstimulation, massive ascites and singleton pregnancy after clomiphene. *JAMA* 207:753, 1969
20. Poland M: Problems of ovulation induction with clomiphene citrate with report of a case of ovarian hyperstimulation. *Obstet Gynecol* 35:55, 1970
21. Macgregor AH, Johnson JE, Bunde CA: Further clinical experience with clomiphene citrate. *Fertil Steril* 19:616, 1968
22. Gemzell CA, Diczfalusy E, Tillinger DG: Clinical effects of human pituitary follicle stimulating hormone (FSH). *J Clin Endocrinol Metab* 18:333, 1958
23. Lunenfeld B, Menzi A, Volet B: Clinical effects of human postmenopausal gonadotropins. *Acta Endocrinol (Kbh) [Suppl]* 51:587, 1960
24. Powers WF: Twin pregnancies—complications and treatment. *Obstet Gynecol* 42:795, 1973
25. Schenker JG, Polishuk WZ: Ovarian hyperstimulation syndrome. *Obstet Gynecol* 6:23, 1975
26. Shapiro AG, Thomas T, Epstein M: Management of hyperstimulation syndrome. *Fertil Steril* 28:3, 1977

27. Engel T, Jewelewicz RM, Dyrenfurth I: Ovarian hyperstimulation syndrome. Report of a case with notes on pathogenesis and treatment. *Am J Obstet Gynecol* 112:1052, 1972
28. Butler JK: Clinical results with gonadotropins in anovulation using two alternative dosage schedules. *Postgrad Med J* 48:27, 1972
29. Taymor ML: Gonadotropin therapy. *JAMA* 203:362, 1968
30. Brown JB, Macleod SC, MacNaughtan C, et al: A rapid method for estimating oestrogens in urine using a semiautomatic extractor. *J Endocrinol* 42:5, 1968
31. Black WP, Coutts JRT, Codson KS, et al: An assessment of urinary and plasma steroid estimations for monitoring treatment of anovulation with gonadotropins. *J Obstet Gynecol Br Common* 81:667, 1974
32. Insler V, Mahmed H, Eichenbrenner I, Serr DM, Lunenfeld B: The cervical score—a single semiquantitative method for monitoring ovarian overstimulation during gonadotropin therapy. *Int J Gynecol Obstet* 10:223, 1972
33. Cabau A, Bessis P: Monitoring of ovulation induction with human menopausal gonadotropin and human chorionic gonadotropin by ultrasound. *Fertil Steril* 36:78, 1981
34. Herlihy C, Evans JH, Brown JB, deCrespigny LJ, Robinson HP: Use of ultrasound in monitoring ovulation induction with human pituitary gonadotropins. *Obstet Gynecol* 66:577, 1982
35. Seibel MM, McArdle CR, Thompson IE, Berger MJ, Taymor ML: The role of ultrasound in ovulation induction: A critical appraisal. *Fertil Steril* 36:573, 1981
36. March CM: Improved pregnancy rates with monitoring gonadotropin therapy by three modulators. *Am J Obstet Gynecol* 156:1473, 1987
37. Shelden R, Kemmann E, Bohrer M, Pasquale S: Multiple gestation with the use of high sperm numbers in the intrauterine insemination in women undergoing gonadotropic stimulation. *Fertil Steril* 49:607, 1988
38. Fedorkow DM, Corenblum B, Pattinson HA, Taylor PT: Septuplet gestation following use of menopausal gonadotropin despite intensive monitoring. *Fertil Steril* 49:364, 1988
39. Birenholz JC, Dmowski WP, Binor Z, Radwanska E: Selective continuation in gonadotropin-induced multiple pregnancy. *Fertil Steril* 48:873, 1987
40. Farquarson DF, Wittman BV, Hansmann M, Yuen BH, Baldwin J, Lindohl S: Management of quintuplet pregnancy by selective embryocide. *Am J Obstet Gynecol* 158:413, 1988
41. Gemzell CA: Induction of ovulation. *Acta Obstet Gynecol Scand (Suppl.)* 47:1, 1975
42. Taymor ML, Berger MJ, Nudemberg F: The combined use of clomiphene citrate and human menopausal gonadotropin in ovulation induction. Hasegawa T (ed): *Fertil Steril Excerpta Medica Int Cong Series* 278:628, 1973
43. Kistner RW: Sequential use of clomiphene citrate and human menopausal gonadotropin in ovulation induction. *Fertil Steril* 27:81, 1976
44. Matsuo HL, Baba Y, Nair RMG, Arimura A, Schally AV: Synthesis of the porcine LH and FSH releasing hormone by the solid phase method. *Biochem Biophys Res Commun* 25:992, 1971
45. Burgus R, Butcher M, Ling N, Monahan M, Rivier J, Fellows R, Amass M, Blackwell R, Vale R, Guillemin W: Structure moleculaire du facteur hypothalamique (LRF) d'origine ovine controlant la secretion d l'hormone gonadotrope hypophysaire du luteinisation (LH). *C R Acad Sci (Paris)* 273:1611, 1971
46. Knobil E: Neuroendocrine control of the menstrual cycle. *Recent Prog Horm Res*, 36:53, 1980
47. Reid RL, Fretts RF, Van Vogt DA: The theory and practice of ovulation induction with gonadotropin-releasing hormone. *Am J Obstet Gynecol* 158:176, 1988
48. Breckwoldt F, Geisthovel, Neuler J, Schillinger H: Management of multiple conception after GnRH/analogue/human menopausal gonadotropin/human chorionic gonadotropin therapy. *Fertil Steril* 49:713, 1988
49. Weinstein FG, Seibel MM, Taymor ML: Ovulation induction with subcutaneous pulsatile gonadotropin-releasing hormone: The role of supplemental human chorionic gonadotropin in the luteal phase. *Fertil Steril* 41:546, 1984

50. Saffan D, Seibel MM: Ovulation inductor with subcutaneous pulsatile gonadotropin releasing hormone in various ovulatory observation. *Fertil Steril* 45:475, 1986
51. Skarin G, Nillius SJ, Wide L: Pulsatile subcutaneous low dose gonadotropin-releasing hormone treatment of anovulatory infertility. *Fertil Steril* 40:454, 1983
52. Lunenfeld B, Vardimon D, Blankstein J: Induction of ovulation with GnRH. In Behrman SJ, Kistner RW, Patton GW Jr (eds): *Progress in Infertility*, 3rd ed. Boston, Little, Brown, 1988, p 513
53. Soules MR, Southworth MB, Norton MS, Bremner WJ: Ovulation induction with pulsatile gonadotropin releasing hormone—a study of subcutaneous route of administration. *Fertil Steril* 46:578, 1986
54. Yen SCC: Clinical applications of gonadotropin-releasing hormone and gonadotropin-releasing hormone analogs. *Fertil Steril* 39:257, 1983
55. Lutterback PM, Pryor JS, Varga L, et al: Treatment of non-puerperal galactorrhea with an ergot alkaloid. *Br Med J* 3:228, 1971
56. Besser GM, Parke L, Edwards CRW, et al: Galactorrhea—successful treatment of plasma prolactin levels by brom-ergocryptine. *Br Med J* 3:669, 1972
57. DelProzo E, Friesen H, Birmeister P: Endocrine profile of a specific prolactin inhibitor, brom-ergocryptine (CB-154). *Schwiez Med Wochenschr* 103:847, 1973
58. Thorner MO, McNeilly AS, Hagan C, et al: Long-term treatment of galactorrhea and hypo-gonadism with bromocryptime. *Br Med J* 2:419, 1974
59. Wuttke W, Cassell E, Meites J: Effects of ergocornine on serum prolactin and LH and hypothalamic content of PIF and LRF. *Endocrinology* 88:773, 1971
60. Backman MT, Peake GT, Stivastava L: Patterns of spontaneous LH release in hormo- and hyperprolactinemia women. *Acta Endocrinol (Copenh)*, 97:305, 1981
61. Mroueh AM, Slier-Khodr TM: Ovarian refractoriness to gonadotropins in cases of inappropriate lactation: Restoration of ovarian function with bromcryptine. *J Clin Endocrinol Metab* 42:132, 1975
62. Bohnet HG, Dahlen HG, Wuttke W, et al: Hyperprolactinemia anovulatory syndrome. *J Clin Endocrinol Metab* 42:132, 1975
63. Seppala M, Unnerus HA, Hirvonem E, et al: Bromcryptine increases plasma estradiol-17B concentration in amenorrhea with normal serum prolactin. *J Clin Endocrinol Metab* 43:474, 1976
64. Van der Steeg, HJ, Bennini HJT: Bromcryptine for induction of ovulation in hormoprolactinemic post-pill anovulation. *Lancet* 1:502, 1977
65. Corenblum B, Taylor PJ: A rationale for the use of bromcriptine in patients with amenorrhea and hormoprolactinemia. *Fertil Steril* 34:239, 1980
66. Crosignani PG, Reschini E, Lumbruso GC, Arosio M, Peracchi M: Comparison of placebo and bromcriptine in the treatment of patients with hormoprolactinemic amenorrhea. *Lancet* 1:502, 1977
67. Seibel MM, Oskowitz S, Kamrava M, Taymor ML: Bromcryptine response in hormoprolactinemic patients with polycystic ovary disease—a preliminary report. *Obstet Gynecol* 64:213, 1984
68. Buttram VC, Vaquero C: Post-ovarian wedge resection adhesive disease. *Fertil Steril* 26:874, 1975
69. McArthur JW, Ingersoll FM: Urinary excretion of FSH and ICSH activity by women with diseases of the reproductive system. *J Clin Endocrinol* 18:1202, 1958
70. Kamrava MM, Seibel MM, Berger MJ, Taymor ML: Reversal of persistent ovulation in polycystic ovarian disease by administration of low dose follicle stimulating hormone. *Fertil Steril* 37:520, 1982
71. Claman P, Seibel MM, McArdle C, Berger MJ, Taymor ML: Comparison of intermediate dose purified urinary FSH with and without hcG for ovulation induction in polycystic ovary disease. *Fertil Steril* 46:518, 1986

CHAPTER 27

Microsurgical Techniques and Pelvic Adhesions

The 1970s was an era of revolution in infertility surgery, and in particular in surgery of the fallopian tubes. The development and the use of magnifying techniques, the understanding of the cause of and the development of techniques for the prevention of adhesion formation led to a marked improvement in results. A number of specialists have gained renown in the last decade with the excellence of their technique and their results. However, there is no reason why a well-trained gynecologic surgeon with an understanding of the pathophysiology involved and a knowledge of the principles of microsurgery, as well as some specialized training in the technique, cannot accomplish excellent results. In recent years a number of comprehensive reviews and texts have been published.[1-4]

PRINCIPLES OF MICROSURGERY

The term microsurgery applies not only to the use of the microscope or operating loupes, but to the delicate handling of tissues and the use of other measures that result in minimal tissue damage and a minimum of postoperative adhesions. These principles should be utilized not only in tuboplastic procedures, but whenever possible in all infertility surgery. Indeed, whenever pelvic surgery is carried out in any woman in her reproductive years, microsurgical techniques should be utilized.

Causes of Adhesions

Peritoneal adhesions are the result of an injury to peritoneal surfaces, an injury that can be mechanical, thermal, or chemical. Deprivation of blood supply, foreign bodies, or infection can aggravate the condition. As a result of the injury, there is an inflammatory response and release of an inflammatory exudate. Fibrin coats the tissues. Later, the fibrin is invaded by fibroblasts with a subsequent development of fibrous adhesions. The way to prevent adhesions is to prevent the inflammatory response and the subsequent release of a fibrin-rich exudate. The procedures described below are designed to reduce injury to the tissue and to reduce the inflammatory response.

Adequate Exposure

The incision should be large enough so there is a minimum of pulling on, and retraction of, the pelvic organs and of the abdominal wall. Excessive use of retractors can injure the peritoneum with subsequent adhesion formation. For this reason, a Kirshner retractor with fixed blades is better than movable retractors. Furthermore, when using the microscope, adequate exposure allows the uterus and fallopian tubes to be packed in such a way that they are near the level of the abdominal incision. Adequate exposure also allows a pack to be placed beneath the uterus and a silastic platform to be put in place beneath the tubes and ovaries so that there is a fixed focal plan for the microscope without additional movement of the organs (Fig. 27-1).

Atraumatic Handling of Tissues

All tissues, including tubes, uterus, and ovaries, should be handled delicately. Glass or Teflon® rods should be utilized to lift the tubes and ovaries as much as possible. The extensive packing described above helps in this regard. Adhesions and other tissues for the most part are cut with a unipolar microcautery[4] or laser.[5] These techniques produce minimal tissue damage and at the same time seal off small blood vessels. If knife or scissors are to be used they should be exceedingly sharp.

Hemostatis and Irrigation

If bleeding is anticipated, such as in myomectomy, tubocornual resection, or salpingostomy, a dilute Pitressin® solution (20 units diluted to 80 ml of saline) will reduce bleeding, and the smaller blood vessels will be easier to coagulate with a microcautery or a defocused laser beam. It is important not to leave blood on peritoneal surfaces. Such blood can lead to adhesion formation.[6] Furthermore, the peritoneal surfaces should not be wiped with sponges, which

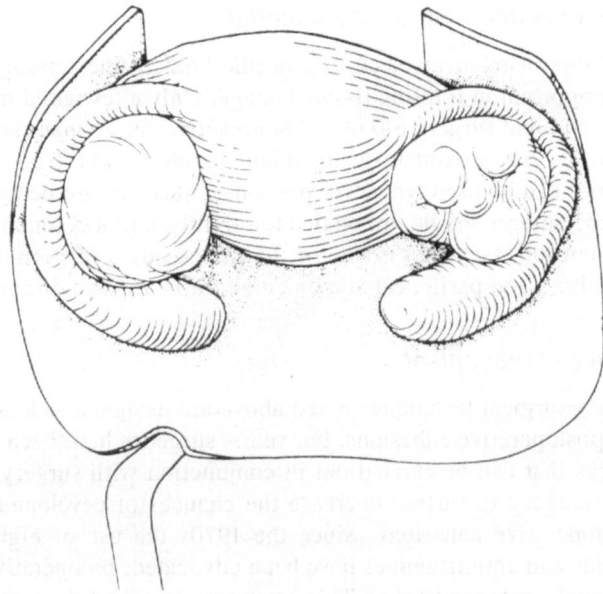

Figure 27-1. The use of packing and a silastic platform to stabilize the fallopian tubes during surgery (from Hunt,[3] with permission from Year Book Publishers).

only add to the irritation. Rather, constant irrigation with lactated Ringer's solution containing 1000 units of heparin per liter should be used.

Magnification and Accurate Approximation of Tissue Edges

The details of the use of the microscope in infertility surgery have been presented in the excellent reviews that have been published.[2-4] The major purpose of magnification is so that accurate approximation of tissue edges can be carried out. This provides primary healing. Magnification is also necessary in order to handle the fine suture material that is used and for pinpoint hemostatis. Many surgeons find that binocular loupes, with magnification ranging from two to eight times, are adequate for most work. The major drawback to the loupes are the fixed focal length and weight as well as lack of illumination and the fixed magnification. Loupes are probably adequate for lysis of adhesions and salpingostomy, which are relatively short procedures. However, tubal reanastamosis procedures, which are lengthy and require variations in magnifications with excellent lighting, are better performed with an operating microscope.

Fine Instruments and Fine Suture Material

Special fine instruments such as a needle holder, fine scissors, and fine forceps are important in limiting tissue damage. Only a few good instruments are required. In tubal surgery 8-0 or 9-0 nonreactive suture materials are used in the muscularis to approximate the tubal lumen. Sutures of 6-0 nonabsorbable suture material can be used whenever peritoneal surfaces are being closed or approximated. Sutures should not be tied too tightly, and it is important not to close under tension. Ischemia is one of the main causes of peritoneal adhesions.[7] For this reason peritoneal and omental grafts are also discouraged.

Postoperative Management

The microsurgical techniques noted above are designed to lessen the occurrence of postoperative adhesions. For years, surgeons have been concerned with measures that can be carried out in conjunction with surgery or immediately after surgery to further decrease the chances of development of significant postoperative adhesions. Since the 1970s the use of high doses of corticosteroids and antihistamines have been advocated, preoperatively, intraoperatively, and postoperatively.[8] This treatment was based on experiments originally carried out in animals and later extended to pediatric surgery.[9] The purpose of the antihistamines is to reduce the initial inflammatory response to trauma consisting of hyperemia, increased vascular permeability, and exudate formation. The corticosteroids delay fibroplasia.

The regimen calls for 20 mg of dexamethasone and 25 mg of promethazine in separate syringes, to be administered intramuscularly 2 hours postoperatively. The same dose is instilled into the pelvis at the time of closure of the abdomen, and then it is given every 4 hours for 12 doses postoperatively. Because of the delayed healing, it is important to use nonabsorbable sutures in the critical areas and not to remove skin sutures for at least 10 days.

In a collaborative study, Horne reported a 61% pregnancy rate using this program.[8] Because of the difficulty in controlling all factors, it is impossible to say that this regimen played a significant role in the results reported. A study from Scandinavia has given some objective confirmation as to the beneficial effect on postoperative adhesions, if not fertility.[9] A laparoscopy was carried out postoperatively in two groups of patients, one in which the antihistamine-corticosteroid regimen was used and in a control group without medication. Adhesion formation was significantly reduced by the treatment. More recent reports, however, have thrown doubt on the effectiveness of this approach. According to a recent review, clinical studies are scant in reporting the use of glucocorticoids.[10] One recent study failed to demonstrate any advantage of glucocorticoids and promethazine over the instillation of 400 ml of lactated Ringer's solution.[11] High-dose corticosteroid therapy is not without risk, and this factor should be weighed against the somewhat questionable effects when considering its use.[12]

In recent years a high-molecular-weight glucose solution (dextran 70) has been widely utilized. Its effectiveness in preventing adhesions in animal experiments is well documented.[13–15] As far as human application is concerned, there has been a difference in the reported results. Some have claimed that there is no significant effect on the development of adhesions,[11] while others have found a beneficial effect.[16] The most recent approach to the prevention of adhesions is the use of a fabric composed of oxidized, regenerated cellulose. A multicenter study concluded that the product did indeed reduce the incidence, extent, and severity of postoperative adhesions.[17]

PERITUBAL AND PERIOVARIAN ADHESIONS

Etiology

Previous pelvic infection, often of a low-grade nature, can result in adhesions that interfere with tubo-ovum pickup. Low-grade salpingitis, which does not result in serious damage to the fimbria, but is accompanied by a perisalpingitis, is one of the more common causes. This is likely to be the end result of a nongonococcal infection, due to either colon bacilli, streptococci, or anaerobic bacteria, which has been treated fairly promptly before severe damage has been done. Low-grade salpingitis usually occurs postpartum or postabortal, but can follow almost any type of intrauterine intervention, such as a dilation and curettage, endometrial biopsy, or even tubal insufflation. The increasing numbers of therapeutic abortions may result in a higher incidence of the peritoneal factor since the rate of infection after therapeutic abortion has been estimated at 2%. Intrauterine insemination, whether advertent or planned, can lead to endometritis and salpingitis with a similar end result. The intrauterine device (IUD) has been incriminated in many overt tubal infections,[18] as well as the cause of adhesions. For this reason, the therapist should look cautiously upon the use of the IUD in the nulliparous female if other methods are available and acceptable.

A ruptured appendix is a major cause of peritubal and periovarian adhesions.[19] This is why the surgeon should make every effort to (or should not neglect to) remove the appendix in the young girl, even in questionable cases. Any pelvic surgery can lead to adhesions; the elective removal of ovarian cysts in a young girl is a common practice, even though the majority of these cysts turn out to be functional. Accumulation of blood in the pelvis incident to ruptured ectopic pregnancy, ruptured follicle, or surgery can lead to adhesion formation. For these reasons, if pelvic surgery has been carried out for tubal pregnancy, thorough irrigation of the peritoneal cavity should be carried out before closure.

It is difficult to identify the bacteria involved in most infections, particularly at the end stage of pelvic adhesions. Recent interest in the role of mycoplasma in infertility has centered around the cervix, but some therapists suggest that some low-grade pelvic infections also may be due to mycoplasma. My own experience tends to support this view. However, because of the general prevalence of mycoplasma in an asymptomatic population, to assign it an etiologic role must remain speculative. A number of studies have incriminated *Chlamydia trachomatis* as a cause of salpingitis, and if such an infection were treated early, only peritubal adhesions might persist.[20]

Despite a large number of potential causes listed above, the woman often has no history of a previous overt infection or intrauterine manipulation, yet the adhesions are still there.

Findings at Laparoscopy and Laparotomy

The findings at endoscopy, and later at laparotomy, vary anywhere from a few adhesions between the ovary and the pelvic wall to a pelvis in which the genital organs are covered and interconnected in a mass of adhesions. In fertility, anything that interferes with normal ovum pickup by the fallopian tube is significant, particularly if it is bilateral. Normal ovum pickup requires that the fimbria be in intimate contact with the surface of the ovary, that the fimbria be freely movable and have access to the major portion of the ovary. Sometimes there are actually bands or coverings of adhesions separating the fimbria from the ovary (Fig. 27-2), and in such cases, the defect is obvious. In other cases, however, there may be free access of both the surfaces of the ovary to the fimbriated end of the tube, but either because of adhesions of the ovary to the side of the pelvis or because of adhesions between the tubes and the structures above the pelvic brim, there is a relative inadequacy of the tubo-ovum pickup.

TREATMENT OF PELVIC ADHESIONS

Laparotomy

The management of pelvic adhesions has been reviewed by Holtz.[15] The principles of microsurgery outlined earlier in this chapter should be utilized. Adhesions can be divided either by a unipolar microcautery over glass rods or with the laser over titanium rods[21] (Fig. 27-3). Constant irrigation is utilized and blood and clots are rapidly removed by suction. Magnification with loupes may be helpful, but is not always necessary. Bleeding points are controlled with the bipolar cautery or nonreactive fine suture material. If relatively large pieces or large sections of omentum need to be freed from the pelvic organs, small

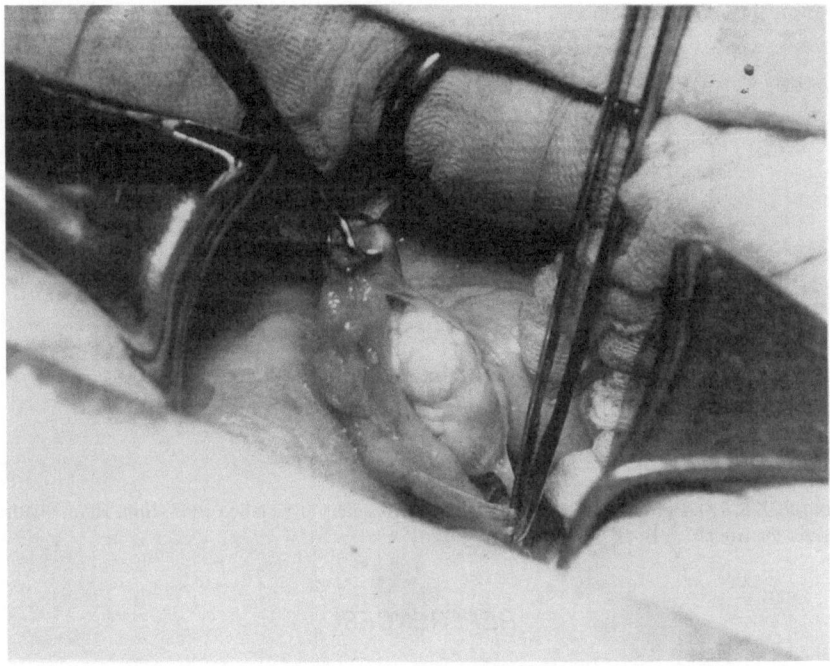

Figure 27-2. Peritoneal adhesions.

bites should be taken and ligated with nonreactive suture material. The various modalities used to reduce the redevelopment of adhesions should be utilized postoperatively.

Laparoscopy

The laparoscope, with its potential for multiple punctures, provides an excellent approach to the lysis of minimal or moderate adhesions. With two or, if necessary, three incisions the operative site can be viewed, the tissue can be kept under traction away from vital structures, and adhesions can be cut and cauterized. The surgeon can handle one or two adhesions holding an ovary or tube out of the normal position in this way, but the temptation to do more should be avoided. Extensive cauterization may simply be an invitation for the reformation of adhesions. Extensive adhesions are better divided at laparotomy where microsurgical techniques can be utilized. It is still to be shown that extensive pelviscopic surgery can provide the results obtained by delicate microsurgery performed through an open laparotomy.

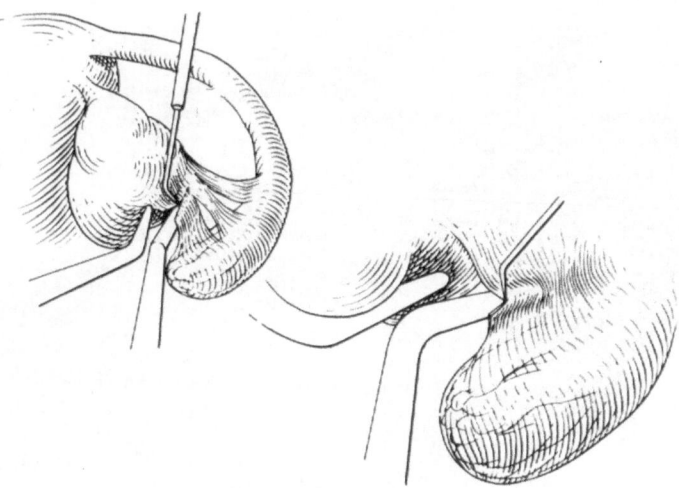

Figure 27-3. Lysis of adhesions with unipolar microcautery over teflon rods (from Hunt,[3] with permission from Year Book Publishers).

REFERENCES

1. Winston RW: Microsurgery of the fallopian tubes. In Taymor ML and Nelson JH Jr (eds): *Progress in Gynecology.* New York, Grune and Stratton, 1983, p 399
2. Gomel V: *Microsurgery in Female Infertility.* Boston, Little, Brown, 1983
3. Hunt RB: *Atlas of Female Infertility Surgery.* Chicago, Year Book, 1986
4. Patton GW Jr: A concept of gynecologic microsurgery. In Behrman SJ, Kistner RW, Patton GW Jr (eds): *Progress in Infertility,* 3rd ed. Boston, Little, Brown, 1988, p 107
5. Baggish MS, Chong AP: Carbon dioxide laser microsurgery of the uterine tube. *Obstet Gynecol* 58:111, 1981
6. Nissell H, Larsen B: Role of blood and fibrinogen on the development of intrafallopian adhesions in rats. *Fertil Steril* 30:470, 1978
7. Holtz G: Prevention and management of peritoneal adhesions. *Fertil Steril* 41:497, 1984
8. Horne HW Jr, Clyman M, Debrovner C, et al: The prevention of post-operative adhesions following conservative operative treatment for human infertility: A final 3-year follow-up report. *Int J Fertil* 18:109, 1973
9. Replogle RL, Johnson R, Gross RS: Prevention of post-operative intestinal adhesions with combined promethazine and dexamethasone therapy: Experimental and clinical studies. *Am Surg* 163:580, 1966
9a. Swolin K: Die einwirkung von grossen intraperitonealen dosen glukokortikoid auf die bildung von postoperativen adhesionen. *Acta Obstet Gynecol Scand* 46:204, 1967
10. Pfeiffer WH: Adjuvants in tubal surgery. *Fertil Steril* 33:245, 1980
11. Fayez JA, Schneider PJ: Prevention of pelvic adhesion formation by different modalities of treatment. *Am J Obstet Gynecol* 157:1184, 1987
12. Holtz G: Current use of ancillary modalities for adhesion prevention. *Fertil Steril* 44:174, 1985
13. Di Zerega GS, Hodgen GD: Prevention of postsurgical tubal adhesions. Comparative study of commonly used agents. *Am J Obstet Gynecol* 136:173, 1980

14. Utian WH, Goldfarb JM, Starks GC: Role of Dextran 70 in microtubal surgery. *Fertil Steril* 31:68, 1979
15. Holtz G: Management of peritoneal adhesions. In Behrman SJ, Kistner RW, Patton GW Jr (eds): *Progress in Infertility*, 3rd ed. Boston, Little, Brown, 1988, p 155
16. Adhesion Study Group: Reduction of post-operative adhesions with intraperitoneal 32% dextran 70, a prospective randomized clinical study. *Fertil Steril* 40:612, 1983
17. INTERCEED (TC7) Adhesions Barrier Study Group: Prevention of post-surgical adhesions by INTERCEED (TC7), an absorbable adhesion barrier: A prospective, randomized multicenter clinical study. 51:933, 1989
18. Taylor SS, MacMillan JH, Greene BE, et al: The intrauterine device and tubo-ovarian abscess. *Am J Obstet Gynecol* 119:388, 1974
19. Powley PH: Infertility due to pelvic abscess and pelvic peritonitis in appendicitis. *Lancet* 1:27, 1965
20. Sweet RL: Pelvic infection in infertility. In Behrman SJ, Kistner RW, Patton GW Jr (eds): *Progress in Infertility*, 3rd ed. Boston, Little, Brown, 1988, p 25
21. Martin DC: Laser surgery for adhesions. In Baggish MS (ed): *Basic and Advanced Laser Surgery in Gynecology*. Appleton-Century-Crofts, Norwalk, CT, 1985, p 331

CHAPTER 28

Tubal Microsurgery

The microsurgical techniques described in the previous chapter find their greatest application in reconstructive surgery of the fallopian tube. Microsurgical technique should be used throughout. Some surgeons use an operative microscope, but when only a brief period of magnification is required, loupes are usually sufficient. It is best to perform the surgery in the preovulative phase of the cycle so that a hemorrhagic corpus luteum will not interfere with the surgery. Prophylactic antibiotics are usually prescribed. Dye instilled into the tube is helpful in identifying the end of the tube and in proving patency at the end of the procedure. A pediatric catheter or a uterine manipulator* of transcervical cannula with sterile tube and syringe leading up to the operating field will allow the surgeon to control the flow of fluid into the fallopian tube from the uterus during the surgery. The techiques of fimbrioplasty, salpingostomy, tubocornual anastamosis, and tubal reversal have been described in detail in various texts and reviews, and only the highlights will be reviewed here.[1-4] Either a unipolar microcautery or a laser cutting beam can be used to divide tissues. Studies to date show no advantages of one over the other.

SURGERY FOR DISTAL TUBAL OBSTRUCTION

To provide the patients with a fairly accurate prognosis, and also to be able to compare results from one report to another, the type of surgery to be per-

*Ziunanti Surgical Instruments, Inc., Woodland Hills, CA.

formed should be accurately labeled. The types of surgery performed are listed in Table 28-1 in order of severity and prognosis. Salpingolysis and fimbriolysis obviously give an excellent result and have been dealt with in chapter 27.

Fimbrioplasty

When there is only agglutination of the fimbria to pelvic surfaces or to each other, or when there is a partial closure of the tube squeezing the fimbria (phimosis), excellent release of the fimbria can be obtained by microsurgical techniques. A glass rod is placed beneath the area of adherence and cut with the cautery laser. When phimosis is present, the rod is placed beneath the scar, which is divided, releasing the fimbria (Fig. 28-1). The results of fimbrioplasty are generally quite good and range from 20% to 60% in intrauterine pregnancies.

Salpingostomy

Distal tube obstruction results from a serious infection with bacterial invaders similar to those described as the cause of pelvic adhesions. However, infection with gonococcus is more likely to result in complete obstruction, and chlamydia has been recently incriminated as a cause of complete obstruction as well. Before opening the fallopian tubes, all adhesions are divided. It is also very important to dissect the distal end of the tube off the ovary. A salpingostomy carried out at the true end of the tube, the site of the previous ostium that is now recognized by pucker point, is one most likely to remain open. Occasionally, the tissues at the distal end of the tube are so thickened that it is necessary to make an ostium elsewhere. The results will not be as satisfactory. Once the pucker point has been identified, it is opened with the cautery

Table 28-1. Classification of Distal Tubal Surgery

Salpingolysis
 An operation that frees peritubal adhesions where the tube and fimbria appear to be healthy

Fimbriolysis
 An operation that frees the fimbria of the tube of adhesions

Fimbrioplasty
 An operation that frees partial occlusion of the tubal opening, including the division of adhesions between opposing walls of the mucosa and the division of adhesions between agglutinated fimbria

Salpingostomy
 An operation that creates a new opening in a completely occluded tube

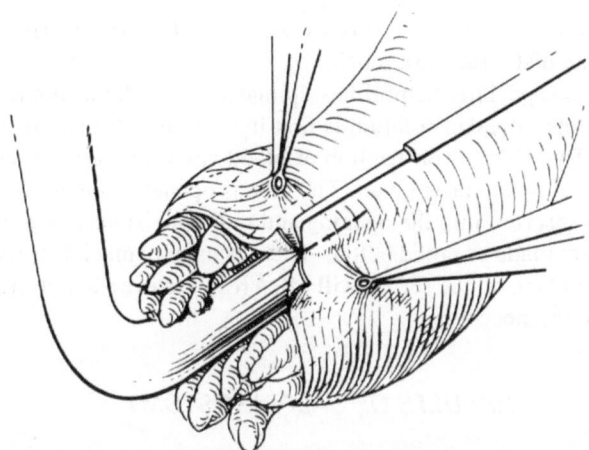

Figure 28-1. Fimbrioplasty. Excision of fibrous tissue that occludes the end of the fallopian tube (from Hunt[3]).

(Fig. 28-2). Dye will be seen to escape from the opening. A glass rod is inserted and radial incisions are made enlarging the tubal lumen. Incisions are made over avascular areas and along scarlines (lines of agglutinated fimbria) if these can be identified. Three or four radial incisions are made sufficient to allow eversion of the flaps that are produced. Bleeding points are coagulated with the bipolar cautery. The flaps are kept everted by suturing to the peritoneum sur-

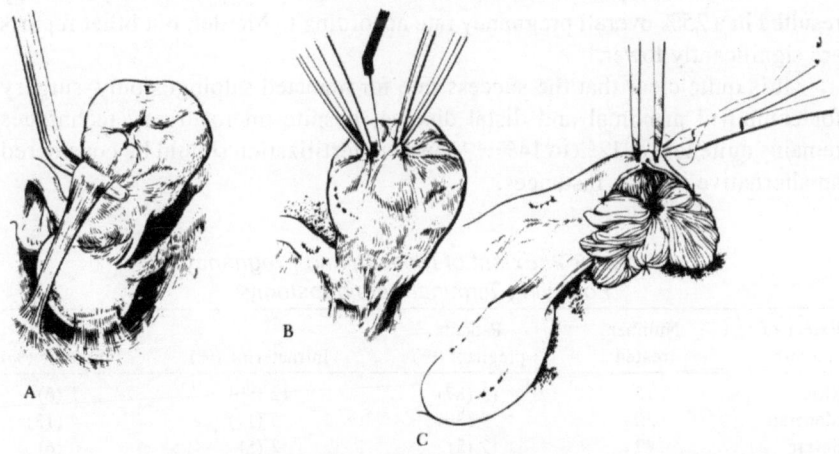

Figure 28-2. Salpingostomy. A. Lysis of adhesions to free end of tube. B. Opening tube at pucker point with a microcautery. C. Sewing mucosal flaps to peritoneal surface of tube (from Patton[4]).

face of the tube with 6-0 prolene sutures. Any defects in the ovaries caused by dissection of the distal tube are repaired.

The laser is especially helpful in salpingostomy, as far as the technique is concerned. Dilute pitressin solution is first injected into the tissue around the pucker point. This causes constriction of blood vessels that will then be more effectively sealed by the laser beam. The tube is opened at the pucker point. A titanium rod is inserted into the opening and radial incisions along the lines of agglutination are made as noted before. There is usually much less bleeding. A defocused laser beam on the serosa will often result in eversion of the flaps and sutures may not be necessary.

RESULTS OF SALPINGOSTOMY

As noted above, results of surgery for complete distal blockage of the fallopian tube are influenced by the extent of disease. Another consideration is the effect of microsurgical techniques on success rates. In a report by Rock and co-workers, shown in Table 28-2, the pregnancy rate was 80% with mild disease, 17% with moderate disease, and 5% with severe disease, with an overall pregnancy rate of 22%.[6]

Table 28-3 compares the results of macrosurgery and microsurgery. It would appear that the pregnancy rates are higher with microsurgery but that there is a slight increase in the incidence of ectopic pregnancy, negating some of the benefits of microsurgery.[13]

When utilizing laser for salpingostomy the results appear to be no better (21%) than those reported for non-laser techniques.[12] Operative laparoscopy resulted in a 25% overall pregnancy rate according to Mettler, but other reports are significantly lower.[14]

It is quite clear that the success rate for repeated salpingostomy, surgery for combined proximal and distal disease, despite microsurgery techniques remains quite low at 12% to 14%.[4,11] In vivo fertilization should be considered an alternative in such instances.

Table 28-2. Extent of Disease and Pregnancy
Following Terminal Salpingostomy[a]

Extent of disease	Number treated	Patients pregnant (%)	Intrauterine (%)	Ectopic (%)
Mild	15	13 (87)	12 (80)	1 (6)
Moderate	30	9 (30)	5 (17)	4 (13)
Severe	42	2 (5)	2 (5)	0 (6)
Total	87	24 (18)	19 (22)	5 (5)

[a]From Rock et al.[6]

Table 28-3. Results of Salpingostomy[a]

Author	Year	Number of patients	Intrauterine pregnancies (%)	Ectopic pregnancies (%)
		Macrosurgery		
Palmer[7]	1968	123	34 (28)	16 (13)
O'Brien et al.[8]	1969	57	15 (26)	1 (2)
Fjallbrandt	1975	35	6 (17)	3 (2)
Roland and Leister[9]	1970	25	4 (16)	0 (0)
Rock et al.[6]	1978	99	16 (16)	6 (16)
Total		339	75 (22.1)	25 (7.3)
		Microsurgery		
Swolin[10]	1975	33	15 (45.0)	6 (18)
Marik	1977	82	12 (23.0)	2 (3)
Gomel[16]	1983	89	40 (45.0)	4 (11)
Winston[2]	1983	241	65 (26.9)	23 (9.5)
Total		415	132 (31.8)	35 (8.4)

[a]Adapted from Winston.[2]

SURGERY FOR PROXIMAL TUBAL OBSTRUCTION

Etiology and Diagnosis

The cause of proximal tubal obstruction is not always clear. Indeed, when resected tubes or cornual segments are examined by a pathologist, often no disease process can be found. However, severe bacterial salpingitis can result in obstruction and can be caused by the same bacterial invaders that cause distal disease. This often manifests itself grossly as salpingitis isthmica nodosa. Endometriosis, adenomyosis of the fallopian tube, has also been incriminated as a cause of proximal tubal obstruction.[15] Congenital narrowing is another cause.

However, obstruction at the interstitial portion of the tube can be due to spasm. For this reason, when proximal obstruction is seen at hysterosalpingography the x ray should be repeated before proceeding with laparoscopy. If there is a failure to demonstrate tubal patency after two tubograms and tubal lavage at laparoscopy, laparotomy can be planned. However, the tube should not be divided until obstruction has also been demonstrated by attempted lavage through the uterus at the time of laparotomy.

Surgical Technique

Prior to development of the technique of microsurgery the surgical approach to proximal obstruction was resection of the obstructed cornual portion of the uterus. Results of microsurgical anastomosis, and of in vitro fertilization if tubal anastomosis is not possible, are so surperior to cornual implantation that there is little place for this procedure at the present time. However, it has recently been redescribed by Hunt.[3]

An excellent description of microsurgical tubocornual anastomosis has been presented by Gomel.[16] Briefly, the technique involves division of the tube close to the tubocornual junction. Dilute Pitressin solution into the cornual portion of the uterus will minimize bleeding. Dye is injected through a catheter placed in the uterus to determine patency. Not only should patency be demonstrated, but the tubal mucosa should appear pink and healthy under the operating microscope. Cuts through the cornua can be made with a sharp knife, iris-type scissors, or a special curved blade developed by Gomel to minimize loss of cornual musculature (Fig. 28-3).

When the proximal side has been completed, attention is directed to the distal tube. Successive cuts taken through the isthmus are made until patency and healthy tissue is noted. With salpingitis a large portion of the isthmus must be sacrificed before healthy tissue is reached.

Winston prefers to carry out the anastomosis over a plastic stent and has developed stents and instruments to facilitate this procedure. The stents are removed at the end of the procedure.

Prior to carrying out the anastomosis, a stay suture of 6-0 prolene is placed in the mesosalpinx and through the musculature of the cornua just below the tubal muscularis (Fig. 28-4). This is kept untied while tubal sutures are being placed, but it will be tied when all sutures are in place in order to remove tension from the fine muscularis sutures. Sutures of 8-0 or 9-0 nonabsorbable or non-reactive suture material are then placed in the muscularis of tube at 6, 3, 9, and 12 o'clock. These are serially tied. A layer of 6-0 sutures is now placed in the seromuscularis layer to complete the anastomosis (Fig. 28-5).

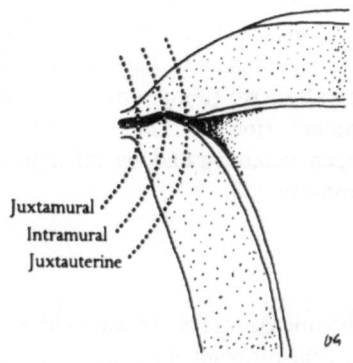

Juxtamural
Intramural
Juxtauterine

Figure 28-3. Successive cuts through cornua until patency and healthy tissue is reached (from Gomel[1]).

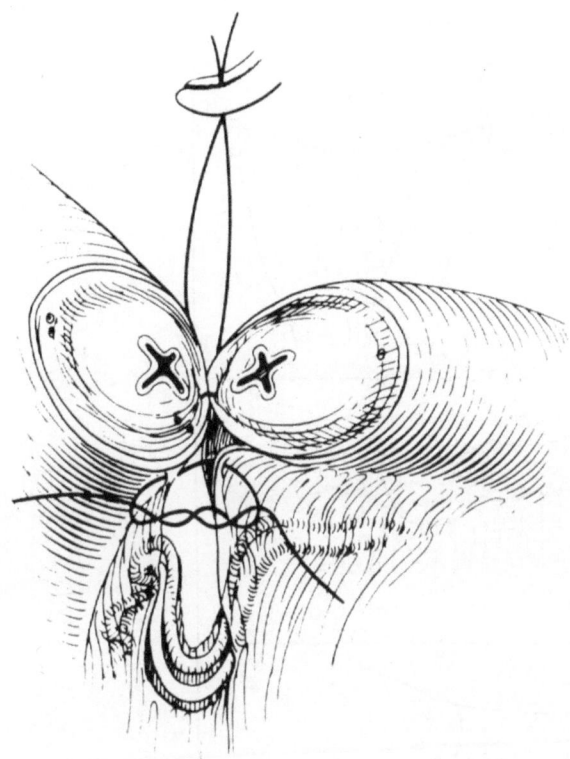

Figure 28-4. Stay suture of 6-0 prolene and 6 o'clock suture of 8-0 nylon in place (from Hunt[3]).

Results

Winston reported a 37% pregnancy rate for tubocornual anastomosis with only one ectopic pregnancy. Cornual implantation during the same time period resulted in a pregnancy rate of only 21%. Success rates as high as 56% have also been reported with few ectopic pregnancies.[17] Patients with multiple sites of occlusion, however, have a very poor prognosis.[18]

TUBAL REANASTOMOSIS

The best results from tubal microsurgery occur when performing tubal reanastomosis for tubes that have been surgically divided, ligated, or clamped. Success rates as high as 75% have been reported.[2] Success rates are related to the length of the tubes that are to be brought together and thus to the type of

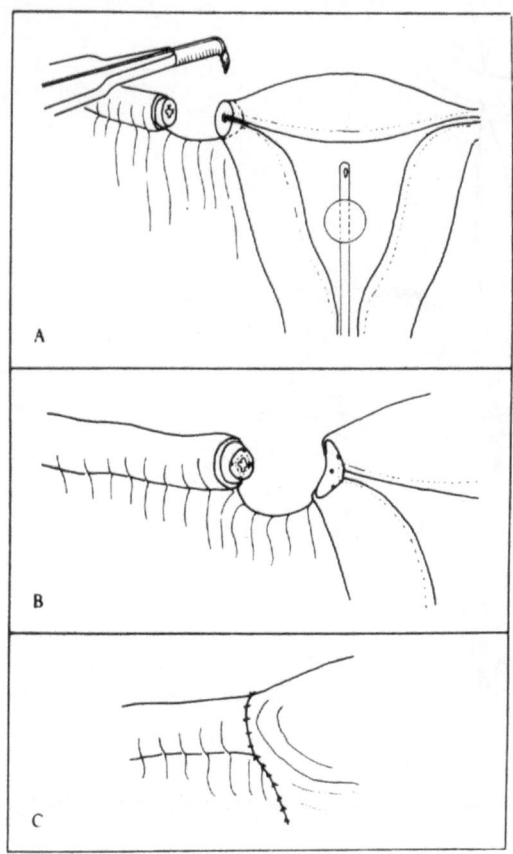

Figure 28-5. A and B: The Gomel knife. C: The completed anastomosis (from Gomel[1]).

tubal ligation that had been utilized. Anastomosis resulting in tubes less than 4 cm bring relatively poor results. An isthmic anastomosis brings about the best results.[19] Thus a simple clamping of the isthmus will destroy little tissue and allow for this excellent prognosis. On the other hand, surgical removal of segments of tubes or extensive cauterization will often destroy the entire isthmus and cornua-ampullary anastomosis will be required. The success rates dropped to approximately 50%. If ligation was carried out through the ampulla, ampullary anastomosis will be required. This results in a still lower success rate.

Surgical Technique

The technique of reanastomosis is similar to that described for tubo-

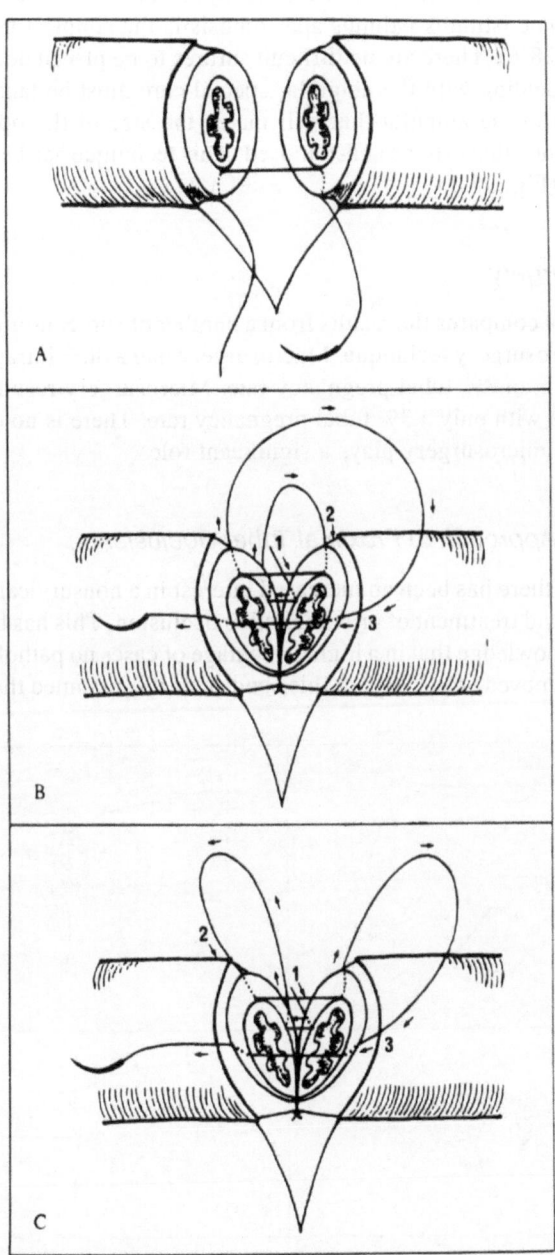

Figure 28-6. Tubal–tubal anastomosis. Placement of sutures (from Gomel[1]).

cornual anastomosis. Many of the procedures are indeed a tubocornual anastomosis. The isthmus-isthmus anastomosis is the simplest for the microsurgeon (Fig. 28-6). There are no difficult sutures to be placed deep in cornual tissue. When dealing with the ampulla, special care must be taken to make a small opening in the ampulla that will match the size of the opening in the isthmus or cornua that is to be anastomosed. This technique has been described by Gomel[1,16] (Fig. 28-7).

Results of Surgery

Table 28-4 compares the results from a number of surgeons utilizing either macro- or microsurgery technique. Macrosurgery had a 36% intrauterine pregnancy rate with an 8% tubal pregnancy rate. Microsurgery resulted in a 61% pregnancy rate with only a 3% tubal pregnancy rate. There is no doubt that in this procedure microsurgery plays a significant role.

Nonsurgical Approach to Proximal Tubal Occlusion

Recently, there has been an increased interest in a nonsurgical approach to the diagnosis and treatment of proximal tubal occlusion. This has been brought about by the knowledge that in a high percentage of cases no pathology is found in the tissue removed at surgery for this condition. It is assumed that congenital

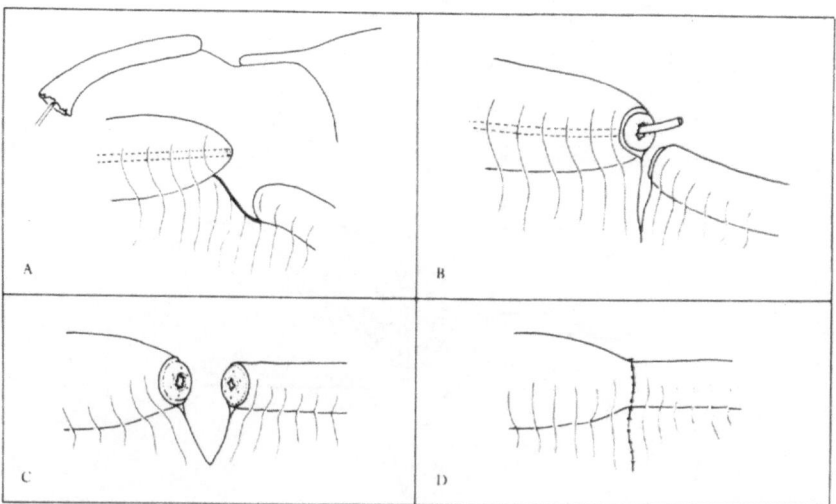

Figure 28-7. Isthmic–ampullary anastomosis. Demonstration of a method to keep opening in the ampulla small (from Gomel[1]).

Table 28-4. Tubal Reanastomosis for Reversal of Sterilization[a]

Author	Year	Number of patients	Intrauterine pregnancies (%)	Ectopic pregnancies (%)
		Macrosurgery		
Williams[20]	1973	16	4 (25)	0 (0)
Siegler and Perez[21]	1975	46	17 (37)	2 (4)
McCormick and Torres[22]	1976	14	4 (29)	3 (21)
Hudari et al.[23]	1977	13	8 (52)	1 (8)
Diamond[24]	1977	12	3 (25)	1 (25)
Total		101	36 (36)	9 (8)
		Microsurgery		
Diamond[24]	1977	28	16 (57)	2 (7)
Daniell[13]	1979	16	10 (63)	2 (13)
Wilson	1980	3	2 (67)	0 (0)
Winston[2]	1983	126	73 (58)	3 (2)
Gomel[16]	1980	118	76 (64)	1 (.8)
Total		291	177 (61)	8 (3)

[a]Adapted from Winston.[2]

narrowing or inspissated mucus is the cause of the apparent blockage seen at hysterosalpingogram. It has been hoped that selective tubal cannulation with or without lavage can diagnose and even treat these occlusions.

One approach is the use of tiny steel probes, or small balloons, passed into the tubal ostium transcervically under fluoroscopic control.[25,28] A high degree of patency is achieved in this manner, which persists. Some pregnancies do occur.

An alternate approach is to pass the wire into the uterine end of the fallopian tube under hysteroscopic and laparoscopic control.[29,30] Similar incidences of patency and pregnancy have been reported. It is still too early to fully evaluate the therapeutic potential of this approach. If some pregnancies do occur, however, it may be a worthwhile procedure and it can thus spare some patients, although not all, an abdominal operation.

REFERENCES

1. Gomel V: *Microsurgery in Female Infertility*. Boston, Little, Brown, 1983
2. Winston RW: Microsurgery of the fallopian tube. In Taymor ML and Nelson JH Jr. (eds): *Progress in Gynecology*, New York, Grune and Stratton, 1983, p 399
3. Hunt RB: *Atlas of Female Infertility Surgery*. Chicago, Year Book, 1986
4. Patton GW Jr: Microsurgical reconstruction of the oviduct. In Behrman SJ, Kistner RW, Patton GW Jr (eds): Boston, Little, Brown, 1988, p 125
5. Patton GW Jr: Pregnancy outcome following microsurgical fimbrioplasty. *Fertil Steril* 37:150, 1982

6. Rock JA, Katayama KP, Martin EJ, Woodruff JD, Jones HW Jr: Factors influencing the success of salpingostomy techniques for distal fimbrial obstruction. *Obstet Gynecol* 52:591, 1978

7. Palmer R: Le traitement chirugical des sterdites tubaise. *Bull Fed Soc Gynecol Obstet* 20:130, 1968

8. O'Brien JR, Arronet GH, Eduljee SY: Operative treatment of fallopian tube pathology in human infertility. *Am J Obstet Gynecol* 103:520, 1969

9. Roland M, Leister D: Tuboplasty in 130 patients. *Obstet Gynecol* 39:57, 1952

10. Swolin K: Electromicrosurgery and salpingostomy: Long-term results. *Am J Obstet Gynecol* 121:418, 1975

11. Winston RL: Microsurgery of the fallopian tube: From fantasy to reality. *Fertil Steril* 34:521, 1988

12. Bateman BG, Nunley WC Jr, Kitchin JD III: Surgical management of distal tube obstruction: Are we making progress? *Fertil Steril* 48:523, 1987

13. Daniel JF, Diamond MP, McLaughlin DS, et al: Clinical results of terminal salpingostomy with the use of the CO_2 laser: Report of the intraabdominal laser study group. *Fertil Steril* 45:175, 1986

14. Mettler L, Giesel H, Semm K: Treatment of female infertility due to obstruction by operative laparoscopy. *Fertil Steril* 33:476, 1983

15. Claman P, Taymor ML, Berger MJ, Seibel MM: Proximal obstruction of the oviduct: A possible role for medical therapy with danazol. J Reprod Med 31:637, 1986

16. Gomel V: Microsurgical reversal of female sterilization: A reapproach. *Fertil Steril* 33:587, 1980

17. Levy G, Diamond MP, DeClerney AH: Pregnancy following tubocornual anastomosis. *Fertil Steril* 46:21, 1986

18. Patton DE, Williams TJ, Cocham CB: Results of microsurgery reconstruction in patients with combined proximal and distal tube occlusion: A double obstruction. *Fertil Steril* 48:670, 1987

19. Rock JA, Guziak DS, Katz E, Sacur HA, King TM: Tubal anastomosis: Pregnancy success following reversal of fallope ring or monopolar cautery sterilization. *Fertil Steril* 48:13, 1987

20. Williams GFJ: Fallopian tube surgery for reversal of sterilization. *Br Med J* 1:599, 1973

21. Siegler AM, Perez RJ: Reconstruction of fallopian tubes in previously sterilized patients. *Fertil Steril* 26:383, 1975

22. McCormick WG, Torres J: A method of Pomeroy tubal ligation anastomosis. *Obstet Gynecol* 43:623, 1976

23. Hudari AA, Vibhasiri S, Isaac AY: Reconstructive tubal surgery for mid-tubal obstruction. *Fertil Steril* 28:620, 1977

24. Diamond E: Microsurgery reconstruction of the uterine tube in sterilized patients. *Fertil Steril* 28:1203, 1977

25. Platio MP, Krudy AG: Transcervical fluoroscopic recanalization of a proximally occluded oviduct. *Fertil Steril* 44:704. 1985

26. Confino S, Friberg J, Gleicher N: Transcervical balloon tuboplasty. *Fertil Steril* 46:963, 1986

27. Thurmond AS, Novy M, Uchida BT, Rosch J: Fallopian tube obstruction: Selective salpingography and recanalization. *Radiology* 163:511, 1987

28. Segars JH, Herbert CM, Moore DE, Hill GA, Wentz AC, Winfield AC: Selective fallopian tube cannulation: Initial experience in an infertile population. *Fertil Steril* 53:357, 1990

29. Sulak PJ, Letteria GS, Hayslip CC, Coddington CC, Klein TA: Hysteroscopic cannulation and lavage in the treatment of tubal occlusion. *Fertil Steril* 48:493, 1987

30. Deaton JL, Gibson M, Riddick DH, Brumsted JR: Diagnosis and treatment of cornual obstruction using a flexible guide wire. *Fertil Steril* 53:232, 1990

CHAPTER 29

Endometriosis

Endometriosis is a common gynecologic problem, and one that is of special significance in infertility. In recent years, there seems to be an increased incidence in the finding of endometriosis associated with infertility. One explanation for this apparent increase is the general use of the laparoscope in infertility diagnosis, and thus the finding of many cases of early endometriosis unassociated with the usual signs and symptoms of the disease. Another cause may be the late onset of marriage, and the discovery of infertility at a later age. Endometriosis is associated more commonly with nulliparous women in their late 20s or 30s rather than with younger age groups.

The primary treatment of endometriosis, unassociated with infertility, is medical, with surgery used only when disease progresses despite the use of medical therapy. On the other hand, when endometriosis is associated with infertility, surgery should often be the primary approach.

Causes of Endometriosis

The various theories about the causes of endometriosis are well known: (1) retrograde menstrual flow, (2) transformation of celomic epithelium, and (3) lymphatic spread. It takes a combination of all three theories to explain the findings of endometriosis in the various parts of the body. Retrograde menstrual flow presents the best explanation for endometriosis in the cul-de-sac and along the uterosacral ligaments. Celomic metaplasia is a better explanation for endometriosis beginning beneath the ovarian capsule and presenting as chocolate cysts.

259

Diagnosis

The therapist should immediately suspect endometriosis when the patient gives a history of secondary dysmenorrhea during the initial interview. Dyspareunia and pain on defecation are other associated symptoms. More extensive endometriosis is often accompanied by pain on either side throughout the cycle, increasing severity not only at the time of menses, but also at midcycle. When these symptoms are accompanied by tenderness, with or without enlargement in the region of one or both ovaries, or by nodularity along the uterosacral ligaments or behnd the cervix, these suspicions are increased. These latter findings are better noted by rectal examination.

Endometriosis, even with severe ovarian fixation, often is asymptomatic, and will only be discovered when endoscopy is part of the infertility workup. With routine use of laparoscopy as part of the diagnostic workup, asymptomatic endometriosis is now being found in a significantly larger number of patients. If symptomology and physical findings are severe enough, endoscopy should be performed without the usual waiting period. There is no doubt about the superiority of laparoscopy over culdoscopy in the diagnosis of endometriosis. Not only does the physician have a more complete view of the pelvis, tubes, and ovaries, but the failures and dangers associated with culdoscopy due to extensive cul-de-sac endometriosis are eliminated. Laparoscopy should always precede laparotomy unless there is significant enlargement of the ovary, which, by itself, would indicate surgery.

During the last few years a number of authors have reported on the findings of elevated levels of CA-125 in a series of patients with endometriosis,[1] although one report indicated that the levels are only significant in dealing with patients with stage 3 and 4 disease.[2]

The association between endometriosis and infertility is well accepted.[3] Indeed it is estimated that 40% of patients with endometriosis are infertile. Whatever the cause, endometriosis as related to infertility deserves special handling as it relates to ovarian or tubal involvement, and as such the extent of disease can be divided into stages of increasing severity. It is very important that the laparoscopist utilize some forms of staging. The one most widely utilized is that of the American Fertility Society (Fig. 29-1).[4] As a result of staging the disease, one can determine whether or not medical or surgical treatment is indicated, and indeed whether any treatment at all is indicated. Furthermore, the prognosis of the disease is directly related to staging.

Mechanisms of Infertility

The mechanism of infertility is obvious when the ovaries or tubes are bound down as in stages 3 and 4. There is interference with normal tubo-ovum

Patient's Name_____ Date_____

Stage I   (Minimal)   — 1–5   Laparascopy_____
Stage II   (Mild)   — 6–15   Laparatomy_____
Stage III   (Moderate)   — 16–40   Photography_____
Stage IV   (Severe)   — >40   Recommended Treatment_____
Total_____

Prognosis_____

Endometriosis	<1cm	1–3cm	>3cm
Superficial	1	2	4
Deep	2	4	6
R Superficial	1	2	4
Deep	4	16	20
L Superficial	1	2	4
Deep	4	16	20
Posterior Cul-de-sac Obliteration	Partial		Complete
	4		40
Adhesions	<⅓ Enclosure	⅓–⅔ Enclosure	>⅔ Enclosure
R Filmy	1	2	4
Dense	4	8	16
L Filmy	1	2	4
Dense	4	8	16
R Filmy	1	2	4
Dense	4*	8*	16
L Filmy	1	2	4
Dense	4*	8*	16

*If the fimbriated end of the fallopian tube is completely enclosed, change the point assignment to 16.

Figure 29-1. The American Fertility Society Revised Classification of Endometriosis.[4]

pickup. However, infertility often co-exists with stages 1 and 2. It is difficult to explain the cause of infertility.

Peritoneal fluids from patients with endometriosis has been described to contain excess prostaglandins, macrophages, and interleuken.[5,6] Interleuken 1 has been shown to have an adverse effect on in vitro gamete function in mice, and it has been theorized that a similar effect might occur in humans in association with minimal and mild endometriosis.[7] However, these theories will have to be looked at with caution until it has been even proven that minimal or mild endometriosis actually causes infertility, and that it is not just an associative finding in many cases of infertility.

Surgical Treatment of Endometriosis

When laparoscopy reveals the existence of adhesions between the tubes, ovary, and peritoneum, when the ovaries are fixed to the posterior leaf of the broad ligament, or when there are enlarged endometriotic cysts of the ovaries, as in stage 3 and stage 4 disease, surgery is the primary treatment. Medical treatment will not dissolve the adhesions or eliminate large cysts of the ovaries. The primary goal of surgery is to preserve as much ovarian function as possible and to improve tubo-ovum pickup. The adhesions to the ovaries are divided with microsurgical techniques (see Chapter 27). The adhesions between the ovary and broad ligament are carefully dissected. It is usually difficult to clamp this area. The cut edges of the broad ligament can be sutured if there is no tension. If the involvement of the ovary is minimal, a small wedge of ovarian tissue can be removed at the site of the previous adherence, and the ovary repaired with fine nonreactive sutures. Adhesions associated with fallopian tubes can be handled easily. Endometrial implants over the peritoneum should be surgically excised if there is not too much deep scarring, and the peritoneum should be sutured, rather than cauterized, because cautery leaves a raw area with a potential for future adhesions.

Large chocolate cysts should be shelled out of the ovary. Deep sutures are then placed in the ovarian tissue for hemostasis and the cortex is closed with a fine nonreactive continuous suture. An anterior suspension is often needed, particularly if the uterus has been freed from its previous third-degree position with adherence to the rectosigmoid. Suspension of the ovary to the uterus prevents it from adhering again to the broad ligament. It is not always necessary to excise all implants, particularly those in surgically dangerous areas, i.e., uterosacral ligaments or bowel. The goal of surgery is improvement of tubo-ovum pickup; other areas can be treated medically.

The use of the laser during a laparotomy provides a significant improvement (see Chapter 18).[8] Adhesions can be lysed quickly and atraumatically, and peritoneal implants can be vaporized. The greatest advantage comes in the treatment of significant endometriotic cysts of the ovaries. With surgery alone, often a great deal of normal tissue had to be sacrificed in attempting a thorough removal of the cyst. With the laser, the cyst can be unroofed with an incision through the ovarian cortex over the cyst. The inner lining of the cyst can be dissected away, and then the base of the cyst can be vaporized with a low-intensity laser beam, thus destroying any remaining endometriotic tissue. The walls of the cyst are approximated with sutures and the capsule closed. Thus, little if any normal tissue is removed.

In surgery for endometriosis, whenever possible, microsurgical techniques should be utilized. Steps to reduce postoperative adhesions should also be taken, such as the use of dextran 70.

Laparoscopic laser and pelviscopic surgery are being used more and more in the surgical therapy for endometriosis.[9,10] For many, laparotomies are being utilized less and less, but the laparoscopic approach is probably best for only the milder degrees of the disease.[11]

Results of Surgical Treatment

The results of pelvic surgery for four studies are shown in Table 29-1. There is a decline in pregnancy rates as the condition becomes more severe. However, a 28% to 40% pregnancy rate for severe endometriosis does seem to indicate that the procedure is worthwhile. Overall success rates for mild endometriosis are at about 61%. It is difficult to know whether or not surgery is really helpful in mild endometriosis because pregnancy rates without any treatment can approximate these numbers.

Medical Treatment of Endometriosis

The medical treatment of endometriosis is based on the observations that certain physiologic states, i.e., anovulation, pregnancy, and the menopause, are associated with a regression of endometriosis. Consequently, various pharmacologic avenues were developed to imitate these states in the treatment of endometriosis. In the 1950s, oral contraceptives were utilized to produce either an anovulatory state or a pseudopregnancy.[12] The results of this form of therapy were quite successful. In the past 10 or 12 years, danazol has been the agent of choice. It has been generally believed that danazol works by inhibiting the hypothalamic–pituitary–ovarian axis, thus creating a pseudomenopausal condition. However, there are some recent studies that question this mechanism of action. Some studies indicate that danazol has a diverse number of pharmacologic actions including a direct effect upon steroidogenesis.[16-18] Another study described an unfavorable shift in lipoprotein levels as well.[21] In any event, a pseudomenopausal condition is produced. The latest approach is to use

Table 29-1. Pregnancy Rates Following Surgical Treatment of Endometriosis

Study	Year	Mild (%)	Moderate (%)	Severe (%)
Garcia[12]	1977	66.7	38.8	28.5
Buttram[13]	1979	73.2	55.9	40.4
Decker[14]	1979	78.0	44.0	28.0
Donnez[15 a]	1987	62.0	52.0	42.0

[a]Laser laparoscopy.

analogues of gonadotropin-releasing hormone to likewise produce a pseudomenopausal state caused by low levels of estrogen.[22]

Indications for Medical Treatment

In general, the less severe degrees of endometriosis are treated medically. In the 1970s, after danazol first became available and when laparoscopy began to be widely utilized in infertility, a number of reports were published describing significant improvement in the appearance of endometriotic lesions along with pregnancy rates varying from 48% to 83% following danazol therapy.[21-23] It was difficult to accurately assess these studies because no controls were available, and it is difficult to know how many of these had only minimal or mild endometriosis without the enlargement or fixation of the ovary. A number of these individuals might have conceived without treatment.

Studies in subsequent years utilizing controls have demonstrated that patients with minimal and even mild endometriosis who are not treated for endometriosis achieve pregnancy rates that are compatible with those achieved by patients receiving danazol.[14,24-28] The results from one study are shown in Table 29-2. It appears from these reports that minimal and even mild endometriosis are only incidental findings in these patients, and treatment with medical methods does not directly help their infertility. Treatment should be withheld until there is further evidence of a beneficial effect.

On the other hand, mild endometriosis should be treated if there is any ovarian involvement. Moderate endometriosis should always be treated, not because there is evidence of a clinical effect on infertility, but to prevent further progression of the disease. Medical treatment is also used preoperatively in severe endometriosis to reduce the size of the lesions and to facilitate surgery. Medical treatment is also used postoperatively in those cases where it is suspected that all the endometriosis has not been removed.[29]

Treatment with Danazol

The starting dosage of danazol is 800 mg/day administered in four sepa-

Table 29-2. Pregnancy Rates for Danazol versus No Danazol in the Treatment of Minimal Endometriosis[a]

	Entered	Completed	Conceiving	Conceiving (%)
Danazol	32	19	6	32
No danazol	30	24	12	50
Total	62	43	18	42

[a]From Bayer et al.[28]

Table 29-3. Side Effects of Danazol

Water retention (weight gain)
Acne
Oily hair
Fatigue
Malaise
Muscle cramps
Restless legs
Night sweats

rate doses. Treatment should begin within the first few days of the onset of a menstrual cycle. The usual length of a treatment course is 6 months, although when it is given preoperatively or postoperatively, the course can be limited to 3 months. If the patient is observed at 2-month intervals and is doing well, the dosage can be reduced to one capsule three times daily and then to one capsule twice daily. Side effects of danazol are listed in Table 29-3. These occur in about 5% to 10% of patients, but most patients tolerate the medication well.

Analogues of Gonadotropin-Releasing Hormone

The use of gonadotropin-releasing hormone (GnRH) analogues for endometriosis is still new and relatively experimental, but numerous studies have been reported.[22,30,31] Since analogues of GnRH have a relatively long life, daily administration results in sustained levels of GnRH, and the pulsatile secretion of natural GnRH is overcome. As a result, pituitary gonadotropin hormone excretion declines, and ovarian secretion of estrogen is diminished. This pseudomenopausal state will result in atrophy of endometriotic tissue.

Depo-type preparations with a potential for once-a-month injection are being readied for the market. There are claims of fewer side effects with GnRH analogues than with danazol. These two facts suggest that some form of GnRH analogue may play a vital role in the medical treatment of endometriosis in the very near future.

REFERENCES

1. Barbieri RL, Niloff JM, Bast RC Jr., Schaetzel E, Kistner RW, Knapp RC: Elevated serum concentrations of CA-125 in patients with endometriosis. *Fertil Steril* 45:630, 1986
2. Fedele L, Arcaini L, Vescillini P, Bianchi S, Candiani A: Serum CA-125 measurements in the diagnosis of endometriosis recurrence. *Obstet Gynecol* 72:19, 1988
3. Kistner RW: Endometriosis and infertility. In Behrman SJ, Kistner RW (eds): *Progress in Infertility*, 2nd ed. Boston, Little, Brown, 1975, 348
4. American Fertility Society Classification of Endometriosis. *Fertil Steril* 43:347, 1985
5. Badawy SZA, Marshall L, Gabal AA, Nussbaum ML: The concentration of 13,14-dihy-

dro-15keto prostaglandin $F_{2\alpha}$ and prostaglandin E_2 in peritoneal fluid in infertile patients with and without endometriosis. *Fertil Steril* 38:166, 1982

6. Badawy SZA, Cuenca V, Marshall L, Munchback R, Rinos AC, Coble DA: Cellular components in peritoneal fluid in infertile patients with and without endometriosis. *Fertil Steril* 42:704, 1984

7. Sueldo CE, Lambert H, Steinleitner AJ, Swanson JA: Effect of peritoneal fluid from endometriosis patients on mucus sperm-ova interaction. Abstract. 1986 Meeting American Fertility Society, p 8

8. Chong AP: Infertility amenable to laser surgery. In Baggish, MS (ed): *Basic and Advanced Laser Surgery in Gynecology*. Norwalk, CT, Appleton-Century-Crofts, 1985, p 279

9. Nezhat C, Crougey SR, Ganison CP: Surgical treatment of endometriosis via laser laparoscopy. *Fertil Steril* 45:778, 1986

10. Keye W, Hansen LW, Astin M, Poulson AM Jr: Argon laser therapy of endometriosis: A review of 92 consecutive cases. *Fertil Steril* 47:208, 1987

11. Nezhat C, Winer WK, Nezhat F: Is endoscopic treatment of endometriosis and endometrioma associated with better results than laparotomy? *Am J Gynecol Health* 2:19, 1988

12. Garcia CR, Davis SS: Pelvic endometriosis and pelvic pain. *Am J Obstet Gynecol* 129:740, 1977

13. Buttram V: Conservative surgery for endometriosis in the infertile female: A study of 206 patients with implications for both medical and surgical therapy. *Fertil Steril* 31:117, 1979

14. Decker WH: Conservative surgical treatment of endometriosis and infertility. *Infertility* 2:155, 1979

15. Donnez J: CO_2 laser laparoscopy in infertile women with endometriosis and women with adnexal adhesions. *Fertil Steril* 48:390, 1987

16. Reyniak JV, Lauerson NH: Danazol: A versatile pharmacologic agent. *Fertil Steril* 37:475, 1982

17. Steingold KA, Lu JKH, Judd HL, Meldrum DR: Danazol inhibits steriodogenesis by the human ovary in vivo. *Fertil Steril* 45:C49, 1986

18. Meldrum DR, Partridge WM, Karow WG, River J, Vale W, Judd HL: Hormonal effects of danazol and medical oophorectomy in endometriosis. *Obstet Gynecol* 62:480, 1983

19. Fahraeus L, Laerson-Cohn U, Ljunberg S, Wallentin L: Profound alterations of the lipoprotein metabolism during danazol treatment in premenopausal women. *Fertil Steril* 45:52, 1984

20. Meldrum DR, Chang RJ, Lu J, Vale W, River J, Judd HL: Medical oophorectomy using a long-acting GnRH agonist: A possible new approach to the treatment of endometriosis. *J Clin Endocrinol Metab* 54:1081, 1982

21. Friedlander RL: The treatment of endometriosis with danazol. *J Reprod Med* 10:197, 1973

22. Dmowski WP, Cohen MR: Antigonadotropin (danazol) in the treatment of endometriosis. *Am J Obstet Gynecol* 130:41, 1978

23. Greenblatt R, Borenstein R, Hernandez-Ayap S: Experiences with danazol in the treatment of infertility. *Am J Obstet Gynecol* 118:783, 1974

24. Portunado JA, Echonojauregui AD, Herran C, Alijarte I: Early conception in patients with untreated mild endometriosis. *Fertil Steril* 39:22, 1983

25. Hull ME, Moghiss KS, Magyar DF, Hayes MF: Comparison of different treatment modalities of endometriosis in infertile women. *Fertil Steril* 47:40, 1987

26. Schenken RS, Malimak LR: Conservative surgery versus expectant management for the infertile patient with mild endometriosis. *Fertil Steril* 37:183, 1982

27. Seibel MM, Berger MJ, Weinstein FG, Taymor ML: The effectiveness of danazol on subsequent fertility in minimal endometriosis. *Fertil Steril* 38:534, 1982

28. Bayer SR, Seibel MM, Saffan DS, Berger MS, Taymor ML: The efficacy of danazol treatment for minimal endometriosis. *J Reprod Med* 33:179, 1988

29. Wheeler JM, Malinak LR: Postoperative danazol therapy in infertility patients with severe endometriosis. *Fertil Steril* 36:460, 1981

30. Schrieck E, Munroe SE, Henzl M, Jaffe RB: Treatment of endometriosis with a potent agonist of gonadotropin-releasing hormone (nafalerin). *Fertil Steril* 44:583, 1985
31. Henzi MR, Corson SL, Moghissi K, Buttram VC, Berquist C, Jacobson J: Administration of nasal nafalerin as compared with oral danazol for endometriosis: A multicenter double-blind comparative clinical trial. *New Engl J Med* 318:485, 1988

CHAPTER 30

Unexplained Infertility

The term *unexplained infertility* is utilized for those couples who have under-gone a *complete* infertility workup, in whom no abnormality has been uncov-ered, and who remain infertile. The completeness of the workup must be emphasized. In too many instances couples are given that diagnosis with only a partial investigation into the causes of their infertility, or with failure to utilize the newest avenues of investigation for infertility diagnosis. A time element must be added to the description as well and there is no way of knowing how long this should be. Certainly, 1 year must pass after the workup to warrant this diagnosis, but many suggest 2 or even 3 years before other therapies are undertaken.

THE COMPLETE INVESTIGATION

It goes without saying that the minimum basic workup should be found negative. The history and examination of both the husband and wife, with special attention to coital habits and potential emotional factors must be com-plete. The postcoital test should reveal an adequate number of progressively motile sperm in the cervical mucus 8 to 16 hours after coitus, with preovulatory cervical mucus. A uterotubogram should reveal no abnormality of the uterus or tubes. An endometrial biopsy should be in phase. Finally, semen quality, in-cluding motility and morphology, should be within normal limits, although a sharp line of normality is difficult to establish. Beyond the basic workup other possible causes of infertility should be evaluated and also found to be negative.

A laparoscopy should demonstrate normal reproductive organs. A dilatation and curettage, or at least sounding of the uterus, to rule out cervical stenosis as part of the infertility workup should be accomplished. Mycoplasma and chlamydia cultures should be carried out and be negative.

NEW ADVANCES IN DIAGNOSIS

In the past 2 years, scientific advances in reproductive endocrinology have opened up a number of new areas for investigation. As a result, the diagnosis of unexplained infertility may shift from physician to physician, depending on whether or not these approaches are available. Furthermore, many of these are still either in the developmental stage or equivocal in their interpretation. At the present time, these provide information when available, but the diagnosis of unexplained infertility should not necessarily be withheld if these tests have not been utilized.

Investigations in the Male

The sperm penetration assay (SPA) described in chapter 12, if available, may be helpful but it is not of absolute value.[1] Adequate penetration does mean that this is not the problem, and zero penetration usually indicates impaired infertility. However, the correlation is not absolute, since one report indicated that 20% of males with a negative SPA were able to fertilize human oocytes.[2] If gamete intrafallopian transfer (GIFT) has been unsuccessful and there has been a negative SPA, in vitro fertilization (IVF) should be utilized to directly assess the fertilizing ability of the sperm on human oocytes. If fertilization fails here as well, further attempts at IVF and GIFT should not be attempted.

Additional study of the fertilizing potential of human sperm are being developed such as fertilization of human oocytes in vitro[3] and the ability to penetrate the zona pellucida of human oocytes.[4] Another approach involves the assay of acrosin, the enzyme contained in the acrosomal cap of the sperm.[5]

Investigations in the Female

Luteinized Unruptured Follicle. In 1978 Marik and Hulka performed laparoscopy in the early luteal phase of the cycle of infertile women with normal ovarian endocrine function, and they described absence of corpora lutea in 30% of the patients. They labeled this condition as the luteinized unruptured follicle syndrome.[6] During the ensuing years many investigators confirmed their findings, and they indicated a 10% incidence.[7] However, more controlled studies suggest that although this condition does exist, it is a relatively uncommon phenomenon.

Periovulatory Dysfunction. Detailed study of the periovulatory period with biochemical measurements and daily ultrasound examination of follicle growth suggests that some cases of unexplained infertility may be due to alteration in normal relationships at this time. Zegers-Hochschild and co-workers found that luteinizing hormone peak occurred within 24 hours before rupturing in conception cycles, but up to 48 hours before rupture in nonconceptive cycles.[8] These findings have been confirmed by Eissa and co-workers who also found poor follicle growth associated with low estradiol levels. [9] Kerin and his co-workers also confirmed the fact that ultrasonic monitoring may provide a reliable measure of follicle growth, and that this correlates with normal or abnormal endocrine function of the ovary.[10]

INCIDENCE

The reported incidence of unexplained infertility is extremely variable because the authors vary so much in the extensiveness of their workup that each may utilize before arriving at this diagnosis. One could also expect that with time, as more diagnostic tests are developed, the percentage of cases falling into this category would decrease. In 1960, Southam reported a 20% incidence.[11] Table 30-1 lists the incidence of this condition from reports of the 1980s. The incidence varies from 3.5% to 28%. This variability is undoubtedly the result of the variability of the workup. According to one report, the use of ultrasound monitoring of ovulation, investigation into sperm antibodies and human leukocyte antigen-B, and the use of the SPA reduced the diagnosis of unexplained infertility by 60%.[16]

SPONTANEOUS PREGNANCIES

The variability of reported incidence of spontaneous pregnancy also reflects the variability of the workup and the variability of the time that has passed since the completion of the workup. Lenton has tabulated the cumulative pregnancy rate in a group of couples in years to pregnancy starting 2 years

Table 30-1. Incidence of Unexplained Infertility

Author	Year	Percent
Templeton and Penney[12]	1982	24
Rousseau et al.[13]	1983	3.5
Hull et al.[14]	1985	28

after a completely negative workup (Table 30-2). Approximately one-quarter of the couples will conceive on their own within the first 3 years, and then there is a plateau effect.[17]

Table 30-3 demonstrates the "spontaneous cure rate" from other reports. At 1 year after workup the results varied from 13% to 71%; after 2 years, 30% to 80%. Even taking into consideration that these figures may be inflated by an incomplete workup, they do indicate that there is a significant spontaneous cure rate over a period of time. This extreme variability must also be taken into account when evaluating the reports of therapeutic approaches. In any event, they suggest that one should not rush into therapeutic maneuvers without some reasonable delay. This is particularly true before recommending such procedures as GIFT or IVF.

THERAPY

The first approach for the therapist is to be certain that a thorough workup has been completed. If available, the use of the new parameters for investigation should be carried out. Once these have been exhausted, as suggested above, time itself should be given a reasonable chance.

Assisted Reproductive Technology is the term given to highly technical procedures that can increase the chances of conception. Very often these procedures do not cure an infertility problem but, on the other hand, they hasten the resolution of the problem. The chances of spontaneous cure versus the possibility of complications including psychological (and economic) burnout should be considered before proceeding.

Intrauterine insemination (IUI) with washed sperm is recommended by many for unexplained infertility after a suitable waiting period. The rationale for its use is speculative. Possibly some problems of sperm migration to the cervix are overcome. Possibly the high concentration of motile sperm in the uterus increases the chance of conception. Most authors now recommend ovu

Table 30-2. Cumulative Pregnancy Rates after 2 Years of Unexplained Infertility[a]

Years	Cumulative pregnancy rate
1	.10
2	.21
3	.27
4	.32
5	.36

[a]From Lenton et al.[17]

Table 30-3. Spontaneous Cure Rate of Unexplained Infertility
of at Least 2 Years' Duration, 1 and 2 Years after Completion of Workup

Author	Year	1 yr (%)	2 yr (%)
Templeton and Penney[12]	1982	13	30
Rousseau et al.[13]	1983	34	53
Hull et al.[14]	1985	71	81
Barnea et al.[15]	1985	50	68
Mean		31	58

lation enhancement along with the IUI.[18-20] The availability of a number of mature oocytes would logically increase the chances of conception, although this increases the chances of complications as well. Serhal reported a cycle pregnancy rate of 2.7% with IUI alone and a 26.4% pregnancy rate with IUI combined with ovulation augmentation.[20] In another report, the conception rate for IUI rose from 2.2% to 14.3% per cycle when gonadotropins were added.[21] With three to six cycles, the pregnancy rates per patient were 41% and 22%, respectively in these two studies. It must be emphasized that high pregnancy rate is accompanied by a high multiple pregnancy rate, and the patient should be so forewarned.

It is difficult to be certain of the significance of these figures because of the previously noted difficulty and variability of defining unexplained infertility and the knowledge of the spontaneous cure rate. Controlled prospective studies are needed.

IVF AND GIFT

For a number of years unexplained infertility has been considered as one of the indications for IVF. Where GIFT is available, this should be the procedure of choice because of the much higher success rate. Both procedures are invasive. A number of studies have reported pregnancy rates approaching those of IVF with IUI combined with gonadotropins.[22] Certainly, then, a number of cycles of IUI with gonadotropins should be attempted before recommending either of these two procedures.

In summary, as far as unexplained infertility is concerned, nowhere in the discipline of infertility is a more total knowledge of the field required: the details of the complete workup, the scientific advances in diagnosis, the new forms of treatment, and a continued understanding of the emotional impact of infertility and its therapy upon the well-being of the patient.

REFERENCES

1. Poland ML, Moghissi VM, Giblin PT, Ager J, Olson JM: Variations of semen measures within normal men. *Fertil Steril* 44:396, 1985
2. Haxton MJ, *Br J Obstet Gynecol* 94:539, 1987
3. Trounson AO, Leeton JF, Wood C, et al: The investigation of idiopathic infertility by in vitro fertilization. *Fertil Steril* 34:341, 1980
4. Hambree WC, Overstreet JW: Defects in human sperm penetration in vitro. In Troen P, Nanlem HR (eds): *The Testis in Normal and Infertile Men*. New York, Raven Press, 1977, p 513
5. Mohsanian M, Syner FN, Moghissi KS: A study of sperm acrosin in patients with unexplained infertility. *Fertil Steril* 37:L23, 1982
6. Marik J, Hulka J: Luteinized unruptured follicle syndrome: A subtle cause of infertility. *Fertil Steril* 29:270, 1978
7. Killick S, Elstein M: Pharmacologic production of luteinized follicles by prostaglandins synthetase inhibitors. *Fertil Steril* 47:773, 1987
8. Zegers-Hochschild F, Lira CG, Parada M, Lorenzini EA: A comparative study of the follicular growth profile in conception and non-conception cycles. *Fertil Steril* 41:244, 1984
9. Eissa MK, Sauers RS, Docker MF, Lynch SES, Newton JR: Characteristics and incidence of dysfunctional ovulation patterns detected by ultrasound. *Fertil Steril* 47:603, 1987
10. Kerin JF, Edmonds DK, Warnes GM, Cox LW, Seamark RF, Matthews CD, Young GB, Baird DT: Morphological and functional relationships of graafian follicle growth to ovulation in women using ultrasonic, laparoscopic and biochemical measurements. *Br J Obstet Gynecol* 88:81, 1981
11. Southam AL: What to do with the "normal" infertile couple. *Fertil Steril* 11:543, 1960
12. Templeton AR, Penney GC: The incidence, characteristics and prognosis of patients whose infertility is unexplained. *Fertil Steril* 37:175, 1982
13. Rousseau S, Lord J, Lepage Y, Compenhaut JV: The expectancy of pregnancy for "normal" fertile couples. *Fertil Steril* 40:768, 1983
14. Hull MGR, Glazener CMA, Kelly NJ, et al: Population study of causes, treatment and outcome of infertility. *Br Med J* 291:1693, 1985
15. Barnea ER, Hulford TR, McInnes DRA: Long-term prognosis of infertile couples with normal basic investigations: A life table analysis. *Obstet Gynecol* 66:24, 1985
16. Coulam CB, Moore SB, O'Fallon WO: Investigating unexplained infertility. *Am J Obstet Gynecol* 158:1374, 1988
17. Lenton EA, Watson GA, Cooke D: Long term follow-up of the apparently normal couple with a complaint of infertility. *Fertil Steril* 28:913, 1977
18. Byrd W, Ackerman GE, Carr BR, Edman C, Guzick DS, McConnell JD: Treatment of refracting infertility by transcervical intrauterine insemination of washed spermatozoa. *Fertil Steril* 48:921, 1987
19. Weiner S, Decherney AH, Polan MC: Human menopausal gonadotropins: A justifiable therapy in ovulatory women with long-standing ideopathic infertility. *Am J Obstet Gynecol* 158:111, 1988
20. Serhal PF, Katz M, Little V, Woronowski H: Unexplained infertility—the value of Pergonal super ovulation combined with intrauterine insemination. *Fertil Steril* 49:602, 1988
21. Kemmann E, Bohrer M, Sheldon R, Fiasconoro G, Beardsley L: Active ovulation management

increases the pregnancy occurrence in ovulatory women who receive intrauterine insemination. *Fertil Steril* 48:916, 1987

22. Avidon A, Avidon B, Lewis A, Zajicek G, Laufer N, Schenker JG: Unexplained infertility — the value of menotropins treatment in comparison to IVF cycles. *Proc VI World Congr In Vitro Fertil,* Jerusalem, 1989, p 76

CHAPTER 31

In Vitro Fertilization and Gamete Intrafallopian Tube Transfer

The birth of the first baby conceived by in vitro fertilization (IVF) in 1978 was a landmark event in the field of reproductive endocrinology and infertility.[1] However, the event itself was the result of at least three decades of intensive scientific investigation. The first attempt at fertilization of the human oocyte was reported by Menkin and Rock in 1948.[2] During the next three decades, advances in embryo culture and use of the laparoscope produced the success of 1978.[3] Since that time, use of ovulatory-inducing drugs to recruit multiple oocytes has brought the pregnancy rates in most centers up to 15% to 20%, and the use of ultrasound retrieval of oocytes has significantly simplified the procedure. As a result, IVF is now a valuable infertility treatment to be offered to many patients, and its benefits and drawbacks can be weighed against other forms of treatment.

IN VITRO FERTILIZATION

Indications

The initial indication for IVF was for women with absent fallopian tubes or blocked tubes not responding to surgery. This still remains the primary indication. However, other problems of infertility may benefit from this procedure as well. Couples in whom the major infertility problem is a deficiency in sperm number or quality may benefit from IVF. Certain minimum measurements of

277

sperm quantity and quality must still be present, and IVF is not the panacea for severe male infertility that was initially hoped. The presence of a hostile cervix, for whatever reason, provides another indication for IVF. Endometriosis, not responding to surgical or medical treatment, is now treated with IVF. Finally, unexplained infertility of 2 or more years' duration is also considered an indication for IVF.

In the indications listed above, male factor, cervical factor, endometriosis, or unexplained infertility, situations where one or both fallopian tubes are normal, centers who carry out gamete intrafallopian tube transfer (GIFT) will utilize that procedure rather than IVF because of its significantly higher success rate. Others still may prefer to utilize IVF because it does not require laparoscopy and is, therefore, less invasive. Also, in conditions of severe male factor, the ability to assess fertilization by IVF is an advantage over GIFT. These are issues that hinge upon the expertise, experience, and clinical judgment of the physicians involved.

Preliminary Studies

In addition to a routine physical examination for good health requirements, a number of fertility screening tests are necessary.

Initially, a screening laparoscopy was considered necessary, and this still may be helpful if laparoscopic retrieval is being utilized. However, most centers now use the transvaginal ultrasound-guided technique, and a preliminary laparascopy is not necessary.

A uterotubogram is still essential in order to demonstrate a normal uterine cavity. The depth of the uterus as well as the direction of the cavity should be ascertained well before the procedure. If there is evidence of cervical stenosis, preliminary dilatation will ensure an atraumatic embryo transfer procedure. A traumatic transfer is considered detrimental to the outcome.

A postcoital test and endometrial biopsy are requested by some centers, but the results really do not affect the decision to perform or not to perform the procedure. Semen analysis is important in order to alert the biologist to the need for special handling of the semen sample.

Oocyte Recruitment

Background. Initially, Steptoe and Edwards utilized ovulation-enhancing drugs in their first IVF attempts. However, because of a lack of success they turned to the natural cycle and did achieve their early successes with this approach.[3] The use of natural cycle is based on the information outlined in chapter 16, that notes that ovulation occurs approximately 36 hours after the onset of the luteinizing hormone (LH) surge in serum or 28 hours after the onset of the LH surge in urine. Rapid, sensitive tests for LH in both serum and urine make this approach possible.

In 1981 Trounson and co-workers demonstrated that a higher pregnancy rate could be achieved utilizing fertility-enhancing drugs and if the addition of the sperm to the oocytes was delayed for 5 to 6 hours after recovery, a time period in which the oocytes could complete maturation.[4] The use of fertility drugs to enhance ovulation is the procedure now utilized by the vast majority of centers, though recently interest in the return to the natural cycle has reawakened in some centers.[5,6]

Rationale of Ovarian Augmentation. During the natural cycle only one follicle grows and only one oocyte matures to be ovulated in the response to natural follicle-stimulating hormone (FSH) and LH stimulation. By continuously adding FSH to the system, either endogenously with clomiphene citrate (CC) or exogenously with human menopausal gonadotropin (HMG), a large number of follicles and oocytes can be brought to various stages of maturation (Fig. 31-1). Ovulation can then be induced by the administration of human

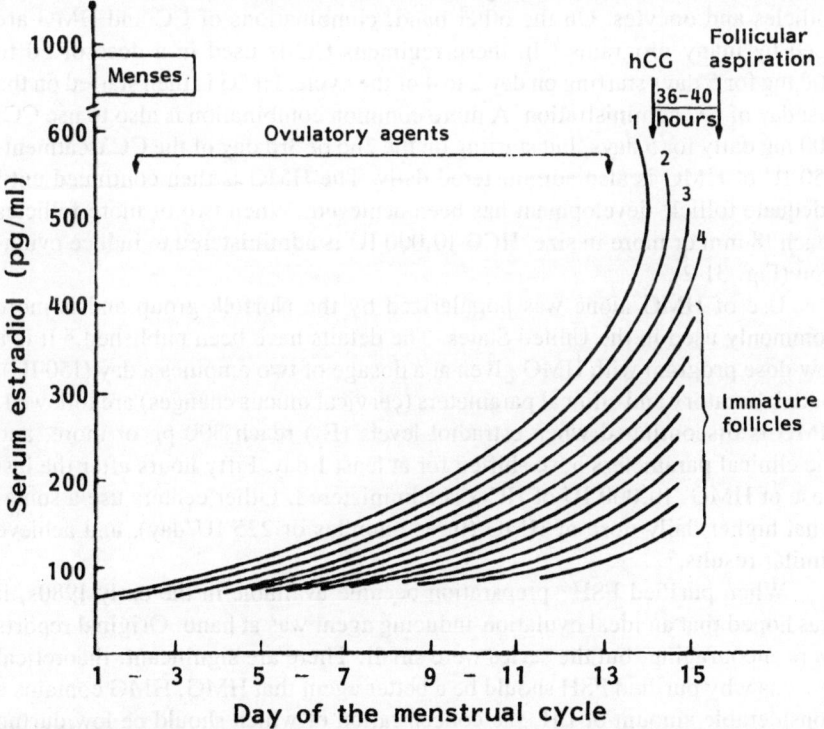

Figure 31-1. Repeated administration of HCG causes a number of follicles to develop to the preovulatory stage (from Hodgens G: *Serono Symposia* 47:126, 1983, reproduced with permission).

chorionic gonadotropin (HCG). This will occur approximately 36 hours after the injection. As a result, a number of oocytes can be retrieved and fertilized. There is no question but that the more embryos transferred, the higher the pregnancy rate. The second advantage of ovarian augmentation is that the timing of ovulation can be controlled. The HCG can be given in the late evening, at a time when ovulation can be expected to occur two mornings later. The procedure can then be planned for an hour or so before the anticipated ovulation when many of the oocytes will be approaching maturity. This ability to plan the procedure well in advance removes a tremendous strain from the facility's personnel and patients.

Regimens for Ovulation Enhancement. At the present time, the majority of centers follow one of a number of regimens that include the use of, singly or in combination, CC, HMG, and agonists of gonadotropin-releasing hormone (GnRH).

CC was initially utilized alone, but superior results with other combinations have resulted in its being discarded as an agent alone for recruiting follicles and oocytes. On the other hand, combinations of CC and HMG are used by many programs.[7] In these regimens CC is used in a dose of 50 to 100 mg for 5 days starting on day 2 to 4 of the cycle. HMG is then started on the last day of CC administration. A more common combination is also to use CC, 100 mg daily for 5 days, but starting on the 2nd or 3rd day of the CC treatment, 150 IU of HMG is also administered daily. The HMG is then continued until adequate follicle development has been achieved. When two or more follicles reach 18 mm or more in size, HCG 10,000 IU is administered to induce ovulation (Fig. 31-2).

Use of HMG alone was popularized by the Norfolk group and is more commonly used in the United States. The details have been published.[8] It is a low-dose program with HMG given at a dosage of two ampules a day (150 IU). Both laboratory and clinical parameters (cervical mucus changes) are followed. HMG is discontinued when estradiol levels (E_2) reach 300 pg or more, and the clinical parameters have shifted for at least 1 day. Fifty hours after the last dose of HMG, 10,000 IU of HCG is administered. Other centers use a somewhat higher daily dose of HMG (three ampules or 225 IU/day), and achieve similar results.[9]

When purified FSH* preparation became available in the early 1980s, it was hoped that an ideal ovulation-inducing agent was at hand. Original reports were encouraging, but the series were small. There are significant, theoretical reasons why purified FSH should be a better agent that HMG. HMG contains a considerable amount of LH, the concentration of which should be low during

---

*Metrodin®, Serono Laboratories, Randolph, Massachusetts.

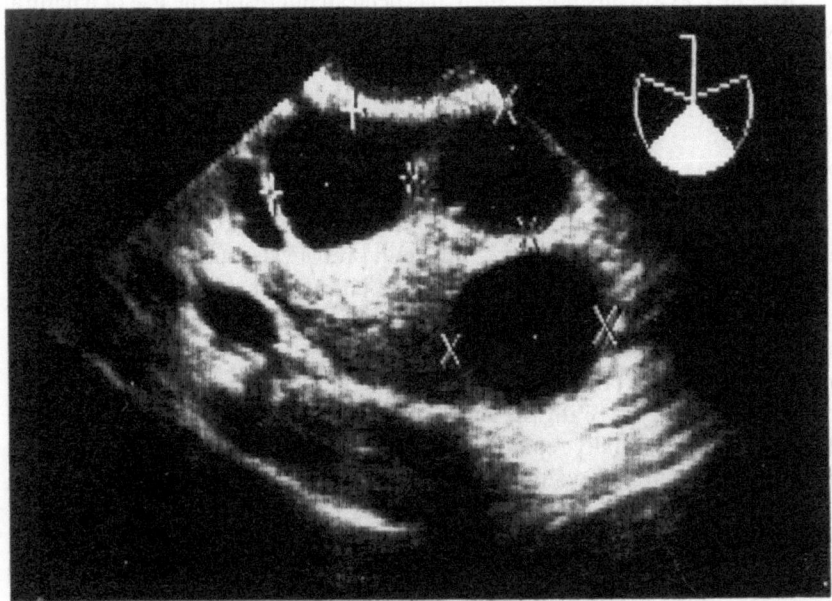

Figure 31-2. Multiple follicular development following clomiphene HMG therapy visualized by vaginal ultrasound.

folliculogenesis. Inappropriate high levels of androgens and progesterone which, in turn, could theoretically have detrimental effects on the health of the follicle or oocyte. Nevertheless, fairly extensive studies to date, some of a collaborative nature, have failed to demonstrate statistically significant differences in pregnancy rates following the use of purified FSH as compared to HMG.

In all regimens utilizing CC and HMG, there is a relatively high rate of failure of appropriate stimulation: spontaneous LH surge, low responders, and high responders. GnRH had been initially utilized as a substitute for CC or HMG, but the results in terms of pregnancies were not encouraging. On the other hand, long-acting agonists of GnRH,* with prolonged half-lives, now play a significant role in ovulation enhancement in many centers.[10] The primary goal is to prevent the occurrence of a spontaneous LH surge. However, with the use of GnRH agonists, rapidly rising estrogen levels (high responders) may be controlled until adequate folliculogenesis has occurred. Some centers claim better overall results with the routine of GnRH agonists, though this still remains to be proved by the use of large prospective controlled studies.

*Lupron®, TAP Pharmaceuticals, Chicago, Illinois.

Recently, as already noted, there has been an interest in the use of a natural cycle, utilizing HCG to trigger ovulation when adequate follicular development of the single follicle has been obtained. It remains to be seen whether or not even improved results can balance out the inconveniences of this approach.

Oocyte Retrieval

Until a few years ago, the way to the follicles and oocytes was through laparoscopy. At the present time, ultrasound retrieval is utilized by probably 90% of centers. The main advantage is the elimination of the need for intratracheal general anesthesia. Some light form of anesthesia is often needed, but the patient still does not suffer from the effects of general anesthesia and pneumoperitoneum. For some centers, the facilities can be simplified, and the cost thereby reduced. With the development of vaginal transducers, vaginal ultrasound has essentially replaced other approaches. It was originally felt that the ultrasound approach would be less efficient in retrieving oocytes. However, with increasing experience, this difference is usually minimized. One study reported an adverse effect of general anesthesia on fertilization and cleavage,[11] and another reported better overall results with transvaginal ultrasound-guided oocyte recovery.[12] Marrs has emphasized, however, that individualization is important. Some patients do better with laparoscopy, and vaginal ultrasound is not without its dangers.[13]

The techniques of both laparoscopic and ultrasound-guided recovery have been described in detail.[14-16] Briefly, whether by laparoscopy or by ultrasound, a large-diameter needle is inserted through the follicle wall and suction is immediately applied, usually by means of a foot pedal. The contents of the follicle are drawn into a collecting tube and then quickly transferred to an adjacent laboratory where a scientist isolates the oocyte from the follicular fluid. The oocyte is readily recognizable, a single cell surrounded by a mass of cumulus cells (Fig. 31-3).

After follicle aspiration, the oocytes are identified in either the initial follicle aspirate or in the subsequent follicular irrigation fluid. Because removal of the cumulus cells surrounding the oocyte may be detrimental, oocyte maturity is judged from the appearance of the cumulus mass rather than by direct observation of the oocyte itself. A tightly clustered cumulus indicates an immature oocyte, whereas an oocyte with loosely expanded cumulus is considered mature. To ensure full maturity, the oocytes that are considered to be mature by cumulus cell criteria are preincubated for 6 to 8 hours, and those considered immature are preincubated 24 to 26 hours prior to adding spermatozoa.[17]

While the oocytes are being preincubated, the semen specimen is being processed. The spermatozoa are separated from the semen, which is unsterile, and the concentration is decreased. A small aliquot of semen is mixed with

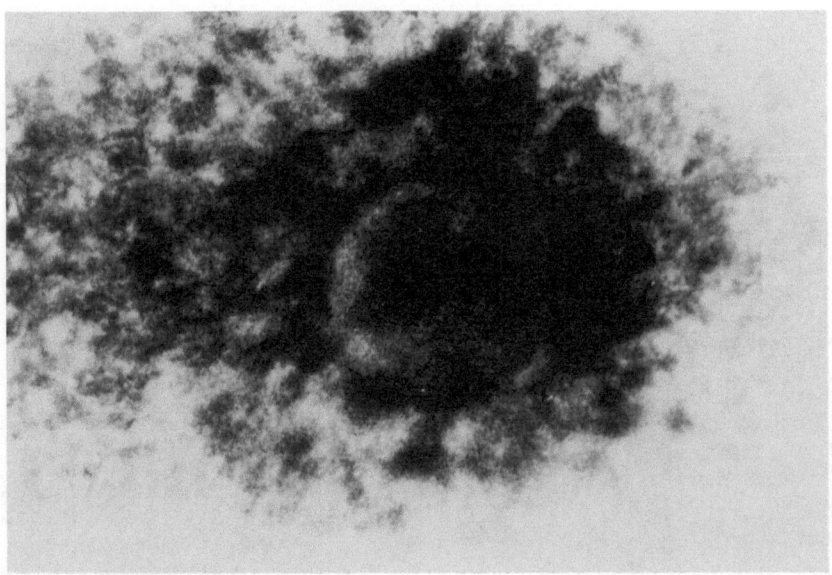

Figure 31-3. The oocyte surrounded by its cumulus mass. The character of the cumulus cells indicates that this is a mature oocyte ready to be fertilized after a few hours of incubation.

sterile culture media in a test tube. By centrifuging the mixture, the washed sperm form a pellet in the bottom of the test tube, and the unsterile wash can be poured off. The sperm pellet is then resuspended in culture media, and the entire process is repeated. The third time the sperm pellet is resuspended, the sperm and culture media are placed into an incubator for 1 hour. The motile sperm that swim away from the pellet are then collected, and these are the ones that will be used for fertilization. This washing process produces bacteria-free sperm and also allows for capacitation, the process by which sperm attain the capacity to fertilize an oocyte.[4] Approximately 50,000 to 100,000 sperm are placed into the culture media containing the oocyte. Special techniques involving multiple tube swim-up or columns of Percoll are utilized to improve the quality of sperm when deficiencies exist.[18,19] After a spermatozoa enters the cytoplasm the oocyte completes its second meiotic division, and the second polar body is extruded. The following morning (11 to 17 hours after insemination) the zygote is visualized, and two pronuclei indicating fertilization are seen (Fig. 31-4). The mean time for the development to the two-cell stage is 37 hours (31 to 43 hours), and the four-cell stage can be identified at 37 to 51 hours (Fig. 31-5). The embryos are usually transferred 42 to 48 hours following insemination.

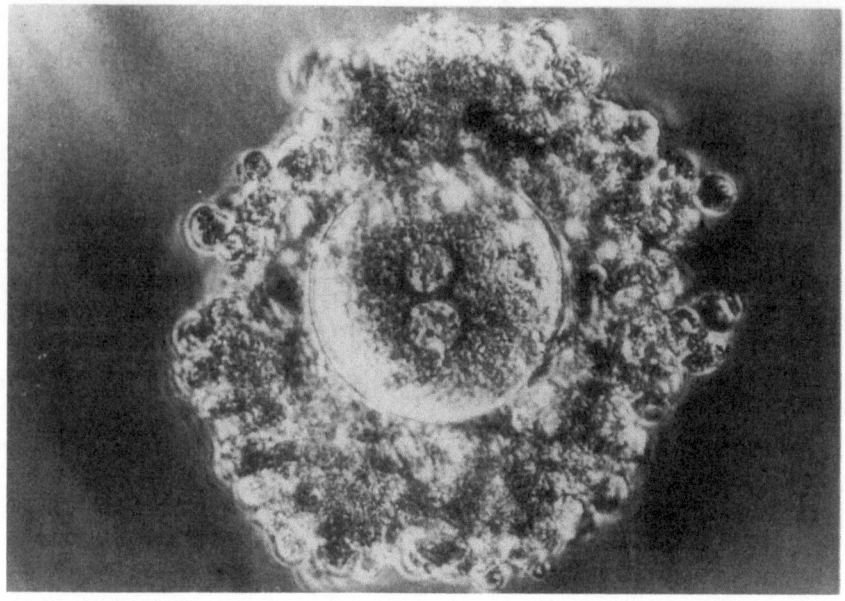

Figure 31-4. The two-pronuclear stage, indicating fertilization has occurred.

Embryo Transfer

Embryo transfer is perhaps the simplest and most straightforward technical aspect of IVF. Yet, it is also the most disappointing, as most of the failures
of IVF appear to occur at this stage. The procedure should be performed in a
procedure room that is next to the culture laboratory. No anesthesia is necessary. A speculum is placed into the vagina and the cervix cleansed with sterile
media. A plastic or metal sheath is placed into the cervix to the level the
internal cervical os. The embryo(s) are preloaded into the tip of a Teflon
catheter, and the catheter tip is then threaded through the cervix to within 1 cm
of the uterus fundus where the embryo(s) are released. The catheter is held in
place for 10 to 20 seconds and then slowly removed. Patients remain in the same
position while the catheter is examined under the microscope to ensure that the
embryo(s) were released. Occasionally they are not, and the process is repeated. After confirming the absence of embryos in the catheter, the speculum
is removed. The patient, still on her hospital bed, lies flat and is taken back to
the recovery room or outpatient area where she remains at total bedrest for
approximately 1 hour. She is then discharged from the hospital and asked to
remain in bed as much as possible for the next 48 to 72 hours. Most centers,
although not all, administer progesterone to support the endometrium following embryo transfer.

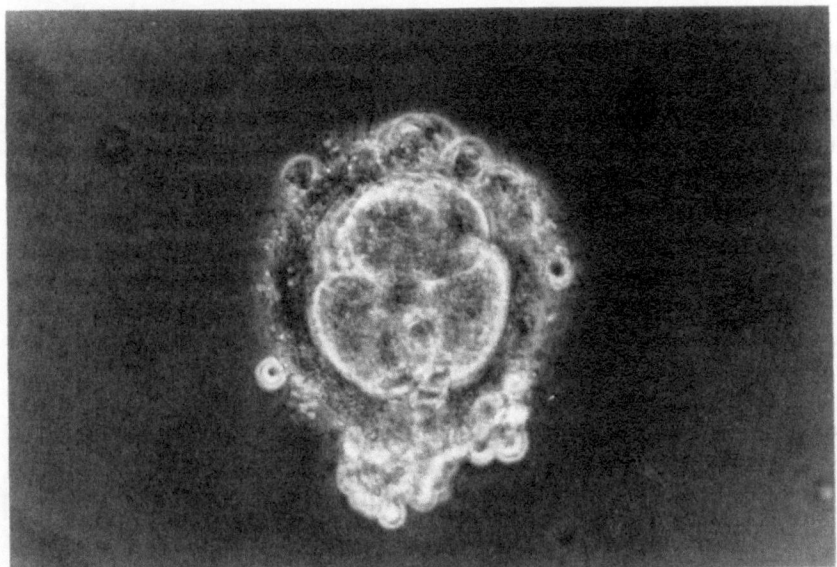

Figure 31-5. A four-cell human embryo just prior to transfer.

Results

The analysis of success rates from different centers is difficult because no standard method of reporting is used. Some list percentages of pregnancies per retrieval cycle, others per transfer; chemical pregnancies may or may not be included. Most disturbing of all is the tendency to report a small section of an overall experience, a section in which the results are especially encouraging. Finally, there is a fairly high spontaneous abortion rate in IVF pregnancies, and it would be more meaningful to present the data as live birth results.

The figures from the Norfolk Center, 1981 to 1985, are shown in Table 30-1. A 24.3% pregnancy per transfer is noted. Removing the 30 chemical pregnancies and doing the calculation by the procedure, the pregnancy rate is 19% per oocyte retrieval, still an excellent rate. Recently the combined Austra-

Table 31-1. IVF Results from Norfolk (1981–1985)[a]

		Number of patients
A.	Cycles	1400
B.	Transfers	1209
C.	Pregnancies	298 (24.3% of B)
D.	Chemical pregnancies	30

[a]From Acosta et al.[20]

lia and New Zealand experience were reported.[21] Since the onset of their program, IVF provided a live-birth rate of 9.5% per procedure. At the present time, IVF at established centers can be expected to achieve a 14% to 18% pregnancy rate and a 10% to 12% live-birth rate per oocyte retrieval. Repeated attempts to increase the chances of success from Norfolk results, utilizing a parametric model, projected a 47.8% pregnancy rate for transfer after four cycles.[22] These figures are important when counseling an infertility couple as to their options.

It must be emphasized that these relatively good results come from using patients younger than 40 years of age and where the husband had semen of reasonably good quality. It was originally hoped that IVF would be a boon to infertility associated with severe oliogospermia. However, it has been reported that if the number of motile sperm per millimeter falls below 5 million ml, there is a significant drop in both the fertilization and cleavage rates.[23] A high incidence of abnormal forms will also affect the outcome adversely.[24] However, in these cases where fertilization and cleavage does occur, there are pregnancies. It is also to be noted that the success rate for women older than 40 years drops sharply as well.[25]

Embryo Freezing

The first report of a pregnancy following cryopreservation, thawing and transfer of a human embryo, was by Trounson and Mohr in 1983.[26] Since that time the procedure has slowly spread to many centers, and the results have gradually improved. Nevertheless, ethical and legal issues play a dominant role in acceptance by patients, physicians, and the public.[27]

Procedure. In IVF it is the practice to transfer from three to five embryos. Most centers will not transfer more than five because of the increased chance of multiple pregnancies: triplet or more. Therefore, it is not the usual practice to fertilize more than five oocytes, or else embryos may have to be discarded. Extra oocytes, with the potential for fertilization, are discarded. Freezing embryos provides an answer to this dilemma. All the oocytes can be fertilized. If more than a suitable number of embryos are obtained, the excess can be frozen. A variety of techniques have been described.[28,29] One to 6 months after an unsuccessful IVF cycle where extra embryos have been frozen, the patients can plan to have two or more embryos thawed and transferred to the uterus during a natural cycle. Daily LH levels are begun on day 6, and the embryos are transferred 1 to 4 days after the LH surge, depending on developmental age.[29]

Results. Analysis of results of implantation of thawed embryos is very complex because not all embryos frozen have as yet been replaced. At the present time, women can only discuss the chances that a thawed embryo may result in a pregnancy. This has generally been accepted to be around 10%, although a recent report had 15% of thawed embryos result in a clinical pregnancy.[30] For many, this is a significant increment because the pregnancy is achieved in a natural cycle without oocyte retrieval.

GAMETE INTRAFALLOPIAN TUBE TRANSFER

GIFT was first described by Asch and co-workers in 1986 as an alternate to IVF.[31]

Indications

GIFT can be utilized in those situations where IVF has been previously utilized but where the fallopian tubes are normal: cervical mucus factor, unexplained infertility, endometriosis not responding to therapy, and male factor infertility. However, GIFT is an invasive and expensive procedure, and the patients should be given every chance to conceive on their own or with less invasive therapy before proceeding to GIFT. A minimum of 2 years of unexplained infertility should be allowed to pass. In most cases, a trial of 3 months of intrauterine insemination with ovulation enhancement should be attempted, because this has been shown to result in a 15% to 25% pregnancy rate in these types of cases (see Chapter 23).

Procedure

Ovarian augmentation as in IVF is utilized to produce a number of mature oocytes and to assure that the procedure will be performed just prior to impending ovulation (34 to 35 hours after an HCG injection). Oocytes are aspirated at laparoscopy under general anesthesia as in IVF laparoscopy. In GIFT, however, the semen specimen is obtained just prior to the start of the procedure and is prepared by sperm washing and swim-up collection of motile sperm. The oocytes are drawn up into a plastic tube. Between four and six oocytes are utilized, and one or both tubes are cannulated. Approximately 200,000 motile sperm are added to the oocytes for each fallopian tube. In oligospermia it has been recommended that higher concentrations of sperm be utilized.[32] The oocytes and sperm in a small plastic tube are threaded through the same cannula that had been used by the ultrasound retrieval needle. The posterior edge of the fimbria is lifted with an atraumatic grasping forceps. The end of the plastic tubing containing the oocytes and sperm is inserted 1 or 2 inches into the distal end of the fallopian tube, and the combination is injected. The procedure is then terminated.

Results

The GIFT procedure is generally twice as effective as IVF in producing clinical pregnancies and live births. For patients younger than age 40 and normal semen parameters, the ongoing clinical pregnancy rate is around 30% per procedure. Oligospermia and age more than 40 years considerably reduce this excellent result. One pitfall is that centers may use GIFT too early in infertility treatment, and many of these patients possibly could conceive with a more conservative approach. This is an area that requires constant self-discipline on the part of centers who do have facilities to perform the GIFT procedure.

REFERENCES

1. Steptoe PC, Edwards RG: Birth after reimplantation of a human embryo. *Lancet* 2:366, 1978
2. Menkin MF, Rock J: In vitro fertilization and cleavage of human ovarian eggs. *Am J Obstet Gynecol* 55:440, 1948
3. Edwards RG, Steptoe PC, Purdy JM: Establishing full-term human pregnancies with cleaving embryos in vitro. *Br J Obstet Gynecol* 87:757, 1980
4. Traunson AO, Mohr LR, Wood C, Leeton JF: Effect of delayed insemination on in vitro fertilization culture and transfer of human embryos. *J Reprod Fertil* 64:285, 1982
5. Duboisson JB, Foulot H, Ranoux C, Aubriot FX, Poirot C, Halouani L, Salesses A: IVF without ovarian stimulation: A simplified protocol. *Proc VI World Congress of IVF*, Jerusalem, 1989, p 7
6. Paulson RJ, Sauer MV, Lobo RA: In vitro fertilization in unstimulated cycles: A new application. *Fertil Steril* 51:1059, 1989
7. Taymor ML, Seibel M, Oskowitz SP, Smith DM, Lee G: In vitro fertilization and embryo transfer: An individualized approach to ovulation induction. *J In Vitro Fert Embryo Transfer* 2:162, 1985
8. Jones HW, Jr, Jones GS, Andrews MC, et al: The program for in vitro fertilization at Norfolk. *Fertil Steril* 44:262, 1985
9. Meldrum DR, Chetkowski R, Steingold KA, de Ziegler D, Cedars MJ, Hamilton M: Evaluation of a highly successful in vitro fertilization program. *Fertil Steril* 48:86, 1987
10. Neveu S, Hedon B, Bringer J, Chinchole JM, Arnal F, Humeau C, Cristol P, Viola JL: Ovarian stimulation by a combination of a gonadotropin releasing hormone agonist and gonadotropin for in vitro fertilization. *Fertil Steril* 47:234, 1987
11. Hayes MF, Succo AG, Savoy-Moore RT, Magyar DM, Endler GC, Moghissi KS: Effect of general anaesthesia on fertilization and cleavage of oocytes in vitro. *Fertil Steril* 48:975, 1987
12. Lavy G, Restropo-Candelo H, Diamond M, Shapiro B, Grumbeld L, Decherney AH: Laparoscopic and transvaginal ova recovery: The effect on ova quality. *Fertil Steril* 49:1002, 1988
13. Marrs RP: Does the method of oocyte collection have a major influence on in vitro fertilization. *Fertil Steril* 46:193, 1986
14. Jones HW Jr: In vitro fertilization. In Behrman SJ, Kistner RW, Patton RW Jr. (eds): *Progress in Infertility,* 3rd ed. Boston, Little, Brown, 1988, p 543–561
15. Wikland M, Nilsson L, Hanson R, Hamberger L, Janson PO: Collection of human oocytes by the use of sonography. *Fertil Steril* 39:603, 1983

16. Dellenbach P, Nisand I, Moreau L, Feger B, Plumers C, Gerlinger P: Transvaginal sonographically controlled follicle puncture for oocyte retrieval. *Fertil Steril* 44:656, 1985

17. Ben Rafael Z, Kopf G, Blasco L, Tureck RW, Mastroianni L Jr: Fertilization and cleavage after reinsemination of human oocytes in vitro. *Fertil Steril* 45:58, 1986

18. Tanphaichitr N, Randall M, Fitzgerald L, Lee G, Seibel MM, Taymor ML: An increase in in vitro fertilization ability of low density sperm capacitated by multiple tube swim-up. *Fertil Steril* 48:821, 1987

19. Tanphaichitr N, Agulnick A, Seibel M, Taymor ML: Comparison of the in vitro fertilization rate by human sperm capacitated by multiple-tube swim-up and Percoll gradient centrifugation. *J In Vitro Fert Embryo Transfer* 5:119, 1988

20. Acosta AA, Rosenwaks Z, Munasher ST, Garcia J: In vitro fertilization. In Gold J, Josimovich JB (eds): *Gynecologic Endocrinology* New York, Plenum, 1987, pp 629–650

21. Saunders DM: Pregnancy rates and perinatal outcome after IVF and GIFT in Australia and New Zealand. *Proc VI World Congress in In Vitro Fertilization,* Jerusalem, 1989, p 4

22. Guzick DS, Wilkes C, Jones HW Jr: Cumulative pregnancy rates for in vitro fertilization. *Fertil Steril* 46:663, 1986

23. Yovitch JL, Stranger JD: The limitations of in vitro fertilization from males with severe oligospermia and abnormal male morphology. *J In Vitro Fert Embryo Transfer* 1:172, 1984

24. Kruger TF, Monkveld R, Stander FSH, Lombard CJ, Van der Mercwe JP, Van Zyl JA, Smith K: Sperm morphologic features as a prognostic factor in in vitro fertilization. *Fertil Steril* 46:1118, 1986

25. Wilkes CA, Rosenwaks Z, Jones DC, Jones HW Jr: Pregnancy related to infertility diagnosis, number of attempts and age in a program of in vitro fertilization. *Obstet Gynecol* 66:350, 1985

26. Traunson A, Mohr L: Human pregnancy following cryopreservation thawing and transfer of an eight-cell embryo. *Nature* 308:707, 1983

27. Robertson JA: Ethical and legal issues in cryopreservation of human embryos. *Fertil Steril* 47:371, 1987

28. Fehilly CB, Cohen J, Simons RF, Fishel B, Edwards RG: Cryopreservation of cleaving embryos and expanded blastomeres in the human: A comparative study. *Fertil Steril* 44:638, 1985

29. Testart J, Lassall B, Blaish-Allant J, et al: High pregnancy rate after early human embryo freezing. *Fertil Steril* 42:268, 1986

30. Kurt H, Cohen J, DeVane G, Elaner C, Massey J, Mitchell D, Toledo A: Obstetrical outcome of pregnancies from cryopreserved embryos. *Proc VI World Congress of In Vitro Fertilization,* Jerusalem, 1989

31. Asch RH, Balmaceda JP, Elsworth LR: Preliminary experiences with gamete intrafallopian tube transfer (GIFT). *Fertil Steril* 45:366, 1986

32. Matson PL, Blackledge DG, Richardson PA, Turner SR, Yovich JM, Yovich JL: The role of gamete intrafallopian transfer (GIFT) in the treatment of oligospermic infertility. *Fertil Steril* 48:608, 1987

Index